Contents

TX
364
.P58
2000

Part XII • Social Studies   405

Acknowledgments

This has truly been a team effort if ever there was one.

The *Planet Health* curriculum was developed and refined over a seven-year period by a team headed by Steven Gortmaker, Jean Wiecha, and Karen Peterson. Jill Carter, who patiently reviewed countless suggestions and edits resulting from endless discussions among all four authors, is the main writer of the curriculum. But this is just part of the story.

We had a great team at *Planet Health* who all made outstanding contributions: Sujata Dixit, PhD, to the microunits; Kevin Morris, EdM, Eileen C. Sullivan, EdD, and Wendy Santis, MS, to the classroom lessons; and a very special thanks goes to Mary Kate Newell, ALB, for her stellar and steadfast contributions to the production of this curriculum, as well as her drawings.

Initial funding for the *Planet Health* field trial was provided by the National Institute of Child Health and Human Development, National Institutes of Health under grant #R01HD30780-01A1, with additional support from the Centers for Disease Control and Prevention, Prevention Research Centers Grant U48/CCU115807.

We would like to express our appreciation to the school administrators who hosted us while we developed and field-tested *Planet Health*. They are superintendents Mary Lou McGrath, Eugene Thayer, Dr. James Leonard, and Dr. Albert Argenziano; and principals James J. Coady, Margarita Otero-Alverez, Dr. Leonard Solo, James Halliday, Juan Rodriguez, Michael Toomey, Andrew Fila, Cornelius McGreal, John O'Meara, and David Johnston. We also thank all of the teachers involved in our pilot studies.

For their insightful comments on early drafts of these materials, we thank colleagues from Cambridge's Health of the City initiative, including Dr. David Bor, Henrietta Davis, Dr. Rose Frisch, representatives from the Cambridge Public Schools: Dr. Lynne Yeamans, William Bates, Kim DeAndre, and Dr. Robert McGowan, as well as teachers Gail Bastarache, Margo Frechette, Joanne Lowre, Judy McEntegart, Jack Morocco, and Dave Villandry. For eleventh-hour proofreading, thanks to Sherine Brown, Michael D'Agos-tino, Glen Daly, Liza Makowsky, Debra Suckney, and Kelly Wells. For editorial assistance, thanks to Jan Hangen, Janet Renoni Capachietti, Elizabeth Lenart, and Diana Seder Simon.

Acknowledgments are also due to Dr. Lillian Cheung and the staff of the Eat Well & Keep Moving project, including Dr. Ginny Chomitz, Hank Dart, and Marianne Lee, for sharing material from their curriculum. For her early contributions to this educational model, we also acknowledge Karen Morse.

Special thanks to our colleagues at Harvard who worked with us on the field trial: Graham Colditz and Alison Field for their assistance with diet measures, and Nan Laird for advice concerning statistical methods. We thank colleague Walter Willett for his consistent support, and Mary Kay Fox of Abt Associates for managing a first-class data collec-tion staff. We also thank Wendy Santis for her outstanding efforts as field coordinator.

We were fortunate to have a great advisory board for the field trial of *Planet Health*, including William Dietz (chair), Deborah Klein Walker, Maria Bettancourt, Curtis Ellison, Wayne Westcott, Margaret Saidel, Nancy Coville, and Steven Carey.

Kate Crowley provided time, training, and technical assistance in the initial production phase of *Planet Health*. Will Beamer got us started, and Christopher Lavender provided "extreme" word-processing and good cheer. We thank Scott Wikgren, Amy Pickering, and Cynthia McEntire of Human Kinetics for their very professional help in making *Planet Health* an actual book.

Finally, we thank all of our families for those long hours when we seemed to disappear in the vicinity of a video screen, and all the youth and families whose participation made *Planet Health* a reality. We're looking forward to trading this screen time for more active pursuits, and we hope you are too!

A Letter to Teachers

Dear Teacher

Welcome to *Planet Health*, an innovative, interdisciplinary approach to health education. You can use this curriculum to teach students about nutrition and physical activity while building skills and competencies in language arts, math, science, social studies, and physical education. Focusing on this common instructional theme will strengthen connections among academic disciplines for students and teachers. Here's how it works.

Focusing on Wellness

Planet Health encourages students to think holistically about how health behaviors are interrelated. Exercises in self-reflection and skills-building help students choose healthy foods, increase physical activity, and decrease inactivity. Acquiring these habits in adolescence may increase lifelong health and wellness. Wellness, as we all know, makes everything else—including learning—possible.

Achieving Learning Standards

The *Planet Health* curriculum is aligned with the Massachusetts Department of Education Curriculum Frameworks (learning standards) for health, English language arts, mathematics, science and technology, and history and social science.

Emphasizing Literacy Learning Across the Curriculum

Every *Planet Health* lesson incorporates a range of English language arts learning standards. Learning is accomplished through language—whether the subject is health, mathematics, science, or social studies—and literacy learning can be promoted in every major subject.

Fostering Constructivist Teaching and Learning

Planet Health draws upon a constructivist approach to teaching and learning. Constructivist thinking emphasizes that students learn best when they actively construct meaning for themselves. Students come to the classroom with different knowledge and experiences. Constructivism encourages teachers to create learning environments that activate and build on this diversity in a manner that is active, inquiry-based, and student-centered.

Thus, each *Planet Health* lesson begins by activating and assessing prior knowledge. Lessons proceed to inquiry-based activities in which the students read, write, speak, listen, experiment, and reflect in order to answer health-related questions. Planet Health provides a range of teacher and student resources to support this inquiry.

Engaging Discussion and Cooperative Learning

Every *Planet Health* lesson specifies discussion ideas for small and/or large groups to cooperatively learn and solve health-related issues. Higher-level thinking and cognition are encouraged by active discussion, and social development is enhanced by working with peers in groups.

We hope you enjoy *Planet Health!*

Introduction

Poor diet and physical inactivity are the second leading causes of death in the United States, accounting for at least 300,000 deaths each year. These two risk factors contribute to the development of obesity, coronary heart disease, certain cancers, diabetes, and high blood pressure. Although the onset of these conditions may occur in adulthood, their roots may lie in childhood. Poor diet and inactivity are widespread among many children and youth.

Facts About Children's Health

- Only 1 out of every 4 children eats the recommended number of daily servings of fruits.
- Only 1 out of every 2 young people eats the recommended daily servings of vegetables.
- Children are eating more total and saturated fat than experts recommend.
- Only about one-half of young people regularly participate in vigorous physical activity.
- The percentage of young people who are overweight has more than doubled in the last 30 years.
- Many children spend more time watching TV than in any other activity besides sleep.

Planet Health is an interdisciplinary middle-school health curriculum that can counteract these trends by providing children with the knowledge and skills to develop healthy diet and activity habits for life. *Planet Health* is designed to easily fit into your existing math, science, social studies, language arts, health, and physical education curricula. Materials are aligned with the Massachusetts Department of Education learning standards in these subject areas. Through both classroom and physical education (PE) activities, *Planet Health* aims to improve students' fitness and nutritional status by improving dietary patterns, increasing physical activity, and decreasing inactivity, such as watching TV shows and playing computer games. Published research documents the program's effectiveness at changing these health behaviors and reducing obesity (Gortmaker et al. 1999).

Planet Health's success rests on the availability and interaction of its curriculum components. The Planet Health environment includes Section I Physical Education Microunits, including FitChecks, and Section II Classroom Lessons. Section I contains 30 brief lessons and FitCheck, a tool for self-assessment of activity and inactivity. Section II contains 33 classroom lessons. *Power Down*, a TV- reduction campaign is located in appendix D. Although implementing the full curriculum across grades and disciplines will maximize its potential impact on student health, your school may choose to pilot the curriculum on a smaller scale, teaching a selection of lessons in classes in one grade only, teaching the lessons only in health and physical education settings, or even beginning with classes in just one subject area.

Health Messages

Planet Health encourages students to "make space for fitness and nutrition" by reinforcing the four health behaviors below. These messages reflect U.S. Department of

Planet Health Overview

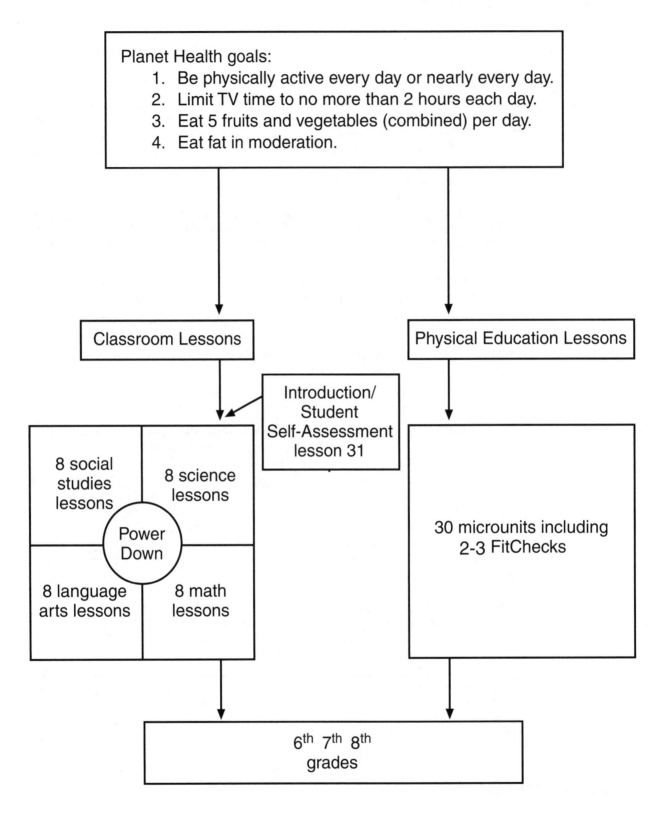

Planet Health goals:
1. Be physically active every day or nearly every day.
2. Limit TV time to no more than 2 hours each day.
3. Eat 5 fruits and vegetables (combined) per day.
4. Eat fat in moderation.

Classroom Lessons

Physical Education Lessons

Introduction/
Student
Self-Assessment
lesson 31

8 social
studies
lessons

8 science
lessons

Power
Down

8 language
arts lessons

8 math
lessons

30 microunits including
2-3 FitChecks

6th 7th 8th
grades

Health and Human Services' Healthy People 2010 goals for nutrition and physical activity (2000) and the American Academy of Pediatrics' recommendation for TV viewing (1986). In addition, our dietary goals are adapted from the U.S. Department of Agriculture's *Dietary Guidelines for Americans* (2000), and also reflect recommendations from the National Cancer Institute (1995).

1. Be active. All adolescents should be moderately physically active for at least 30 minutes daily or nearly every day as a part of their play, chores, transportation, and exercise. Adolescents should participate in vigorous activity three or more sessions per week that last 20 minutes or more per session. They should aim for a total of 60 minutes or more of physical activity on all, or most days of the week (Sallis and Patrick 1994; NASPE 1998; USDHHS 2000).

2. Limit your screen time to no more than two hours per day (American Academy of Pediatrics 1986).

3. Eat five or more servings of fruits and vegetables daily (National Association for Sport and Physical Education 1998; USDHHS 2000).

4. Eat fat in moderation (USDA 2000; USDHHS 2000).

Educational Approach

We use the term "interdisciplinary" to mean key curriculum messages are presented using concepts from multiple subject areas. This approach amplifies opportunities for students to practice the behavioral skills and to reinforce the health messages through diverse learning approaches, developing self-efficacy in making healthy food choices, being physically active, and trading screen time for active time. Self-assessment and goal setting encourage students to reflect on their current behaviors and make plans for change. Teaching these concepts across disciplines highlights their importance and establishes peer and teacher support for "lifestyle" changes in behavior.

Each classroom lesson incorporates subject-specific learning standards (Massachusetts Curriculum Frameworks) so that skills and competencies that are required learning for middle-school students are used as vehicles for conveying *Planet Health*'s messages. This strategy ensures that teachers will not lose valuable class time in implementing *Planet Health*.

Planet Health draws on a constructivist approach to teaching and learning (Phillips 1995). The lessons begin with the activation and assessment of prior knowledge and build on what is known in an active, inquiry-based, student-centered manner. Students read, write, speak, listen, experiment, and reflect to answer health-related questions. They actively engage in brainstorming, debates, case studies, classroom demonstrations, games, group projects, and presentations. The lessons foster critical thinking and responsible decision making, in addition to offering skill-building exercises.

Planet Health also is rooted in social science theories of health behavior change. Behavioral choice theory was utilized by allowing youth to choose among alternative activities, a strategy that both increases sense of control and reinforces healthy behaviors (Epstein et al. 1995). Social cognitive theory also was incorporated into the design of *Planet Health* to provide students with cognitive and behavioral skills that enable healthy change, strengthen competence, and foster support for healthy behaviors from other students, family members, and teachers in different subject areas (Gortmaker et al. 1999).

Program Background

Planet Health was first created under a grant from the National Institutes of Child Health and Human Development (NICHD) to the Harvard School of Public Health to develop, implement, and evaluate a curriculum designed to improve diet and physical activity in middle-school students. The curriculum was implemented by more than 100 teachers with about 2,000 students in four Boston-area school districts. During the two year field-testing period, teachers contributed to curriculum revisions through written evaluations and focus groups. The recommendations made by these teachers helped create the version of *Planet Health* that you hold in your hands.

Planet Health's effectiveness in five intervention schools was evaluated by comparing them with five similar schools that did not receive the curriculum during the field test ("delayed intervention" sites). This research design, a randomized, controlled trial, is the best way to see if an intervention did its job. At the beginning and end of the two-year project, students at the 10 schools completed a questionnaire about their diet and activity patterns and had their height, weight, and body fat measured by a professional team. Results from the intervention and delayed intervention schools were compared at the beginning of the study; students were similar to each other on characteristics important to the project. Project staff were therefore able to compare the results at the end of the study ("follow-up"). With this design, differences at follow-up are likely to be attributable to the *Planet Health* curriculum.

The randomized, controlled trial showed that *Planet Health* decreased obesity among girls over two school years. It reduced daily TV viewing hours in both girls and boys. Likewise, the program increased fruit and vegetable consumption and led to a smaller increase in girls' Caloric intake. *Planet Health*'s impact on obesity seems to be due to reductions in screen time, since girls who reduced their TV time were less likely to be obese at the end of the study. Relative to students in delayed intervention schools, those in the intervention schools showed greater gains in knowledge of diet and of physical activity. We found no evidence for increases in extreme dieting behavior in boys or girls who participated in the *Planet Health* curriculum. Further research is needed to explain the differences in *Planet Health*'s impact on boys and girls. The results of this study were published in the April 1999 issue of the *Archives of Pediatrics and Adolescent Medicine* (Gortmaker et al. 1999).

Curriculum Components

Section 1: Physical Education Microunits

The PE curriculum contains the following:

- *30 Physical Education Microunits.* Microunits are simple, five-minute lessons introduced by PE teachers during the warm-up or cool-down period of PE class. The microunits teach students about the health benefits of physical activity and motivate students to work toward their personal fitness potential. They encourage students to "make space" for physical activity in their lives by decreasing TV viewing and other "screen time" activities.

- *Physical Education FitCheck Sheets.* This self-assessment tool coaches students to reflect on their current activity and inactivity levels and set goals for improvement or maintenance of healthy behaviors. Students are encouraged to create goals that trade their inactive time for active time. They evaluate progress in meeting their personal goals by completing a FitCheck at least two or three times during the school year.

Each microunit includes

- A fitness tip
- Fitness lesson
- How-to
- Questions for students

The microunits are designed to be taught during the warm-up or cool-down period of PE class. They take only five minutes to deliver, leaving as much time as possible for physical activity in PE class. The 30 lessons can be taught over two to three years and repeated in greater depth by using the lesson extensions provided in each microunit. We recommend that students complete FitChecks at least two or three times each school year.

For more information on how to use the PE Curriculum, including the microunits and FitCheck, refer to the Teacher Introduction to the Microunits on page 2. Material in many of the microunits has been adapted from other sources (see page 6).

Section 2: Classroom Lessons

The classroom curriculum contains the following:

• An introductory lesson *Do You Make Space for Fitness and Nutrition?* This lesson should be used to introduce students to the *Planet Health* Curriculum and health messages. Students will assess their own nutrition and activity behaviors using a short questionnaire and demonstrate their understanding of these concepts by answering an open-ended or "key" question. The self-assessment can be repeated at the end of the school year to help students and teachers reflect on changes in students' knowledge and behaviors. This lesson can be taught in any subject area but is well-suited for health and other classes that practice answering open-ended and key questions as part of their curriculum.

• Units in four major subjects. The Language Arts, Math, Science, and Social Studies units each contain eight lessons, 32 lessons total. Two lessons in each subject address each *Planet Health* theme: eating fat in moderation, eating five or more fruits and vegetables daily, participating in regular, preferably daily, physical activity, and limiting TV, videos, and computer games to no more than two hours per day. At the beginning of each unit, a *Planet Health* At A Glance chart identifies for each lesson the subject area theme, level of difficulty, subject-specific skills, materials, and estimated teaching time.

• *Power Down*, a television reduction campaign. This lesson is a two-week exercise appropriate for use in a math, science, or health education class and is adaptable as a school-wide campaign. *Power Down* asks students to assess and reflect on their current television, video, and computer habits in order to set goals for reducing their "screen time." This campaign compliments the Physical Education FitCheck.

• Resources. Additional background information is located in the appendixes at the back of this book:

Appendix A Nutrition Resources

Appendix B Physical Activity Resources

Appendix C Social Studies Resources

Appendix E Curriculum Frameworks

All lesson plans provide

• a summary paragraph
• behavioral objectives
• learning objectives
• materials
• teaching procedure
• student activity sheets
• teacher resources follow

Some lessons also include student resources and overhead transparency masters.

The *Planet Health* curriculum offers schools great flexibility in deciding which lessons are grade-appropriate and when each lesson should be inserted into the ongoing academic curriculum. Ideally, each sixth-, seventh-, and eighth-grade teacher should teach two to three classroom lessons per year. However, schools new to the program may choose to pilot the curriculum on a smaller scale, teaching a selection of lessons in one grade only, teaching lessons only in health and physical education settings, or even beginning with classes in just one subject area. We strongly recommend that clusters or departments coordinate to ensure that students first complete the introductory student self-assessment lesson, followed by Language Arts lesson 32 on the Food Guide Pyramid (this lesson is also well-suited for a health or consumer science class). If this is not possible, spend a few minutes reviewing *Planet Health*'s four health messages and the FGP before teaching one of the other lessons. (See below for ideas on how coordinate the program.)

The lessons within each subject area can be taught in any sequence. Some *Planet Health* teachers in the field test preferred teaching two, three, or four lessons consecutively, while others preferred spreading them throughout the year. The choice is yours. For the most part, this decision will be driven by your own curriculum. Because the *Planet Health* lessons infuse health and fitness topics into middle-school competencies and skills, you can teach them when you focus on skills they address. For example, a social studies lesson on the democratic process can be taught when you are teaching about citizen participation and lawmaking.

Even though these lessons include subject area skills, some teachers may feel uncomfortable or frustrated about incorporating health topics into their already packed curriculum. Support and understand these feelings. Encourage them to stick with the curriculum for at least two years. Teachers who piloted the lessons reported that things generally seemed easier the second time through. Some felt that the curriculum strengthened their connections with students, which made it easier to teach other subject matter as well. For more information on how to use the *Planet Health* Classroom curriculum refer to the Introduction to Classroom Lessons on page 98.

School-Wide Coordination

Planet Health's impact depends on how many opportunities students are given to learn in the program's environment. Ideally, students should experience the entire curriculum over two to three years. However, be creative in starting *Planet Health* at your school. If interdisciplinary teaching is new to your school, you may want to start small by beginning with just one or two subject area teachers and the physical education teacher. Additional subjects and teachers can then be added, building on your initial success.

As is true with all interdisciplinary curricula, implementing *Planet Health* in your middle school will take some initial planning. You may wish to appoint one person to coordinate the initial planning process. We recommend that each department (language arts, math, science, social studies, and physical education) meet to review the lessons specific to their subject areas and decide which lessons should be taught at each of the three grade levels. Several planning tools have been included to help you with this process. Examine the *Planet Health* At A Glance charts located at the beginning of each unit in Section 2. These provide an overview including a list of classroom lessons, *Planet Health* themes, level of difficulty, subject specific skills, materials, and estimated teaching time. We recommend that individual clusters or departments decide how (as a unit or spread throughout the year) and when during the year they plan to insert the lessons into the curriculum. Interdisciplinary coordination among physical education and major subject teachers can enhance the *Planet Health* experience for students and teachers alike.

At the end of the first year of implementation, teachers should meet to reevaluate their lesson choices and sequencing. Were they graded appropriate? Did they complement the existing curriculum?

Using the Planet Health Curriculum Guide

After reading the book introduction, proceed to the Teacher Introduction to the Microunits or the Introduction to Classroom Lessons located at the beginning of their respective sections. These will provide you with tips on how to coordinate, select, and teach the *Planet Health* lessons. Further implementation and training ideas can be found on the *Planet Health* Web site **www.hsph.harvard.edu/prc/**.

References

American Academy of Pediatrics. 1986. *Television and the family.* Elk Grove Village, IL: American Academy of Pediatrics.

Bandura, A. 1986. *Social foundations of thought and action.* Inglewood Cliffs, NJ: Prentice- Hall.

Epstein, L.H., Valoski, A.M., Smith, J.A., Vara, L.S., McCurley, J., Wisniewski, L., Kalarchian, M.A., Klein, K.R., and Shrage, L.R. 1995. Effects of decreasing sedentary behavior and increasing activity on weight change in obese children. *Health Psychology* 14:1-7.

Gortmaker, S.L., Peterson, K.E., Wiecha, J., Sobol, A.M., Dixit, S., Fox, M.K., and Laird, N. 1999. Reducing obesity via a school-based interdisciplinary intervention among youth: Planet Health. *Archives of Pediatrics and Adolescent Medicine* 153(4):409-418.

Massachusetts Department of Education. 1996-1999. Massachusetts Curriculum Frameworks in Health, English Language Arts, Mathematics, Science and Technology, and History and Social Science. Malden, MA: MDOE. **info.doe.mass.edu**

National Association for Sport and Physical Education. 1998. *Physical activity for children: A statement of guidelines.* Reston, VA: NASPE.

National Cancer Institute and National Institutes of Health. 1995. *Time to take five: Eat 5 fruits and vegetables a day.* DHHS, NIH Publication No. 95-3862.

Phillips, D.C. 1995. The good, the bad, and the ugly: The many faces of constructivism. *Educational Researcher* 24(7):5-12.

Sallis, J.F., and Patrick, K. 1994. Physical activity guidelines for adolescents: Consensus statement. *Pediatric Exercise Science* 6:302-314.

U.S. Department of Agriculture and U.S. Department of Health and Human Services. 2000. *Nutrition and your health: Dietary guidelines for Americans* 2000, 5th edition. **www.usda.gov/cnpp**

U.S Department of Health and Human Services. 2000. Healthy People 2010, conference edition, vols. I and II. **www.health.gov/healthypeople**

Incorporating Planet Health
Into Your School

Hold a training workshop.

Departments meet to decide:
Which lessons will be taught in the 6th, 7th, and 8th grades?

Clusters meet to decide:
Will the lessons be taught as a unit or spread throughout the year?

Teacher decides:
How will I teach the lesson?
If there is more than one activity, which activities fit my students' skills and my time constraints?

Middle School Planner

Subject area	Lesson	Teacher	Grade		
			6th	7th	8th
Introduction	Introduction to the Microunits				
Part I Introducing Exercise and Fitness	1 Thinking About Activity, Exercise, and Fitness				
	2 Warm Up Before You Exercise				
	3 Cool Down After You Exercise				
Part II FitCheck	4 Charting Your FitScore, Fit ★ Score, and SitScore				
	5 What Could You Do Instead of Watching TV?				
	6 Making Time to Stay Fit				
	7 Setting Goals for Personal Fitness				
Part III Getting Started	8 Let's Get Started on Being Fit				
	9 More About the Three Areas of Physical Fitness				
	10 Frequency, Intensity, Time, and Type				
	11 Choose Activities You Think Are Fun				
	12 How Often Should I Exercise?				

(continued)

Middle School Planner *(continued)*

Subject area	Lesson	Teacher	Grade		
			6th	7th	8th
Part IV Improving Fitness	13 Improving Cardiovascular Fitness				
	14 Improving Muscular Strength				
	15 Improving Flexibility				
Part V Measuring Fitness	16 Improving Your Overall Physical Fitness Levels				
	17 Knowing Your Resting Heart Rate				
	18 Exercise Makes Your Heart Beat Faster				
Part VI Be Active Now!	19 Be Active Now for a Healthy Heart Later				
	20 Be Active Now for Healthy Bones Later				
	21 Be Active Now to Stay in Shape				
Part VII Get Ready to Exercise	22 Energy for Exercise				
	23 Weather and Exercise				
	24 Getting Enough to Drink				
	25 Food and Supplement Myths				
Part VIII Fitness Can Be Fun!	26 Aerobics				
	27 Calisthenics				
	28 Running, Jogging, and Fitness Walking				
	29 Swimming				
	30 Cycling				

Subject area	Lesson	Theme	Teacher	6th	7th	8th
Introduction	31 Do You Make Space for Fitness and Nutrition?	Student self-assessment				
Part IX Language Arts	32 Pyramid Power	Balanced diet				
	33 Carbohydrates: Energy Food	Balanced diet				
	34 The Language of Food	Fruits and vegetables				
	35 Keep it Local	Fruits and vegetables				
	36 Write a Fable: Important Messages About Activity	Activity				
	37 Go for the Goal Describe One, Try One!	Activity				
	38 Lifetime Physical Activities	Lifestyle				
	39 Choosing Healthy Foods	Lifestyle				
Part X Math	40 Problem Solving: Making Healthy Choices	Balanced diet				
	41 Figuring Out Fat	Balanced diet				
	42 Looking for Patterns: What's for Lunch?	Balanced diet				
	43 Apples, Oranges, and Zucchini: An Algebra Party	Fruits and vegetables				
	44 Plotting Coordinate Graphs: What Does Your Day Look Like?	Activity				
	45 Survey the Class	Activity				

(continued)

Middle School Planner (continued)

Subject area	Lesson	Theme	Teacher	Grade 6th	7th	8th
	46 Circle Graphs: Where Did the Day Go?	Lifestyle				
Part XI Science	47 Energy Equations	Lifestyle				
	48 Mighty Minerals: Calcium and Iron	Balanced diet				
	49 Fat Functions	Balanced diet				
	50 Smart Snacks	Balanced diet				
	51 The Plants We Eat	Fruits and vegetables				
	52 Foods for Energy	Activity				
	53 Muscle Mysteries	Activity				
	54 The Human Heart	Lifestyle				
	55 How Far Can You Jump?	Lifestyle				
Part XII Social Studies	56 Food Through the Ages	Balanced diet				
	57 Democracy and Diet	Balanced diet				
	58 Global Foods	Fruits and vegetables				
	59 Around the World With Five a Day	Fruits and vegetables				
	60 Map Maker	Activity				
	61 Free to be Fit	Activity				
	62 Impact of Technology	Lifestyle				
	63 Food Rituals and Society	Lifestyle				
	Charting TV Viewing Time	Power Down				

Monthly Planner

Month	Language arts		Math		Science		Social studies	
	Theme	Lesson	Theme	Lesson	Theme	Lesson	Theme	Lesson
September								
October								
November								
December								
January								
February								
March								
April								
May								
June								

Weekly Planners

Month of

Week	Language arts	Math	Science	Social studies
1: Theme Lesson				
2: Theme Lesson				
3: Theme Lesson				
4: Theme Lesson				

Month of

Week	Language arts	Math	Science	Social studies
1: Theme Lesson				
2: Theme Lesson				
3: Theme Lesson				
4: Theme Lesson				

Month of

Week	Language arts	Math	Science	Social studies
1: Theme Lesson				
2: Theme Lesson				
3: Theme Lesson				
4: Theme Lesson				

Month of

Week	Language arts	Math	Science	Social studies
1: Theme Lesson				
2: Theme Lesson				
3: Theme Lesson				
4: Theme Lesson				

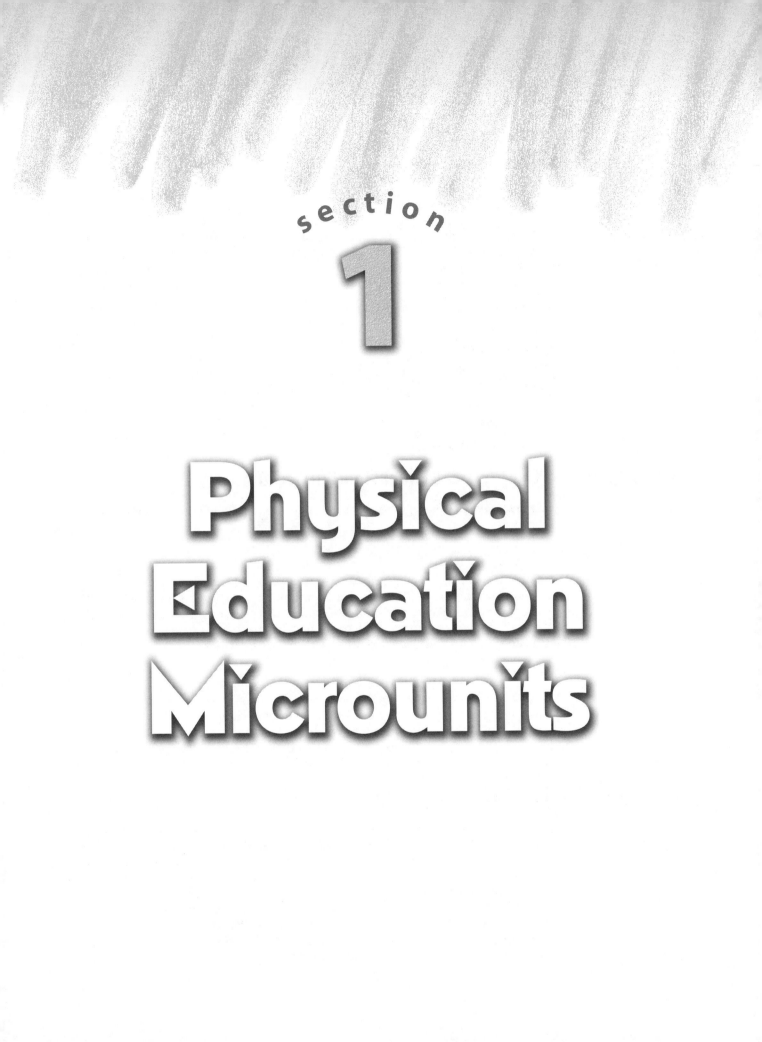

1

Physical Education Microunits

Teacher Introduction to the Microunits

The *Planet Health* physical education curriculum is composed of two components: Microunits and FitChecks. This introduction will describe these components and provide you with guidance on how to teach the PE curriculum and incorporate it into your classroom. Following this introduction you will find seven physical education parts:

- Introducing Exercise and Fitness
- FitCheck
- Getting Started
- Improving Fitness
- Measuring Fitness
- Be Active Now!
- Get Ready to Exercise
- Fitness Can be Fun!

Components of the Physical Education Curriculum

The *Planet Health* physical education curriculum includes PE microunits and FitCheck sheets.

PE Microunits

Microunits are simple, five-minute lessons introduced by PE teachers during the warm-up or cool-down period of PE class. The microunits teach students about the health benefits of physical activity and motivate students to work toward their personal fitness potential. They encourage students to make space for physical activity in their lives by decreasing TV viewing and other screen time activities.

FitCheck Sheets

FitCheck is a self-assessment tool that encourages students to reflect on their current activity and inactivity levels and set goals for improvement or maintenance of healthy behaviors. Students are encouraged to create goals that trade their inactive time for active time. They evaluate progress in meeting their personal goals by completing a FitCheck at least two or three times during the school year.

Using the Physical Education Curriculum

You can teach the microunits at the start of PE class or during the cool-down period at the end of class. Start with lessons 1-7 so that students learn how to do FitCheck as early as possible in the school year. After this, you may wish to change the order of the microunits to better coordinate with your own sports and fitness curriculum.

The units are written in a read-aloud style. While some teachers may find this convenient, others may feel uncomfortable with the script-like quality. Feel free to paraphrase if it makes you more comfortable; however, first familiarize yourself with the key elements of the lesson in order to include the main concepts. We also encourage you to personalize the lessons with your own fitness-related experiences.

You can easily vary the pace and complexity according to student interest and other considerations. In some classes, you may have time to combine lessons or elaborate; in other classes, you may need to slow down by either simplifying a lesson, splitting it up over two classes, or repeating the same information in two or more classes. We recommend that at least one lesson be included each week. You may use all of the microunits in one year, or spread them out over two years.

Most microunits include extensions, which appear in shaded boxes. Extensions add depth when students are ready for more advanced information. You can include them or not include them as you see fit. For example, if you will be teaching the same students for more than one year, you can leave the extensions out the first year you teach the units, and add them in the second year.

Structuring the Presentation

Here is a suggested format for presenting the microunits:

1. At the start of class, tell students the day's fitness tip (located at the beginning of each microunit).
2. Teach the fitness lesson and how-to sections (or do so at the end of class).
3. Complete your scheduled activity for the class.
4. Teach the fitness lesson and how-to if you did not do so at the beginning of class.
5. Reiterate the fitness tip.

To make the microunits more interactive, you can get students to discuss the how-to section with you and to respond to the questions for students as time permits. Their answers will help you know if students understand the lesson or if you need to slow down or elaborate on the concepts you present.

FitCheck Overview

FitCheck is a self-assessment tool that physical educators can use to help children identify, understand, and reflect upon their own patterns of physical activity and inactivity. Use it if it matches your students' abilities and fits into your curriculum.

FitCheck components are:

• FitScore and SitScore sheets. Students keep track of their physical activities and screen time activities over a seven-day period and translate their results into FitScores and SitScores. This is completed at home.

• Goal-setting sheet. Students set activity goals based on their FitScores and SitScores.

• FitScore and SitScore progress charts (bar graphs). Students graph their scores when they complete each FitCheck or two to three times during the year. (Try to make one time close to the end of the school year.)

Using FitCheck

Microunits 4-7 introduce FitCheck to students.

• Lesson 4 *Charting Your FitScore, Fit ★ Score, and SitScore*. This lesson introduces FitCheck.
• Lesson 5 *What Could You Do Instead of Watching TV?* This is one of two lessons preparing students for goal setting (lesson 7). It presents recommendations for limiting TV use and offers alternatives to TV, video and computer games, and video tapes and movies.

- Lesson 6 *Making Time to Stay Fit.* This is the second lesson preparing students for goal setting (lesson 7). Students make a group goal for class that day and evaluate their progress at the end of class. You may want to do this lesson several times with students until they are comfortable with goal setting and evaluation.
- Lesson 7 *Setting Goals for Personal Fitness.* Students set goals to improve their FitScores and SitScores. At the next FitCheck they evaluate their progress.

For more information, see the Teacher's Guide to FitCheck on page 20.

Coordinating With Classroom Teachers

Planet Health implementation can be enhanced by coordination among teachers from different subject areas including PE. Having one or two teachers that can take the lead in this regard really helps. PE and classroom teachers have assumed this role in the past. To enhance your understanding of *Planet Health*'s classroom component, and in case you are interested in being a coordinator at your school, read the Introduction to Classroom Lessons (page 98).

Microunit Summaries

The following sections briefly summarize what is covered in each part. The lessons can be read like a script or adapted to fit your own teaching style.

Part I Introducing Exercise and Fitness

The lessons in this section introduce students to the concept of physical fitness and the benefits of living an active lifestyle.

- Lesson 1 Thinking About Activity, Exercise, and Fitness
- Lesson 2 Warm Up Before You Exercise
- Lesson 3 Cool Down After You Exercise

Part II FitCheck

Lessons 4-7 teach students how to use the *Planet Health* FitCheck to reflect on their activity and inactivity patterns and set goals for becoming more active. Students are encouraged to increase their activity and decrease their inactivity by trading screen time (TV and computer time) for more active types of play. Before teaching these lessons, be sure to read the Teacher's Guide to FitCheck on pages 18-20.

- Lesson 4 Charting Your FitScore, Fit ★ Score, and SitScore
- Lesson 5 What Could You Do Instead of Watching TV?
- Lesson 6 Making Time to Stay Fit
- Lesson 7 Setting Goals for Personal Fitness

Part III Getting Started

The lessons in this section introduce students to the F.I.T. & T. rule for improving physical fitness.

- Lesson 8 Let's Get Started on Being Fit
- Lesson 9 More About the Three Areas of Physical Fitness
- Lesson 10 Frequency, Intensity, Time, and Type

- Lesson 11 Choose Activities You Think Are Fun
- Lesson 12 How Often Should I Exercise?

Part IV Improving Fitness

This section teaches students how to improve their cardiovascular endurance, muscular strength, and flexibility.

- Lesson 13 Improving Cardiovascular Endurance
- Lesson 14 Improving Muscular Strength
- Lesson 15 Improving Flexibility

Part V Measuring Fitness

This section teaches students how to modify their own fitness programs and how to assess whether their fitness is improving.

- Lesson 16 Improving Your Overall Physical Fitness Levels
- Lesson 17 Knowing Your Resting Heart Rate
- Lesson 18 Exercise Makes Your Heart Beat Faster

Part VI Be Active Now!

The three lessons in this section discuss the long-term health benefits of living an active lifestyle.

- Lesson 19 Be Active Now for a Healthy Heart Later
- Lesson 20 Be Active Now for Healthy Bones Later
- Lesson 21 Be Active Now to Stay in Shape

Part VII Get Ready to Exercise

The lessons in this section discuss factors that affect optimal performance: nutrition, fluid replacement, proper clothing, and drug and food supplement use.

- Lesson 22 Energy for Exercise
- Lesson 23 Weather and Exercise
- Lesson 24 Getting Enough to Drink
- Lesson 25 Food and Supplement Myths

Part VIII Fitness Can be Fun!

The lessons in this section discuss the benefits, locations, equipment, and safety tips for six popular physical activities: calisthenics, running, fitness walking, swimming, bicycling, and aerobic dance.

- Lesson 26 Aerobics
- Lesson 27 Calisthenics
- Lesson 28 Running, Jogging, and Fitness Walking
- Lesson 29 Swimming
- Lesson 30 Cycling

References for the Microunits

American Academy of Pediatrics. 1986. *Television and the family*. Elk Grove Village, IL: American Academy of Pediatrics.

American College of Sports Medicine. 1996. Position of the American College of Sports Medicine: Exercise and fluid replacement. *Medicine and Science in Sports and Exercise* 28:i-vi.

American Heart Association. 1996. Cardiovascular disease in the black population. **www.amhrt.org/biostat/fsblks.htm**

Anderson, B., and Anderson, J. 1980. *Stretching*. Bolinas, CA: Shelter Publications.

Ashton, D., and Davies, B. 1986. *Why exercise?* Oxford, UK: Basil Blackwell LTD.

Buss, R. 1993. *The ABSEF guide for teaching physical fitness to kids: An exercise and nutrition manual for instructors and parents*. LeMars, IA: ABSEF.

Corbin, C.B., and Lindsey, R. 1985. *Concepts of physical fitness with laboratories: Instructor's manual*. Dubuque, IA: William C. Brown.

Corbin, C.B., and Lindsey, R. 1994. *Concepts of physical fitness with laboratories* (8th ed.). Dubuque, IA: William C. Brown.

Dairy Council of California. 1998. *Exercise your options: A food choice and activity program for middle-school students*. **www.dairycouncilofca.org**

Gortmaker, S.L., Dietz, W.H., and Cheung, L. 1990. Inactivity, diet and the fattening of America. *Journal of the America Dietetic Association* 90(9):1247-1255.

Haskell, W.L. 1994. Health consequences of physical activity: Understanding and challenges regarding dose-response. *Medicine and Science in Sports and Exercise* 26(6):649-660.

Jackson, D., and Pescar, S. 1981. *The young athlete's health handbook*. New York: Everest House Publishers.

Jonas, S. 1995. *Regular exercise: A handbook for clinical practice*. New York: Springer Publishing Co.

Katch, F., and McArdle, W.D. 1993. *Introduction to nutrition, exercise, and health* (4th ed.). Philadelphia: Lea & Febiger.

Martin, L.I. 1978. *The parent's book of physical fitness for children*. Saddle Brook, NJ: American Book, Stratford Press.

McSwegin, P., Pemberton, C., Petray, C., and Going, S. 1989. *Physical best instructor's guide*. Reston, VA: American Alliance for Health, Physical Education, Recreation, and Dance.

Merki, M.B. 1996. *Teen health: Course 2* (teacher's wraparound ed.). New York: Glencoe and McGraw-Hill.

National Athletic Trainers Association. 1971. *Fundamentals of athletic training. A joint project of the National Athletic Trainers Association, the Athletic Institute, and the Medical Aspects of Sports Committee of the American Medical Association*. Chicago: American Medical Association.

National Cancer Institute and National Institutes of Health. 1995. *Time to take five: Eat 5 fruits and vegetables a day*. DHHS, NIH Publication No. 95-3862.

National Dairy Council. 1994. *Food power: A coach's guide to improving performance*. National Dairy Council.

National Osteoporosis Foundation. 1996. Risk factors. **www.nof.org**

National Research Council. 1989. *Diet and health: Implications for reducing chronic disease risk*. Washington D.C.: National Academy Press.

President's Council of Physical Fitness. 1991. *Get fit! A handbook for youth ages 6-17*. Washington D.C.

Sallis, J.F., and Patrick, K. 1994. Physical activity guidelines for adolescents: Consensus statement. *Pediatric Exercise Science* 6:302-314.

U.S. Department of Agriculture and U.S. Department of Health and Human Services. 2000. *Nutrition and your health: Dietary guidelines for Americans 2000*, 5th edition. **www.usda.gov/cnpp**

U.S. Department of Health and Human Services. 2000. Healthy People 2010, conference edition, vols. I and II. **www.health.gov/healthypeople**

U.S. Department of Health and Human Services, Public Health Service, Centers for Disease Control and Prevention, National Center for Chronic Disease Prevention and Health Promotion, Division of Nutrition and Physical Activity. 1999. *Promoting physical activity: A guide for community action*. Champaign, IL: Human Kinetics.

Wilmore, J.H., and Costill, D.L. 1993. *Training for sport and activity: The physiological basis for conditioning process*. Champaign, IL: Human Kinetics.

Student Introduction to the Microunits

Introduction

This year I'd like you to [continue to] work toward being physically active on a regular basis and achieving fitness levels you feel good about. I will be introducing you to some basic facts about physical fitness and physical activity through microunits. Microunits are made up of a fitness tip and fitness lesson and will take about five minutes at the beginning of class. The information provided on physical activity is for everyone, whether or not you are an athlete.

In addition to the microunits, you'll also get some practice setting and working on personal activity goals. To do this, two or three times this year you will have a FitCheck, which will help you measure how active and inactive you are. The goals you set will help to maintain or increase your current activity level.

Before we start, it is important to understand that being fit means being physically conditioned, which gives you the energy to do things without feeling very tired or drained. It is not about being an athlete or team star. If you work on being more active, you will become more fit, feel good about yourself, look good, and be healthier. Remember, all of you have a personal physical fitness potential that you can achieve. Being fit will help you to do your best, not only in sports and exercise, but in all activities throughout your life.

[In the next class,] we will begin with a lesson on being physically active.

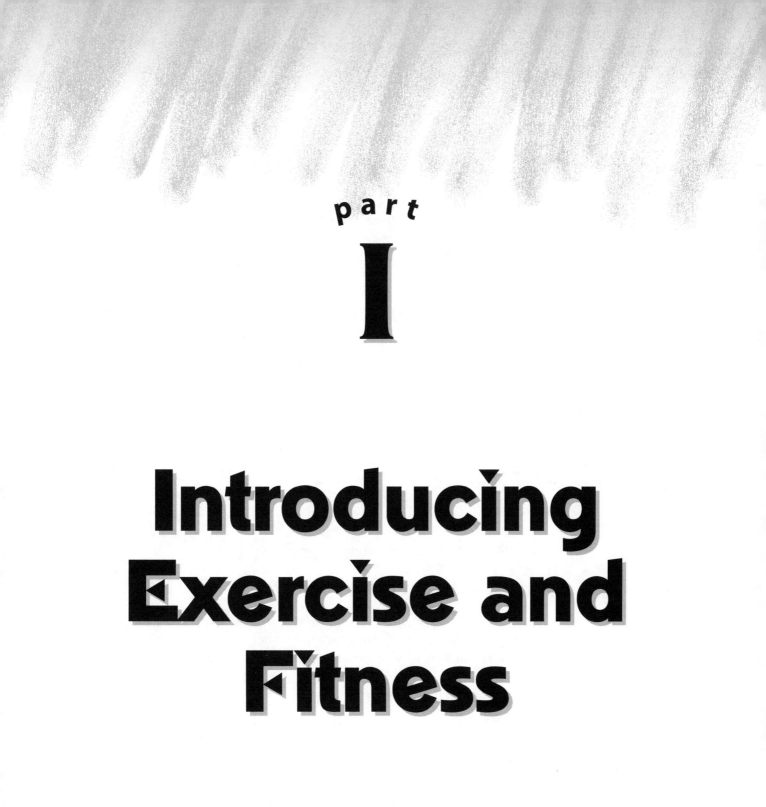

part

I

Introducing Exercise and Fitness

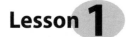

Thinking About Activity, Exercise, and Fitness

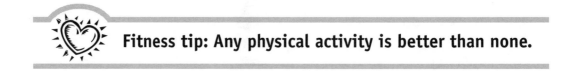

Fitness tip: Any physical activity is better than none.

A Brief Introduction to Physical Fitness

- Being fit means you have the energy you need to
  - work,
  - exercise,
  - play, and
  - get from place to place without easily tiring.
- To get fit, you need to be physically active.

Any Physical Activity Is Better for You Than None

- Exercise is physical activity that is planned and structured, like running a mile or playing soccer for an hour. Many people think that only exercise improves fitness.
- In fact, many kinds of movement can improve your health and fitness level:
  - Dancing
  - Jumping rope
  - Walking the dog
  - Throwing a ball
  - Climbing stairs
  - Swimming
- But, the more active you are, the more fit you will become.

  In addition to physical activity, healthy eating will also help you stay fit. We'll discuss more about this aspect of fitness later.

Positive Effects of Physical Fitness

- Being physically fit
  - makes you healthier,

- helps you build a positive self-image, and
- helps you feel better about yourself.
- Fitness is fun, and it feels great!

Long-Term Health Benefits of Physical Activity

Learning to be active now will help you become an active adult. If you become fit now and stay active as you get older, you'll lower your risk of having certain health problems as an adult, such as obesity, heart disease, broken bones, bone loss, diabetes, and certain types of cancers. Moderate amounts of physical activity will help you prevent these health problems.

Physical Activity Recommendations for Adolescents

Adolescents should be moderately active for at least 30 minutes every day, or nearly every day, as part of their play, exercise, chores, and transportation. Adolescents should also engage in three or more sessions per week of vigorous activities that last 20 minutes or more. They should aim for a total of 60 minutes or more of physical activity nearly every day.

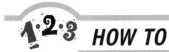 ## HOW TO

1. Start thinking about the physical activities you do and the things you do that are not active, like
   - watching TV,
   - playing video and computer games, and
   - watching movies.
2. Next, think about ways to increase your activity level. You can do this by replacing inactive time with active time. For instance, you can
   - ride bikes instead of watching a show on TV that you don't really like, and
   - play basketball instead of playing a video game.
3. Remember, being active will help you stay healthy now, and as you grow up.

 ## QUESTIONS FOR STUDENTS

1. What are some of the things that you do to be physically active?
2. What can you do to increase your physical activity?
3. What are the benefits of being fit?
4. What kinds of things get in the way of you being more physically active?

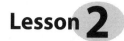

Warm Up Before You Exercise

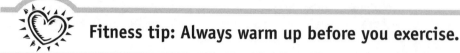 Fitness tip: Always warm up before you exercise.

How Warm-Ups Work

- Warm-ups heat up your body by gradually increasing your heart rate.
- Warm-ups also prepare your muscles and joints for strenuous activity.

Benefits of Warming Up

- Warm-ups help to
  - stretch and soften muscles,
  - increase joint flexibility, and
  - improve circulation.
- Warming up will help you do better when you start your exercise or game.
- Warm-ups reduce the chances of muscle and joint injuries.
- Warming up can take less than 5 minutes.

Determining Warm-Up Length and Intensity

In general, the length and intensity of the warm-up should increase when you prepare for an activity that is either very strenuous or is going to require a sudden and great output of energy (like a sprint). However, if the activity can be started gradually, a shorter warm-up is sufficient because the exercise itself will act as a warm-up.

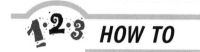 *HOW TO*

1. Before you participate in endurance or strength-training activities, warm up with 2 to 5 minutes of
   - bicycling,
   - walking, or
   - jogging in place.

2. Follow your cardiovascular warm-up with stretching.
- Flexibility exercises should be done slowly and smoothly until you feel mild tension on your muscles.
- Always stretch muscles until they are taut (pulled or drawn tight), not beyond.
- To warm up, hold the stretch for 10-60 seconds for 1 to 3 repetitions.
- Remember to breathe while you stretch.
- Concentrate on lengthening the time of the stretch.

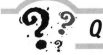

QUESTIONS FOR STUDENTS

1. How do warm-ups benefit exercise?
2. How much time should you spend on warm-ups?
3. What exercises can you do to warm up?

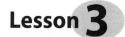

Cool Down After You Exercise

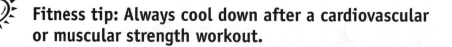

Fitness tip: Always cool down after a cardiovascular or muscular strength workout.

When to Cool Down

- Cool down when you are done with your cardiovascular and strength-training workouts with stretching and gentle walking.
- Cooling down generally takes 5-10 minutes.

Benefits of Cooling Down

- Cooling down helps you to get your breathing and circulation back to normal.
- It also helps keep your muscles from becoming sore and stiff.

Cooling Down Is Important

A gradual cool-down can help you maintain flexibility and bring your breathing and circulation back to normal. If you don't cool down, you may get dizzy or nauseated. You may even faint because less blood is circulating to the heart and brain.

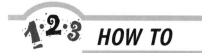 *HOW TO*

1. After exercising for 30 minutes or so (in a typical PE class), allow 5-10 minutes to cool down.
2. Walk around for a few minutes, relax your muscles, and breathe deeply until breathing returns to normal.
3. Once you have relaxed, stretch all of the major muscle groups you used during your workout—it is safer and more effective to stretch warm muscles.
4. Cool-down stretches can be the same as warm-up stretches.

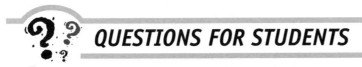

QUESTIONS FOR STUDENTS

1. Why should you cool down after exercising?
2. What can happen if you don't cool down?
3. How much time should you spend on cooling down?
4. What exercises can you do to cool down?

FitCheck

Teacher's Guide to FitCheck

FitCheck is a self-assessment tool that physical educators can use to help children identify, understand, and reflect upon their own patterns of physical activity and inactivity. Use it if it matches your students' abilities and fits into your curriculum.

FitCheck components are:

- FitScore and SitScore sheets. Students keep track of their physical activities and screen time activities over a seven-day period and translate their results into FitScores and SitScores. This is completed at home.

- Goal-setting sheet. Students set activity goals based on their FitScores and SitScores.

- FitScore and SitScore progress charts (bar graphs). Students graph their scores when they complete each FitCheck or two to three times during the year. (Try to make one time close to the end of the school year.)

The following sections will prepare you to present FitCheck to your students.

- *Using the FitScore and SitScore Progress Charts*

- *Interpreting FitScores and SitScores*

- *Tips for Teaching FitCheck:* These points summarize the main ideas to review before teaching the FitCheck sheet.

- *FitCheck Questions:* We have anticipated some of the questions students might have. It may be helpful to keep this set of questions handy the first few times you teach FitCheck.

- Coordinating the Microunits and FitChecks

You may choose to keep scoring and goal setting as activities done in separate classes so they take as little time as possible. We recommend that you complete at least five FitChecks throughout the school year.

Using FitCheck

Microunits 4-7 introduce FitCheck to students.

- Lesson 4 *Charting Your FitScore, Fit ★ Score, and SitScore*. This lesson introduces FitCheck.

- Lesson 5 *What Could You Do Instead of Watching TV?* This is one of two lessons preparing students for goal setting (lesson 7). It presents recommendations for limiting TV use and offers alternatives to TV, video and computer games, and video tapes and movies.

- Lesson 6 *Making Time to Stay Fit*. This is the second lesson preparing students for goal setting (lesson 7). Students make a group goal for class that day and evaluate their progress at the end of class. You may want to do this lesson several times with students until they are comfortable with goal setting and evaluation.

- Lesson 7 *Setting Goals for Personal Fitness*. Students set goals to improve their FitScores and SitScores. At the next FitCheck they evaluate their progress.

Using the FitScore and SitScore Progress Charts

There is no microunit to accompany the progress charts. After each FitCheck, or at two or three times during the school year, teachers should have students graph their scores so they can see their progress over time. This is an activity that could be coordinated with a math teacher or even carried out in math class.

Interpreting FitScores and SitScores

FitCheck encourages students to aim for a total of at least 60 minutes of physical activity on five to seven days a week (a FitScore of 5-7) and to aim for at least 20 minutes of vigorous activity on 3 or more days each week (a Fit ★ Score of 3 or more). It also encourages them to shoot for a total screen time of no more than 2 hours each day (a SitScore of 5-7). However, since children of this age have difficulty tracking time on tasks, students are asked to record what they do for activity and inactivity and to estimate whether it is more or less than these time recommendations, rather than recording the exact number of minutes.

We are asking students to aim for a total of 60 minutes nearly every day, rather than the minimum of 30 minutes listed in the Healthy People 2010 physical activity goals for adolescents. The 60 minute time recommendation seems reasonable since the National Association for Sport and Physical Activity (NASPE 1998) recommends that "elementary school-age children should accumulate at least 30-60 minutes of activity from a variety of activities on all or most days of the week." *Planet Health* users are only one to three years older than these students, and there is no evidence that middle–school-aged children need to be less active than younger children.

Expert recommendations for physical activity and inactivity for adolescents:

• Healthy People 2010 Physical Activity Goals include the following:
  1. 22-6: Increase the proportion of adolescents who engage in moderate physical activity for at least 30 minutes on 5 or more of the previous 7 days.
  2. 22-7: Increase the proportion of adolescents who engage in vigorous physical activity that promotes cardiorespiratory fitness 3 or more days per week for 20 or more minutes per session.

• The American Academy of Pediatrics recommends children and teens spend no more than two hours per day on leisure-time screen media: watching TV and movies and playing video and computer games.

Tips for Teaching FitCheck

1. Read through all the FitCheck units (4-7) first.
2. Plan a schedule of FitChecks for the year. We recommend doing at least two or three during the school year. You can spread out scoring, goal-setting, and charting assignments over several classes to maximize physical activity time in your classes. If your students are not able to handle goal setting and evaluation, you can still do the scoring sheets.
3. Set up a filing system. The easiest method is to set up a manila file folder for each student and to store these in a box or drawer.
4. You may want to coordinate with a math teacher to do the bar graph exercise (FitScore and SitScore Progress Charts).
5. Youth have difficulty tracking time on tasks. So rather than having them record the exact number of minutes of activity and inactivity, encourage students to record what they do and estimate whether it is more or less than the time recommendations.
6. Students may have difficulty estimating how much of their activity was vigorous or hard. To help them with this, review the examples of vigorous activities listed in lesson 4 and ask them which of their activities made them breathe hard.

7. Help students be realistic about their goals. Physical activity must fit in with other daily activities and family schedules and must be safe and supervised according to family rules. Students don't need to trade all their excess sit activity time for fit activities. Trading 1-2 hours per week is probably realistic.

FitCheck Questions

What kind of physical activities should students choose for a goal?

Whatever they like. They can select an activity to get better at, or they can pick an activity they are totally unfamiliar with and develop skills in that area.

Do students have to choose a vigorous activity or a sport?

No. They can choose any physical activity to trade with their inactive time. This includes unstructured outdoor play.

What happens if a student's goal is unmet by the next FitCheck?

The student can explore what prevented goal attainment in the evaluation section of the goal-setting sheet. If this process is pursued in a non-critical fashion, it can help students modify their expectations and learn to set realistic goals.

Is losing weight by the end of the school year a reasonable goal?

No. FitCheck sheets should not be used as weight-loss tools. Many young people who think they need to lose weight really don't need to. Weight loss can be unhealthy while children are growing. Encourage students who want to lose weight to talk with their parents, the school nurse, and their physicians.

Coordinating the Microunits and FitChecks

At the start of the year, determine how often you will teach microunits and how often students will have FitChecks. We recommend teaching one microunit per class or per week, and having a FitCheck at least two or three times per year. On FitCheck days you do not need to teach a microunit.

Start with lessons 1-7 so that students learn how to do FitCheck as early as possible in the school year. After this, you may wish to change the order of the microunits to better coordinate with your own sports and fitness curriculum.

Explaining the scoring and completing the goal-setting sheet of the FitCheck will take about 20 minutes the first time, so you may need to set aside the better part of a class for this when you begin. These sections should take less time as students become more familiar with them.

The FitCheck may present challenges to your PE classes. Some students have difficulty setting goals and remembering to work on them. You may want to send students home with reminder cards that they can post in obvious places. If time and student abilities continue to be barriers to FitCheck implementation, try to keep doing the scoring activities even if it means cutting back on goal setting. Goal setting and evaluation are difficult concepts for some students in middle school.

Introduction to FitCheck

 Fitness tip: FitChecks will help you increase your activity level. Regular FitChecks will allow you to chart your progress in reaching your activity goals.

Fitness Lesson

[Next week] you will begin *Planet Health*'s FitCheck. The FitCheck measures your FitScore, the time you spend in moderate activities like walking, your Fit ★ Score, the time you spend in vigorous activities like running, and your SitScore, the time you spend in screen activities like watching TV. Based on these scores, you can create goals to improve your fitness. After the FitCheck week, the FitCheck sheets will remain in [location] at all times. Only you will have access to your FitCheck sheet. You will use the FitCheck sheet every ___ weeks *(we recommend an interval of 4-8 weeks)*. If you need to look at your folder at a time other than during a FitCheck week, ask me to get it for you.

To chart your progress, you will keep track of your FitScore, Fit ★ Score, and SitScore.

- A FitScore reflects the time you spend in moderate physical activities.

- A Fit ★ Score reflects the time you spend in vigorous activities, such as basketball, aerobics, and walking.

- A SitScore reflects the amount of time you spend in screen activities like watching TV or movies or playing video or computer games. A SitScore represents time when you are not moving around.

A FitCheck consists of:

- totaling your FitScore, Fit ★ Score, and SitScore,
- setting a goal, and
- reflecting on your progress in reaching your goal.

Progress evaluation begins at the second FitCheck.

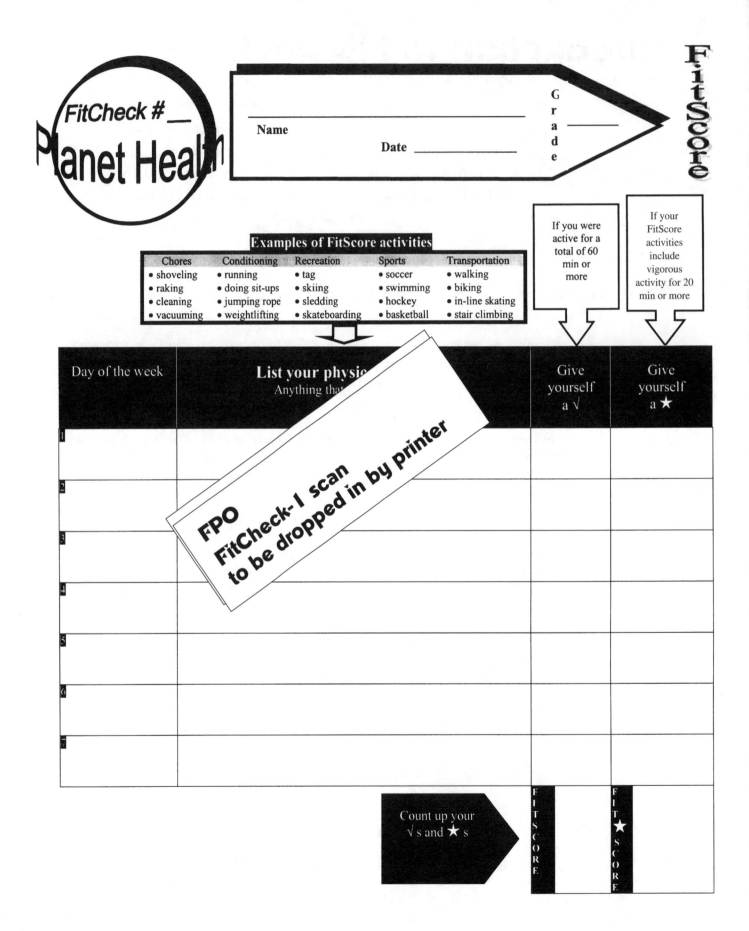

FitCheck # __

Planet Health

Name _____

Date _____

Grade _____

FitScore

Examples of FitScore activities

Chores	Conditioning	Recreation	Sports	Transportation
• shoveling	• running	• tag	• soccer	• walking
• raking	• doing sit-ups	• skiing	• swimming	• biking
• cleaning	• jumping rope	• sledding	• hockey	• in-line skating
• vacuuming	• weightlifting	• skateboarding	• basketball	• stair climbing

If you were active for a total of 60 min or more

If your FitScore activities include vigorous activity for 20 min or more

Day of the week	List your physic... Anything that...	Give yourself a √	Give yourself a ★
1			
2			
3			
4			
5			
6			
7			

FPO
FitCheck-I scan
to be dropped in by printer

Count up your √ s and ★ s

FITSCORE

FIT★SCORE

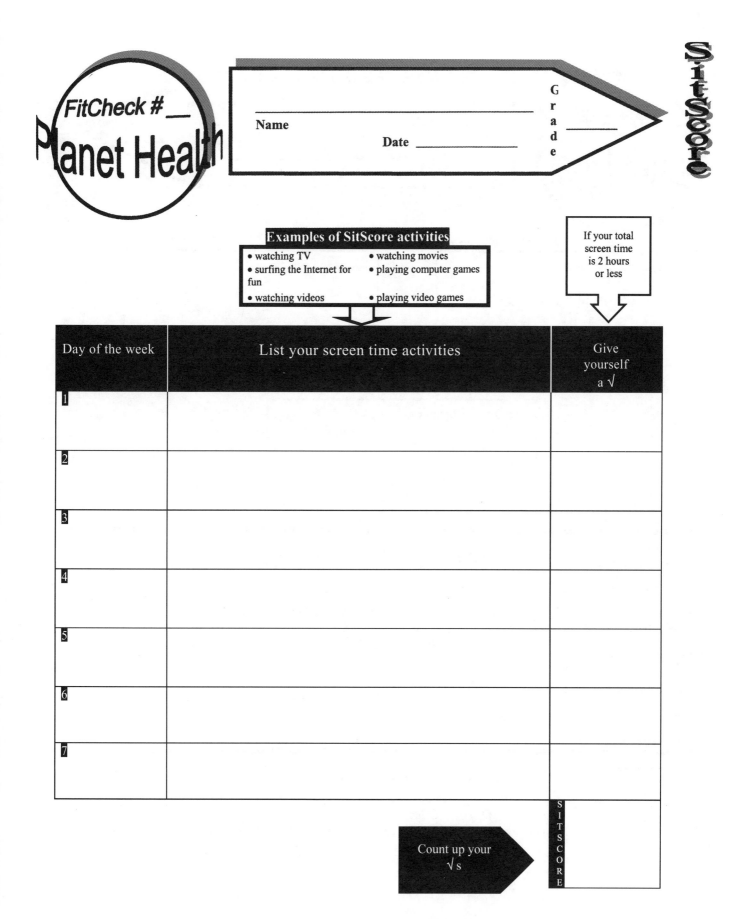

FitCheck #__
Planet Health

SitScore

Name _____

Date _____

Grade _____

Examples of SitScore activities

- watching TV
- surfing the Internet for fun
- watching videos
- watching movies
- playing computer games
- playing video games

If your total screen time is 2 hours or less

Day of the week	List your screen time activities	Give yourself a √
1		
2		
3		
4		
5		
6		
7		

Count up your √s

SITSCORE

FitCheck #___

Planet Health

Name _____

Date _____

Grade _____

My FitScore was _____

I need to (circle one)

	Score
keep it up!	5-7
be more active.	0-4

My Fit ★Score was _____

I need to (circle one)

	Score
keep it up!	3 or more
add more vigorous activities.	0-2

My SitScore was _____

I need to (circle one)

	Score
keep it up!	5-7
trade screen time for active time.	0-4

Set a goal to improve your fitness

You could:
- trade some screen time for active time, like riding your bike instead of watching TV.
- do more of what you're already doing, like in-line skating for 30 minutes instead of 15.
- work harder at what you're already doing.
- add new activities. Check to see if you can walk to school instead of getting a ride.

For example:

I will _____ *ride my bike instead of watching TV* _____
(for how long?) _____ *for 30 minutes* _____
(when?) _____ *after school on Tuesdays and Fridays* _____

I will _____
(for how long?)_____
(when?)_____

Date: [_____]

Reflect on your progress

Did you meet your goal?   **O** Yes   **O** No
Why/why not? Explain how you reached your goal, or why you did not reach your goal.

_____
_____
_____

Graph your FitScore below

Graph your Fit ★ Score below

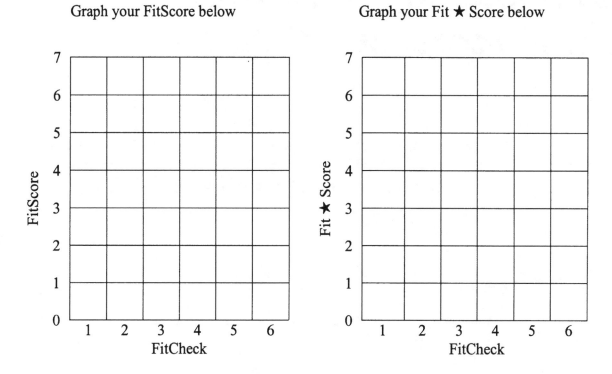

Graph your SitScore below

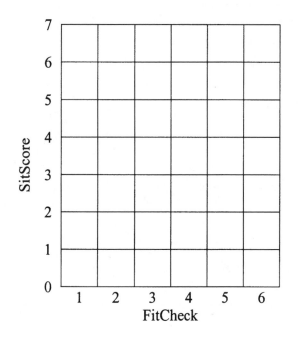

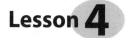

Charting Your FitScore, Fit ★ Score, and SitScore

 Fitness tip: The FitChecks will help you think about your activity and inactivity patterns. You can use this information to set personal goals.

What is FitCheck?

- You will use FitCheck to find out how often you are active as well as how much time you spend being inactive.
- Doing a FitCheck consists of
  - recording your physical activities and screen time (TV, computer and video games, movies, etc.) for a week, totaling your FitScore, Fit ★ Score, and SitScore at the end of the FitCheck week,
  - graphing your scores,
  - setting fitness goals, and
  - evaluating your progress toward your goals.

Use FitCheck to Chart Your FitScore

- Your FitScore represents the time you were physically active during the past week. It is the number of points you earn for time spent participating in moderately intense AND vigorous activities.
- You will keep track of your moderately intense physical activities like
  - brisk walking,
  - biking on level terrain,
  - dancing,
  - recreational swimming, and
  - mowing the lawn.
- You will also keep track of vigorous physical activities like
  - running,
  - jumping rope,
  - biking up a hill,

- swimming laps, and

- playing soccer and basketball.

• Vigorous activities make you breathe hard.

Use FitCheck to Chart Your Fit ★ Score

• Your Fit ★ Score tracks the amount of time you spend engaged in vigorous physical activities.

• If your FitScore activities included vigorous acitvity for 20 minutes or more, you get a ★.

Use FitCheck to Chart Your SitScore

• Your SitScore represents the time you were not moving around during the past week.

• To get an idea of how much time you spend being inactive, you will record your screen time activities like

- watching TV,

- playing computer or video games,

- playing hand-held computer games,

- surfing the Internet for fun, and

- watching videos and movies.

Defining Moderate and Vigorous Exercise Intensities

You should be able to carry on a conversation while participating in an activity of light to moderate intensity. Some examples of moderately intense activities are brisk walking, mowing the lawn with a motorized mower, dancing, recreational swimming, and biking on level terrain.

Vigorous activities make you breathe hard. You should still be able to talk, but you may not want to have an extensive conversation. Some examples of vigorous activities are race walking, mowing the lawn with a nonmotorized push mower, high-impact aerobic dancing, continuous swimming, and biking uphill.

1·2·3 HOW TO

Teachers, pass out one FitCheck sheet and a pencil to each student. Go over the instructions and use an example (possibly yourself) to demonstrate how to complete the FitCheck sheet.

1. You will complete the FitCheck for homework this week.

2. Complete the headings on pages 1 and 2.

3. You will use the FitScore sheet (page 1) to track your physical activities, in- and outside of school, for 7 days.

4. At the end of each day, write the day of the week in column 1. List all your physical activities in column 2. Include activities you participate in as part of PE classes, chores, sports, transportation, recreation, and conditioning.

5. Estimate how long you were physically active. If you were active 60 minutes or more, put a check mark in column 3. If you engaged in vigorous activity for 20 minutes or more, put a star in column 4. Begin filling this out tonight and continue for the next 7 days.

6. Use the SitScore sheet (page 2) to track your screen time, time spent watching TV or videos or playing computer or video games (time spent on the computer doing homework does not count). This is inactive time. Of course, there are other times during the day when you are not moving around, like when you sit in class at school. You can't decrease your class time, but you can choose to decrease your screen time.

7. At the end of each day, write the day of the week in column 1. List all your screen time activities in column 2. Estimate your screen time for the day. If your screen time is 2 hours or less, put a check mark in column 3.

8. At the end of the week, you will figure out your FitScore, Fit ★ Score, and SitScore by counting your checks and stars.
   • Aim for a FitScore of 5-7. To achieve this, you will need to be physically active for 60 minutes or more 5 to 7 days this week.
   • Aim for a Fit ★ Score of 3 or more. To achieve this, you will need to be vigorously active for at least 20 minutes 3 or more days this week.
   • Aim for a SitScore of 5-7. To achieve this, you will need to limit your screen time to 2 hours or less on 5 to 7 days this week.

9. Bring your completed FitCheck to school on [day of the week]. We will graph our scores in class that day.

10. You will repeat the FitCheck two or three times during the school year. This will allow you to compare your scores and see whether your activity and inactivity patterns have changed. I will keep your completed FitCheck sheets. Only you will have access to them.

 ## QUESTIONS FOR STUDENTS

1. What do your scores tell you about your lifestyle?
2. How might the FitCheck help you change your lifestyle?

Lesson 5

What Could You Do Instead of Watching TV?

 Fitness tip: Watching less than 2 hours of TV each day can help you get fit!

TV Cuts Down on Your Time to Be Active

- Many children your age spend a lot of their free time doing things that require sitting down.
- For some kids, this includes watching TV for about 5 hours a day.
- Think about how this cuts into your activity time.

Watching Too Much TV Can Make You Less Fit

- Being inactive day after day can quickly make you lose
  - flexibility,
  - muscle strength, and
  - cardiovascular endurance.
- When you sit still, you burn fewer calories than you would if you were moving around.

Watching Too Much TV Can Be Harmful to Your Health

When you sit in front of the TV, you lose a chance to be active and to improve your fitness level. Likewise, many people snack more than they need to while they are watching TV. Studies show that the kids who watch the least TV are the kids who are least likely to be overweight. The combination of eating too much and moving less can cause people to gain too much weight over time. People who are overweight are more likely to develop health problems, making it harder to lead a happy, active life.

Warning!!

Remember, you need plenty of healthy food for being active and growing, especially when you are growing fast. Never make a decision to cut back on the amount of food you eat without talking it over with your parents, your school nurse, or doctor.

HOW TO

1. Doctors recommend that children and teens watch no more than 2 hours of TV each day.
2. This means you can watch up to four half-hour shows every day—but you can watch less, too.
3. Watch only shows you like.
4. Take note of the times when you watch TV but you aren't really interested—when you channel surf or watch reruns—and use that time to be physically active instead.
5. Try to limit your TV viewing to no more than 2 hours each day.

QUESTIONS FOR STUDENTS

1. What is the maximum amount of TV that doctors recommend children watch per day?
2. What could happen if you watch too much TV?
3. Why is being active better than watching TV, movies, or playing video games?
4. What are some activities that you can do instead of watching TV?

Lesson **6**

Making Time to Stay Fit

 Fitness tip: It's the regular in regular activity that's important. Make space for fitness!

Making Space for Fitness

- Find the time to be active.
- Set aside a specific time to exercise.
- Small increases in physical activity add up over time, and can produce long-term health benefits.

Never Pass Up the Opportunity to Be Physically Active

- Stretch when you wake up in the morning.
- Take the stairs instead of the escalator or elevator at the mall.
- If it is safe for you, walk or bike instead of getting a ride or taking the bus.

Goal Setting

- It's important to set goals for increasing your physical activity.
- Today we will practice setting activity goals.
- We'll begin by trying to write a goal that will motivate each of you to be more active during today's class.

Exercise With Others

Exercising with others can make doing an activity more fun. Make a plan to exercise with a friend. You can also do active things you like with your parents, brothers, or sisters. Finally, you may want to join a team.

Finding Active Time at School

Think about times during the day when you can trade inactive time for physical activity. Try to be more active during PE, and walk briskly to your classes.

Finding Active Time Away From School

In addition, you can be more active while you are away from school. Invite friends over to play active games, practice dance, aerobics, gymnastics, or lift weights. Clean your room (and your house). Vacuuming, cleaning out closets, and other tasks require bending, stretching, and lifting. Have fun with it! Listen to music!

Quick Ideas to Become More Fit

- Help a younger sister or brother get started in an activity or sport.
- Learn how to baby-sit and play with young children.
- Try to be as active as a two- or three-year-old—it just might tire you out.
- Watch TV only if it's your favorite show.
- Exercise while you watch your favorite shows on TV.
- Borrow an exercise video from the video store or library.
- Take up an after-school activity or sport.
- Go for a walk or bike ride with a friend.
- Try to stay outside for an hour after school with your friends if your parents approve.

1·2·3 HOW TO

Make one goal to be completed by all students in gym class today. For example, "I will warm up for 5 minutes before exercising, actively participate (break a sweat) in PE today, and spend 5 minutes cooling down at the end of class." You may want to discuss the goal with students and come up with one together.

1. Write the goal on the chalkboard (or in large print on sheets of paper hung on the wall), so students can see it throughout class.
2. At the end of class, leave time for students to evaluate whether they reached their goal.
3. Ask students the following:
   - Did you reach the class goal?
   - For those of you who reached the goal, how do you know you reached your goal?
   - For those you who didn't reach your goal, what could you have done to reach your goal?
4. You may want to repeat this lesson in PE class until students are comfortable with goal setting and evaluation.

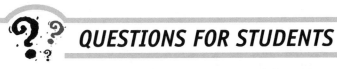

QUESTIONS FOR STUDENTS

1. What are some ways you can make time to stay fit?

2. It's important to set realistic goals for yourself—ones that you have a reasonable chance of reaching. Which of the following goals is realistic for a student who currently gets a ride to school from her mom? Goal 1: I will walk to and from school instead of getting a ride every day for the next month. Goal 2: I will walk to school three mornings a week for the next month.

Planet Health's language arts curriculum also includes a goal-setting lesson. You may want to coordinate timing with the language arts teachers at your school. If you do, be sure to tell the students they'll have another opportunity to work on this topic.

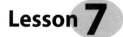 **Lesson 7**

Setting Goals for Personal Fitness

 Fitness tip: Set fitness goals that fit your life. Trade some sit time for fit time.

Setting Personal Fitness Goals

- Setting fitness goals is a good first step to getting fit.
- Today you will learn more about goal setting.
- You will use FitCheck to set a personal fitness goal.
- While setting goals, keep in mind how much time you spend in front of a screen. If you have a lot of inactive time, set a goal to trade inactive time for active time.

Trading Bored Time With Fun Time

How much of your screen time is spent channel surfing, watching shows you don't like, watching reruns, or playing video games because you have nothing better to do? You should trade that time for active time. Play a sport, do an aerobics tape with a friend, or walk the dog. (See Lesson 5 for more ideas.)

Planet Health Fitness Goals

Be moderately physically active for at least 30 minutes every day or nearly every day as part of chores, play, transportation, and exercise. Participate in vigorous activity at least three times each week for 20 minutes or more per session. Aim for a total of 60 minutes of plysical activity per day. Spend no more than 2 hours per day watching TV and playing video or computer games.

1·2·3 *HOW TO*

Before discussing the Goal-Setting section of FitCheck, have students review their most recent FitScore and SitScore sheets. Then read these instructions to students:

1. Write your most recent FitScore, Fit ★ Score, and SitScore above the appropriate box in the top section of the Goal-Setting sheet.

2. To figure out how you are doing, compare your scores to the ones listed in the boxes. Complete the sentence, "I need to" by circling the phrase next to the range that includes your score. For example, say you have a SitScore of 2; that means that on 2 days during the FitCheck week, you watched 2 hours or less of TV each day. On 5 days, your screen time exceeded 2 hours. You would circle "trade screen time for active time."

3. You should
   - aim for a FitScore of 5-7. To achieve this, you will need to be physically active for 60 minutes or more 5 to 7 days this week.
   - aim for a Fit ★ Score of 3 or more. To achieve this, you will need to be vigorously active for at least 20 minutes 3 or more days this week.
   - aim for a SitScore of 5-7. To achieve this, you will need to limit your screen time to 2 hours or less on 5 to 7 days this week.

4. Now use this information to set a fitness goal.

5. If your SitScore was low, consider trading screen time for active time. How about riding your bike instead of watching TV?

6. Other goal options may be to
   - participate more often in an activity you enjoy, such as in-line skating for 30 minutes instead of 15.
   - work harder at the activities you already do.
   - add new activities, such as walking to school instead of getting a ride.

7. Whatever you do, choose an activity you like. Remember that making a plan with a friend could make the activity more fun and help you do it more often.

8. [Give students time to complete their goals, then collect the FitCheck sheets.] You will check your progress toward your goal the next time we do a FitCheck.

Goal Evaluation

1. Read your goal from the previous FitCheck.
2. Think about your progress toward the goal.
3. Fill in today's date in the section *Reflect on Your Progress*.
4. Answer the question, "Did you meet your goal?"
5. In one or two sentences, explain why you did or did not reach your goal. If you reached your goal, explain how you reached your goal.

Pass out a new FitCheck sheet to students and have them assess their FitScore, Fit ★ Score, and SitScore (lesson 4, page 23-24).

QUESTIONS FOR STUDENTS

1. Have you written a realistic goal? If not, how can you modify it to make it more reasonable to achieve?

2. What kinds of things might keep you from achieving your goal? How can you overcome these obstacles?

part

III

Getting
Started

Lesson 8

Let's Get Started on Being Fit

 Fitness tip: For total physical fitness, work on cardio-vascular endurance, muscle strength, and flexibility.

What Is Physical Fitness?

- Being physically fit means you have the energy and strength to handle the everyday demands of your life:
  - Walking to school
  - Playing a game of soccer during gym
  - Actively listening and participating in class
  - Completing daily chores
  - Participating in after-school activities
  - Doing a good job on your homework
  - Sprinting to escape the jaws of the neighborhood dog
- You can complete all of your daily activities without feeling overly fatigued.

Overall Physical Fitness

- Many factors contribute to your overall physical fitness.
- The factors that are most important to your health are
  1. cardiovascular endurance (or cardiovascular fitness),
  2. muscle strength, and
  3. flexibility.

The Three Areas of Physical Fitness

- Physical fitness consists of cardiovascular endurance, muscle strength, and flexibility.
- Each one of these components helps your body to be physically fit in different ways.
- Cardiovascular endurance helps you do physical work or play for a long time without getting tired.
- Muscle strength helps you lift and move yourself and heavy stuff.
- Flexibility helps you reach, bend, twist, and move without injury.

A Closer Look at the Three Areas of Physical Fitness

- Cardiovascular endurance: Enables you to do continuous physical activity for long periods of time. This requires your heart, blood vessels, lungs, and muscles to efficiently carry and use oxygen.
- Muscle strength: Allows you to exert a force, such as lifting or moving yourself or a heavy object.
- Flexibility: Enables you to move your muscles and joints through the full range of motion without discomfort or injury.

Bone Integrity and Body Composition Are Two Other Components of Health-Related Fitness

Regular physical activity will help you build strong bones and maintain a healthy body composition. A fit person has strong bones and muscles and a healthy amount of body fat.

Skill-Related Components of Physical Fitness

Success in sport and other physical activities may require you to develop some other abilities, such as

- agility,
- balance,
- power,
- speed,
- coordination, and
- reaction time.

1·2·3 HOW TO

1. To improve your cardiovascular fitness, do physical activities that increase your heart and breathing rate:
   - Walk briskly
   - Hike
   - Swim
   - Play dodge ball
   - Jump rope
   - Play soccer
   - Dance
   - Ride your bike
   - Do in-line skating

2. To improve your strength and muscular endurance, do work, play, or exercise that makes you repeatedly lift or move a load (an object, your body, a weight) that is heavier than you are used to.

- Do push-ups, pull-ups, and sit-ups.
- Pedal your bike up an incline.
- Shovel snow.
- Ask your physical education teacher to help you design a safe weight-training program.

3. Performing these activities in sets of repetitions will improve your muscle strength and endurance.

4. To improve your flexibility, stretch regularly. Activities like gymnastics, dance, and figure skating require good flexibility.

5. To best improve your overall physical fitness, participate in a variety of physical activities.

6. Be sure to do activities that work and stretch the upper and lower body parts.

 QUESTIONS FOR STUDENTS

1. Can you name some activities that will improve each component of physical fitness?

2. Which area of fitness do you think you need to improve the most?

More About the Three Areas of Physical Fitness

 Fitness tip: To get fit, choose a mixture of activities that you can do regularly to build your cardiovascular fitness, muscle strength, endurance, and flexibility.

Physical Fitness

- We learned that in order to be physically fit and to meet the daily demands of work and play, a person must possess an adequate level of
  - cardiovascular fitness,
  - muscular strength, and
  - flexibility.
- To be fit, you need to work in all three areas of fitness because each area has a different effect on our bodies.

Some Activities Address One Area of Fitness, While Others Address More Than One

- To be fit, you need to participate in a variety of physical activities.
- It is important that you be able to identify which activities belong to different fitness areas.
- Then you need to identify activities in each area that you enjoy and do them.

No One Type of Physical Activity Improves All Components of Fitness

Aerobic activities generally increase cardiovascular and muscle endurance, but not strength and flexibility. Similarly, many activities that build muscular strength and flexibility don't do much for endurance. These activities also improve only the body part being worked. Therefore, strength and flexibility exercises must be performed for each muscle group and at each joint.

HOW TO

1. Let's think about some daily activities and exercises you do, and figure out what areas of physical fitness they address. For example: what area of physical fitness do you work on when you

   • carry heavy boxes or grocery bags? (improves upper-body strength)

   • bike to your friend's house? (increases your cardiovascular endurance)

   • shovel snow? (improves muscle strength and endurance and cardiovascular endurance)

Ask students to name a few activities. Involve the class in identifying the components of physical fitness being addressed.

QUESTIONS FOR STUDENTS

1. Name three components of physical fitness.

2. Which component do you need to work on the most?

3. During class today we will play (or do) [activity]. What components of fitness will we be working on during this activity?

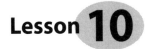 **Lesson 10**

Frequency, Intensity, Time, and Type

 Fitness tip: To be fit, keep the F.I.T. & T. rule in mind. How long, how hard, and how often you are active will determine how fit you are!

Designing a Program for Overall Fitness

- When you plan a fitness program for yourself, think about frequency, intensity, time, and type of activities. This is the F.I.T. & T. rule.
  - Frequency is how often you do something.
  - Intensity is how hard you do something.
  - Time refers to how long the activity lasts.
  - Type refers to including a variety of activities in your routine.
- Here is more information.

Frequency

- Frequency refers to
  - how often you exercise, or
  - the number of times you are active per week.
- Frequency recommendations for each fitness component vary.

Intensity

- Intensity refers to how hard or strenuously you exercise—for example:
  - how fast your heart beats,
  - how much you stretch, or
  - how much weight you lift.
- The peak intensity at which you can do an activity will depend on your physical condition.
- As your fitness level improves, you can do more intense activities.

Time

- Time refers to how long you spend being active.
- Time recommendations for each component of fitness vary.

Type

- Type refers to the kind of exercise you choose to do—namely,
  - cardiovascular or aerobic exercise (prolonged, nonstop, repetitive activity),
  - muscle strength or anaerobic exercise (short bursts of high-intensity activity like sprinting or lifting heavy weights or other objects), and
  - stretching.

Health and Fitness Benefits

Following the F.I.T. & T. formula will improve your

- level of fitness in each fitness component,
- performance in sports and physical activities, and
- overall health.

The health benefits of physical activity can occur at levels less than those required for improving performance. Regularly doing even low-intensity activities like leisure walking for 30 minutes or more can reduce your risk for heart disease and helps you maintain a healthy body weight.

1·2·3 HOW TO

1. How often should you exercise?
   - Be moderately active for at least 30 minutes daily or nearly every day as part of play, transportation, chores, and exercise.
   - Do vigorous activities at least three times per week.
   - Aim for a total of 60 minutes or more of physical activity nearly every day.
2. How hard should you exercise?
   - Increase the intensity of physical activity gradually.
   - Try to include activities of low, moderate, and vigorous intensity in your routine.
   - If you increase the intensity of your activities or exercises, you can reduce the duration of your activities.
3. For how long should you exercise?
   - Moderately intense activities should be done more frequently and for a longer time than vigorous activities
   - Do moderately intense activities like brisk walking for at least 30 minutes.
   - Do more vigorous activities like jogging for at least 15-20 minutes.
   - Even low-intensity activities have health benefits if they are done regularly for prolonged periods of time.
   - Aim for a total of 60 minutes or more of physical activity nearly every day.

4. What type of exercise should you do?
- Find a combination of exercises you like that improve your overall fitness.
- Aerobic activities like jogging, basketball, and hiking improve your cardiovascular fitness and muscle endurance.
- Carrying heavy objects and lifting weights make your muscles stronger.
- Stretching improves your flexibility.

QUESTIONS FOR STUDENTS

1. What does F.I.T. & T. stand for?
2. What types of physical activities do you like doing? Do you do them with enough frequency, with enough intensity, and for long enough to be fit?
3. Do you include enough variety of activities to work on each of the health-related components of physical fitness?

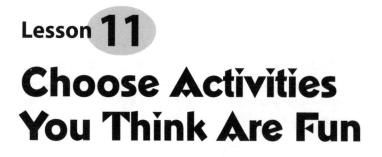

Lesson 11

Choose Activities You Think Are Fun

 Fitness tip: To become fit and stay fit, choose activities you think are fun.

Choose Activities You Like, and Vary Your Workout

- It is easier to stick with something if it is something you enjoy.
- If you do the same thing each time, you may get bored and stop working out. For example, if you choose to walk,
  - try out different safe routes,
  - explore new neighborhoods,
  - walk while you talk with friends,
  - listen to music, and
  - notice your environment.

There Are a Lot of Reasons to Be Active

- Being active may give you a sense of
  - pleasure,
  - self-expression, and
  - personal accomplishment.
- In addition to the personal satisfaction that being active may bring you, it can also help you
  - improve your health,
  - build character,
  - make new friends,
  - release energy, and
  - discover the environment.

Make Reasonable Goals When You Change Your Activity Routine

Improvement in physical fitness can be a slow process. In order to maintain or improve your fitness levels, make sure you do things regularly, and gradually increase your activity intensity. Improvements are seen only if you regularly go beyond what your body is used to. However, too much too soon can lead to frustration, injury, and muscle pain. Remember, change does not happen overnight!

HOW TO

1. Keep in mind *frequency* when planning a fitness schedule.
   - Make sure your activity can be done on a regular basis.
   - If your schedule gets interrupted and you don't exercise for a while, just start again.
2. *Intensity*, *time*, and *type* are also important.
   - Remember to gradually increase the intensity and time of your activity.
   - Likewise, remember to vary the type of exercise you do.
3. Be active regularly. Do moderately intense activity nearly every day and vigorous activity at least three times each week.
4. Increase your activity level *gradually*.

QUESTIONS FOR STUDENTS

1. What are some things to keep in mind while developing your fitness program?
2. What should you do if you stop being active for a week?
3. What are some good reasons to be physically active?

Lesson 12
How Often Should I Exercise?

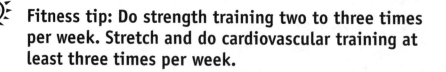 **Fitness tip:** Do strength training two to three times per week. Stretch and do cardiovascular training at least three times per week.

How Often Should You Exercise?

- The frequency, or number of times you work out per week, varies depending on what area of physical fitness you are working on.
- Do strength training two to three times per week.
- Stretch and do cardiovascular (aerobic) training at least three times per week.
- No matter which area of physical fitness you are working on, begin slowly and build up gradually to longer times or harder activities.
- Try to do some physical activity every day, even on the days you don't do planned exercise:
  - Walk to the store instead of getting a ride.
  - Take the stairs instead of the elevator.
  - Play outside with a friend instead of watching TV.

Flexibility Activities

Plan to do flexibility activities at least three times per week. If you are just starting to stretch, gradually increase the number of repetitions and lengthen the duration of the stretch.

Muscle-Strengthening Activities

Plan to do muscle-strengthening activities at least two to three times per week. Begin with one set of 10-15 repetitions, and then increase the number of sets to two and then to three. If you are using weights and can do three sets of 15 repetitions, increase the amount of weight you are using.

> ## Cardiovascular Endurance Activities
>
> Plan to do moderately intense aerobic activity for at least 30 minutes nearly every day and vigorous aerobic activity for at least 20 minutes, three or more days a week. Aim for a total of 60 minutes or more of physical activity nearly every day. Vigorous activities are best for improving cardiovascular endurance. You must work harder or longer than you are used to in order to improve your cardiovascular endurance.

HOW TO

1. Although we talk of physical fitness as a combination of three areas, most of us can integrate all three of these areas in one workout.
2. Start with flexibility exercises to stretch and warm up.
3. Go on to a cardiovascular activity like playing basketball.
4. Then do some muscle strengthing activities like push-ups or sit-ups.
5. Finish by cooling down with some more flexibility exercises.
6. Remember, any activity is better than none.
   - So if you are just getting started with physical activity, don't worry about how hard or how long you are active in the beginning.
   - Just find an activity you like and do it regularly.
   - Even participating regularly in low-intensity activities (like golf, bowling, and leisure walking) can offer some protection against cardiovascular disease, obesity, diabetes, osteoporosis, and certain cancers. However, for optimal health benefits, try to include moderately intense activities nearly every day and vigorous activities three times a week.
7. If you want to excel at an activity, you will likely need to do the activity more often than we've recommended in this lesson. So don't get mad at your coach if he or she has you practice 5 days a week. Not only will you improve your performance, you will improve your fitness and further reduce your risk of developing cardiovascular disease (and the other diseases mentioned above).

QUESTIONS FOR STUDENTS

1. How often should you do flexibility activities in a week?
2. How often should you do muscle-strengthening activities in a week?
3. How often should you do cardiovascular activities in a week?
4. Define repetition and set.

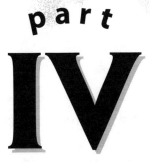

part

IV

Improving Fitness

Improving Cardiovascular Endurance

 Fitness tip: Doing physical activities that build your cardiovascular endurance now will help lower your risk of developing cardiovascular disease later in life. Stay healthy to have more fun!

Learning About Cardiovascular Endurance (Fitness)

- Your ability to do physical work or play for a long time without tiring is called your cardiovascular endurance.
- To have good cardiovascular endurance your heart, blood vessels, lungs, and muscles must efficiently carry and use oxygen.
- People with good cardiovascular endurance can do vigorous physical activity for 20 minutes or more without getting tired.

Aerobic Exercise

- The best way to improve your cardiovascular endurance, or cardiovascular fitness as it is sometimes called, is to do aerobic exercise.
- Aerobic exercise increases your breathing and heart rate by doing nonstop, repetitive exercises.
- Examples of aerobic activities include
  - aerobic dancing,
  - distance running,
  - swimming,
  - cycling,
  - basketball,
  - soccer, or
  - any active game that includes running.
- Increasing cardiovascular endurance now and maintaining it when you grow up will lower your risk of chronic disease in adulthood.

A Closer Look at Aerobic Exercise

The term *aerobic* means "with oxygen." During aerobic exercise, the body is able to supply enough oxygen to continue the activity for long periods of time. Aerobic exercises can be done at low, moderate, or vigorous intensities and should last 20 minutes or more to be effective.

Aerobic exercise improves blood flow and oxygen supply to the heart, helps keep arteries clear, and can lower blood pressure, thus improving cardiovascular endurance and reducing the risk of heart disease later in life.

How Hard Do I Need to Exercise?

Regularly participating in even low-intensity activities (like golf, bowling, and casual walking) offers some protection against cardiovascular disease, diabetes, obesity, and certain types of cancer. However, for optimal health benefits you need to do moderately intense and vigorous activities regularly. Even higher levels of cardiovascular endurance are needed to excel in competitive sports and physical activities.

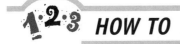 # HOW TO

1. Becoming more fit is not a competitive activity. This is something you are doing to be healthy so you can keep having fun throughout your life!

2. Be moderately active for 30 minutes or more every day, or nearly every day, as part of play, transportation, chores, and exercise.

3. To improve your cardiovascular endurance

   - Do vigorous activities (like running) for at least 20 minutes on 3 or more days a week.

   - Do moderately intense activities more frequently and for a longer time than vigorous activities. Aim for a total of 60 minutes or more of physical activity nearly every day.

   - You must work harder or longer than you are used to in order to improve your cardiovascular endurance.

4. Set your aerobic pace. At your age, you can assume you are getting a good aerobic workout if your heart rate goes up and you begin to breathe faster and deeper, and you are working at a pace you can maintain for at least 20 minutes. Do the talk test: if you can carry on a conversation, you are exercising at a moderate to vigorous training intensity; if you become too out of breath to talk, you may be approaching a pace you cannot maintain.

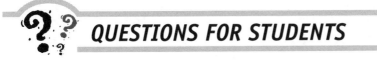 # QUESTIONS FOR STUDENTS

1. How do cardiovascular (aerobic) exercises help us stay fit?

2. What are some examples of cardiovascular (aerobic) activities?

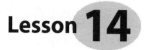

Improving Muscular Strength

Fitness tip: Strength training can build muscle strength and help you avoid shoulder, knee, and back injuries. It can also improve performance in all activities, including sports.

Muscle Strength

- The ability of your muscles to generate force is called strength.
- The most weight that you can lift at one time is a measure of your muscle strength.

Focus on All of Your Muscles

- Exercise all major muscle groups of your body. These include
  - quadriceps,
  - hamstrings,
  - lower back,
  - abdominals,
  - chest,
  - upper back,
  - shoulders,
  - triceps, and
  - biceps.

Benefits of Strong Muscles

- Stronger muscles have more muscular endurance. This means they can work hard over a period of time.
- They will also help you to perform better in other physical activities, sports, and games.

Key Words When Doing Strength Training

- *Repetition:* A repetition is the number of times you can perform a movement without rest.
- *Set:* A set is a group of repetitions for a particular exercise.

Learning About Joints

Every joint has muscles on both sides to do its work and bring it through its range of motion. It is important to exercise the muscles on both sides of every joint. Muscles work by contracting (shortening). When a muscle has done its work, it relaxes back to its resting length.

Preventing Injury and Pain

Strong muscles help prevent certain types of injury and pain. For example, strong thigh muscles (quadriceps) help keep the kneecap lined up properly, which can help prevent knee injuries. Similarly, strong abdominal muscles can help control lower-back problems by keeping the spine in proper position and decreasing the strain on the lower-back muscles. Strength training will make your muscles bigger by increasing the size of your muscle cells.

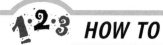 ## HOW TO

1. Strength-training exercises can be done for all of the major muscle groups in the body. Train muscles according to their size.
2. Begin with larger muscles (e.g., leg muscles) and progress to smaller ones (e.g., torso or arms).
3. Do all exercises through a complete range of movement to develop strength.
4. Always warm up before muscle strength (anaerobic) training and cool down afterward.
5. Strength training works best when it is done at a frequency of two to three times per week.
6. Train every other day, and not daily. If strength training is done on the same muscle group every day, you will notice a decrease in strength due to overtraining.
7. Increase your intensity when you can do three sets of 15 repetitions.

 ## QUESTIONS FOR STUDENTS

1. Why is muscle strength important?
2. Is muscle strength needed only by athletes? Why or why not?
3. Identify exercises to strengthen and stretch the muscles at every major joint of the trunk, upper body, and lower body.

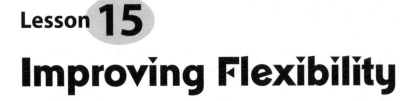
Improving Flexibility

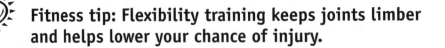

Fitness tip: Flexibility training keeps joints limber and helps lower your chance of injury.

Review of Flexibility

- Your ability to move your muscles and joints through their full range of motion is called flexibility.
- People with good flexibility are able to bend, stretch, and twist with ease.
- To prevent or decrease muscle soreness and stiffness, include stretching exercises in your warming up and cooling down periods.

Benefits of Stretching

- Stretching exercises can help prevent the loss of flexibility.
- Stretching exercises will also lower your chances of injury.
- Stretching can relax overstressed muscles and reduce soreness and cramps.
- However, too much stretching can make muscles sore.

Stretch Regularly

Most young children are very flexible, but lose some range of motion as they grow older. Physical inactivity makes you lose flexibility. So, if you stay active and incorporate stretching into your exercise routine, you may be able to stay flexible long into your adult years. Stretching is relaxing and fun!

 HOW TO

1. Flexibility exercises are muscle specific and should be done for all the major muscles.
2. Flexibility exercises are usually done for only a few minutes, at least three to four times each week.

3. You can do flexibility exercises on their own, or before or after cardiovascular or muscular strength-training exercises.

4. But remember, it's better and safer to stretch warm muscles rather than cold muscles.

5. For each exercise, always stretch to the point where your muscles are taut (drawn tight), not beyond.

6. Hold the stretch for 20-60 seconds for 1 to 3 repetitions.

7. Remember to breathe.

8. Concentrate on lengthening the time of the stretch.

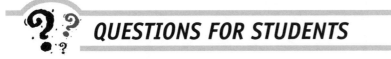

QUESTIONS FOR STUDENTS

1. Why is flexibility important?

2. What are some of the activities you participate in to improve your flexibility?

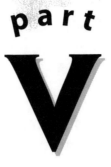

part

V

Measuring Fitness

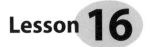

Improving Your Overall Physical Fitness Levels

 Fitness tip: Improve your fitness level by progressing slowly and exercising regularly.

Gradual Improvements

- The way to improve physical fitness is to begin slowly and to gradually build up over time to activities that are harder and last longer.
- Improving gradually will help you to avoid straining or injuring your muscles and joints.

Another Look at F.I.T. & T.

- Remember the F.I.T. & T. rule:
  - Frequency
  - Intensity
  - Time
  - Type
- You can improve fitness by
  - increasing the frequency (if you are not already exercising regularly),
  - increasing the intensity (doing something faster, doing more repetitions or sets, or using heavier weights), and
  - increasing the time you spend on each exercise. You might even choose more types of exercise to do!

Workout Recommendations

Flexibility and cardiovascular (aerobic) exercises should be done at least three times per week, and strength training should be done two to three times per week. When you are doing strength training, remember to gradually build up to three sets of 15 repetitions. If you can do this, you are ready to add more repetitions or sets. If you are using free weights, you add more weight instead of more reps or sets.

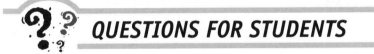

HOW TO

1. Check your frequency!
   - Are you physically active for at least 30 minutes every day or nearly every day as part of play, exercise, chores, and transportation?
   - Do you do moderately intense to vigorous activity at least three times per week for 20 minutes or more?
   - Add more exercises if you need to.
2. Think about the intensity! Can you stretch a little farther, or pick up the pace at aerobics or when running?
   - Slowly increase your intensity over time.
   - Gradually add more time to cardiovascular (aerobic) workouts like running, cycling, or swimming.
   - Try to do moderately intense activities (like brisk walking) for at least 30 minutes.
   - More vigorous activities like running can be done for less time—but aim for at least 20 minutes.
   - Adding more time will increase your endurance and improve your fitness. Aim for a total of 60 minutes or more of physical activity nearly every day.
3. Try new types of exercises for different areas of fitness or for strengthening or stretching different muscles.

QUESTIONS FOR STUDENTS

1. How can you improve fitness?
2. Why is it important to make gradual progress?

Knowing Your Resting Heart Rate

 Fitness tip: As your cardiovascular endurance improves, your resting heart rate goes down.

Resting Heart Rate

- Your resting heart rate is a measure of the number of times your heart contracts (or beats) each minute you are at rest or sleeping.
- It can be measured by taking your resting pulse rate.

Your Heart Rate During Exercise

- Your heart beats faster when you move around and varies depending on how active you are throughout the day.
- The more intense your activity, the faster your heart beats.
- It can go down when your cardiovascular endurance improves, because your heart gets stronger and can pump more blood with each beat.

Heart Rate Varies With Activity and Level of Fitness

An average resting heart rate is around 60-80 beats per minute. Because a stronger heart will pump more blood with fewer strokes, athletes usually have a lower resting heart rate than nonathletes. Some athletes have resting heart rates as low as 35 beats per minute.

1·2·3 HOW TO

1. Take your pulse from inside the wrist.
   - First, turn your left wrist so that your palm faces up.

- Then place two fingers of your right hand on your radial artery. The radial artery is next to the tendons on your wrist, on the side closest to your thumb. Do not use your thumb, because it has its own pulse. Can you feel your pulse?
- Using a stopwatch (or second hand on a clock), count your pulse for 60 seconds. This is your heart rate per minute.

[Or, while you keep track of time, have students count their pulse for 60 seconds.]

2. The best way to measure your resting heart rate is to take your pulse first thing in the morning, before you get out of bed.

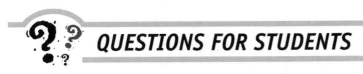

QUESTIONS FOR STUDENTS

1. If you regularly participate in endurance activities, what will happen to your resting heart rate?
2. Why does your heart need to beat faster when you are moving than when you are at rest?

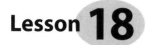

Exercise Makes Your Heart Beat Faster

Fitness tip: Exercise or play can strengthen your heart.

Aerobic Exercises Make Your Heart Stronger

- When you are doing aerobic exercise, you breathe faster and deeper, and your heart contracts faster and with greater force to get more oxygen and nutrients to your working muscles.
- Because your heart is a muscle, it makes sense that in time your heart will get stronger with this kind of exercise.

Knowing When Your Cardiovascular Endurance Is Improving

- As your cardiovascular endurance improves, your heart rate and breathing rate during a given activity (workload) will decrease.
- The activity will feel easier.
- Your heart rate and breathing rate will also return to normal more quickly after exercise, as you become more fit.

Just Move

Any activity or play where you run around for a while is good for you. So move and have fun any way you like.

Aerobic Exercise

Aerobic exercise is nonstop, repetitive exercise that can be continued for a long time. It can be done at low, moderate, and vigorous intensities. Participating regularly in low-intensity aerobic activities provides some health benefits. However, moderately intense to vigorous activities are best for improving cardiovascular endurance. You must work harder or longer than you are used to in order to improve your fitness.

(continued)

Low-Intensity Aerobic Activities

Leisurely walking or strolling, stretching, table tennis, playing catch, bowling, and playing golf (leisurely) are all examples of low-intensity aerobic activities.

Moderately Intense Aerobic Activities

Examples of moderately intense aerobic activities are brisk walking, in-line skating at a leisurely pace, low-impact aerobic dancing, bicycling on level terrain, light calisthenics, weight training (offers aerobic as well as anaerobic benefits when done continuously), shooting baskets, playing softball, recreational swimming, skateboarding, playing hopscotch or four-square, climbing on playground equipment, raking, and scrubbing the floor.

Vigorous Aerobic Activities

Examples of vigorous aerobic activities include running, hiking, or biking up an incline, lap swimming, skating at a vigorous pace, playing basketball, singles tennis, soccer, vigorous calisthenics—push-ups, pull-ups, sit-ups—shoveling snow, climbing stairs, carrying young children, and jumping rope.

1·2·3 HOW TO

1. To improve your cardiovascular endurance, you must work harder or longer than usual.
   - Plan to do vigorous aerobic activities for at least 20 minutes, 3 or more days a week, as these activities are best for improving cardiovascular endurance.
   - Moderately intense activities also improve cardiovascular endurance, but must be done more frequently and for a longer time than vigorous activities.
   - Aim for a total of 60 minutes or more of physical activity nearly every day.
2. One way to measure how hard you're working is to measure your heart rate.
3. To check this out, sit down for a minute and then take your wrist pulse; then take a leisurely walk around the gym for 1 minute and check your pulse rate again.
   - How much did your heart rate change?
   - Repeat these steps for brisk walking and running.
   - What happened to your heart rate as you increased your exercise intensity?
4. The more intense the activity, the faster your heat beats.
5. Remember, any activity is better than none.
   - So if you are just getting started with physical activity, don't worry about how hard or how long you are active at the beginning.
   - Just find an activity you like and do it regularly.

 ## QUESTIONS FOR STUDENTS

1. Why does your heart need to beat faster when you're physically active than when you're at rest?
2. Name some examples of moderately intense and vigorous aerobic activities.
3. How can you tell when your cardiovascular endurance is improving?

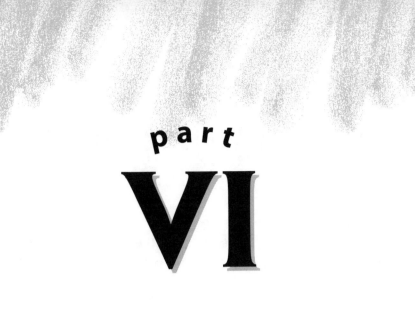

part

VI

Be Active Now!

Lesson 19

Be Active Now for a Healthy Heart Later

 Fitness tip: Being active in your free time can lower your risk of cardiovascular disease later in life.

The Number One Killer

- Cardiovascular disease is a disease of the heart and blood vessels.
- It is the single largest cause of death in the United States for both men and women.

Preventing the Number One Killer

- You can lower your risk of developing cardiovascular disease by starting a lifelong commitment to regular exercise now.
- Maintaining a healthy weight, eating a balanced diet that is low in saturated fat and moderate in total fat, and living smoke-free will also help you prevent cardiovascular disease.

Cardiovascular Disease in the United States

Cardiovascular disease is actually a group of diseases that affect the heart and blood vessels. It includes coronary artery disease (a narrowing of the arteries in the heart that can cause a heart attack, chest pain, or both), high blood pressure, stroke, rheumatic heart disease, and many others. According to 1996 estimates, 58,800,000 Americans have one or more forms of cardiovascular disease. A total of 959,227 Americans died from cardiovascular disease in 1996 (41.1% of all deaths).

Habits That Put Adults at Risk for Cardiovascular Disease Begin in the Teens

Being overweight, high blood cholesterol, stress, high-fat diets, physical inactivity (not moving around), and smoking are all habits that could lead to cardiovascular disease.

1·2·3 HOW TO

1. To prevent cardiovascular disease, develop good physical activity and eating habits at an early age and maintain them throughout your life.
2. Choose activities that make your heart and lungs stronger, like
   • fast walking,
   • running,
   • bicycling,
   • swimming,
   • in-line skating, and
   • hiking.
3. Eat five or more fruits and vegetables a day and a diet low in saturated fat and moderate in total fat.
4. Finally, don't smoke!

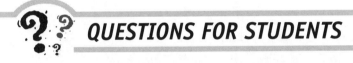

QUESTIONS FOR STUDENTS

1. Name some physical activities that you like to do that will strengthen your heart.
2. Which of these activities do you think you will continue as an adult?

Be Active Now for Healthy Bones Later

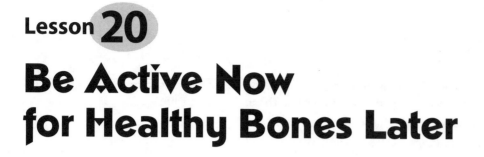

Fitness tip: Building strong bones now can help prevent fractures and bone loss later in life.

Building Strong Bones

- Almost 50% of your bone mass is formed during your teen years.
- Exercising and eating a balanced diet rich in calcium and vitamin D will help you build strong bones.
- Building strong bones now is a critical part of preventing osteoporosis from developing when you are older.
- Living a healthy lifestyle with no smoking and limited alcohol consumption during adulthood will keep your bones strong.
- People with osteoporosis have weak bones that are more likely to break. For example, hip fractures are common among the elderly and are a serious injury because older peoples' bones do not heal easily.

Building Strong Bones With Exercise

- Weight-bearing exercises build strong bones.
- In weight-bearing exercises, your bones and muscles work against gravity; your feet, legs, or arms support your weight as you move. Some examples of this kind of activity are
  - walking,
  - stair climbing,
  - hiking,
  - racket sports,
  - dancing,
  - soccer,
  - push-ups,
  - curl-ups, and
  - basketball, but
  - *not* swimming or biking.

- Weight training also builds strong bones.
- Hitting a ball or landing on your feet after jumping stimulates more calcium to be deposited in your bone. More calcium makes your bones stronger.
- Most sports and daily physical activities require weight-bearing activities. If you participate regularly in a variety of physical activities, you will build strong bones.

Osteoporosis

Osteoporosis literally means "porous bone." While the shape of the bones looks okay, they have fewer minerals in them. The minerals calcium and phosphorus are the major building blocks of bone. Bones that are low in these minerals are brittle and break more easily than healthy bones. It is estimated that 15 to 20 million Americans suffer from osteoporosis. Osteoporosis is more common among women than men (roughly 80% of osteoporosis cases are in women).

Preventing Osteoporosis Also Requires Consuming Enough Calcium

In order to prevent osteoporosis, you need to make sure that you are consuming enough calcium. Persons 9-18 years old require 1300 milligrams of calcium per day, the amount found in four 8-ounce glasses of milk. Milk and other dairy products (yogurt, cheese) offer the largest amount of calcium per serving. Other excellent sources of calcium include

- tofu,
- sardines with bones,
- calcium-fortified foods including orange juice, cereal, and cereal bars.

Spinach, broccoli, and other green leafy vegetables are good sources of calcium, but provide a lot fewer grams per serving than most milk products. If you are unable to consume milk or milk products, you should eat other calcium-rich foods.

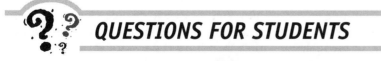

HOW TO

1. To build strong bones and prevent osteoporosis, develop good exercise and eating habits now.
2. Choose physical activities that put some stress on your bones.
3. Eat foods rich in calcium. Have four servings of low-fat dairy products like milk, cheese, and yogurt every day.

QUESTIONS FOR STUDENTS

1. How does exercise help your bones?
2. How can you help prevent osteoporosis and bone fractures?

Lesson 21

Be Active Now to Stay in Shape

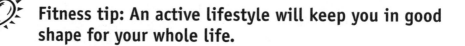 **Fitness tip: An active lifestyle will keep you in good shape for your whole life.**

Energy Balance

- When you eat and drink, the food you take in is used
  - for growing,
  - to give you energy for activities, and
  - for your metabolism.
- Metabolism refers to your internal body functions, such as
  - respiration (breathing),
  - circulation,
  - digestion, and
  - other things.
- Usually, you are in an energy balance, meaning that your body generally uses all of the energy that you take in.

Physical Activity Helps Maintain an Energy Balance

- Energy that is not used for growth, activity, or metabolism is stored as fat.
- Although gaining a certain amount of fat is necessary and normal in a healthy growing teen, excess body fat can build up at any age.
- Physical activity can help regulate your appetite, burn calories, and keep you fit. This helps prevent excessive weight gain.

Normal Weight Gain

Before adolescence, both boys and girls tend to put on some weight. During adolescence, you will continue to gain weight, your body will change shape, and you will grow taller as you enter your final growth spurt to reach adult size and shape. Girls tend to begin this growth spurt earlier than boys (two years earlier, on average). Some teenagers are nervous about these changes and try to diet in response. Remember, it is normal to gain weight during your teens, and dieting can be bad for your health.

> **Warning!**
>
> If you are concerned about gaining too much weight, talk with your parents, school nurse, or health-care provider. They can help you determine if your weight gain is okay. Don't fall into the dieting trap! A balanced diet and active lifestyle will keep your body in shape for your *whole life!*

HOW TO

1. Be active by reducing the time you spend watching TV and movies, and spending less time playing video and computer games—try cutting out an hour a week.
2. Instead, do things like playing active games or exercising.

QUESTIONS FOR STUDENTS

1. Why is it normal for teens to gain weight?
2. What should you do if you are concerned about gaining too much weight?

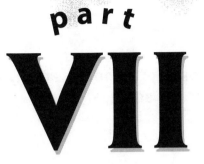

part

VII

Get Ready to Exercise

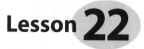

Energy for Exercise

 Fitness tip: Complex carbohydrates are an important source of energy.

When You Exercise, Your Muscles Need Energy

- Your body relies heavily on stored carbohydrates (glycogen) to supply the energy needed by your muscles during exercise.
- You need to replace those carbohydrates by eating healthy foods that have enough calories and are high in complex carbohydrates.
- Otherwise, your muscles will not be able to restock their carbohydrate stores after exercise, and you will feel tired and run-down.

Eat Right for Optimal Performance

Foods like cookies, candy, and soft drinks contain simple carbohydrates and are sometimes eaten before exercising for "quick energy." However, after this energy burst energy falls, and some people become irritable, exhausted, and dragged out. Eating foods that are high in sugar causes a sharp increase in blood glucose, followed by a sharp decrease. Some people are more sensitive to this than others. Although you may have a snack close to when you exercise, plan to wait 2 to 3 hours after a large meal before exercising strenuously. Your pre-activity meal should be high in complex carbohydrates, particularly from whole grain foods, and relatively low in fat and protein. For example, try whole wheat bread with a small amount of peanut butter and a healthy drink (no steak-and-egg pre-game meals).

Stored fat is another important source of energy during exercise. During brief periods of moderate exercise, your body burns carbohydrates and fats equally. As exercise continues for longer than an hour, fat becomes the more important energy source.

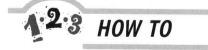 *HOW TO*

1. Get the carbohydrates you need each day, and make them complex carbohydrates whenever you can.

2. Complex carbohydrates are in foods like pasta, rice, bread, cereals, fruits, starchy vegetables (like potatoes), and beans. Try to include foods made from whole grain, like whole wheat bread, brown rice, oatmeal, corn tortillas, tabouli salad, and whole barley soup.

3. Eat the recommended number of servings from the Food Guide Pyramid. For active students your age, this means

   • 9 to 11 servings of grains and cereals each day, and

   • 5 or more servings of fruits and vegetables.

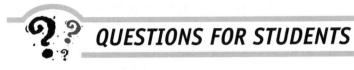

QUESTIONS FOR STUDENTS

1. What types of food are high complex carbohydrates?

2. Why is it important to eat the recommended number of servings of grains daily, especially when you exercise?

Lesson 23
Weather and Exercise

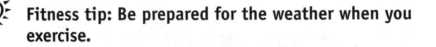 **Fitness tip: Be prepared for the weather when you exercise.**

Preparing for the Weather

Thinking ahead and dressing appropriately for the weather can help you prevent muscle and joint injuries when it's cold, and heat injuries when it's hot. Remember to check the weather before you exercise.

Hot Weather Raises the Risk of Exercise-Related Heat Injuries

- Exercise-related heat injuries are problems that can be traced to dehydration and overheating.
- Since sweat evaporates quickly in hot, dry air, you may not feel sweaty and may not realize how much water you have lost.
- Prevent excessive fluid loss by drinking water before, during, and after exercise. This is important for good performance, and for avoiding
  - heat cramps,
  - heat exhaustion, and
  - heat stroke.
- When your body loses a lot of water, you sweat less. Since it's the evaporation of sweat that cools you off, heat builds up and your body temperature rises.
- Dehydration also causes your blood volume to decrease. As a result, your heart must beat faster to deliver oxygen to your working muscles.

Humidity on Top of Heat Increases the Risk of Heat Problems

- Sweat does not evaporate well in humid environments. Without evaporation your body can't cool itself.
- If you are exercising and sweat is "dripping" from your skin, you may be missing the cooling benefit of sweat.

Be Careful in Cold Weather, Too!

- In cold weather, you need to keep your muscles warm.
- Cold muscles are stiff and raise your risk of strains and other injuries.

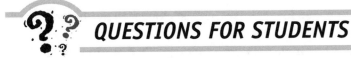

HOW TO

1. In the heat:
   - Exercise at the coolest time of the day.
   - Avoid exercise or practice when the temperature peaks (usually from about noon to 3 P.M. when the weather is hot).
   - If you must work out then, build up your heat tolerance by slowly increasing the amount of time you work out each day.
   - Wear the lightest clothing possible. Loose-fitting cotton is coolest. Consider jerseys with mesh on them, lightweight shorts, and low-cut socks. Wear sunscreen of SPF 15 or higher on exposed skin.
   - Drink plenty of water before, during, and after you exercise.
2. When it's cold:
   - Wear several layers of loose clothing, and when the temperature is below 40 °F wear a hat or an ear-band.
   - By wearing layers, your body heat is trapped—but sweat can be absorbed by the clothing.
   - Wear synthetic fibers designed for sports or cotton next to your skin. Many synthetic fabrics don't absorb sweat well and will leave you cold and damp. Read labels to find clothes that will wick away moisture.
   - As you warm up, you can always remove a layer or two to avoid overheating.

QUESTIONS FOR STUDENTS

1. How should you dress when you exercise in hot and humid weather?
2. How should you dress when you exercise in cold weather?
3. What can you do to avoid excessive fluid loss (dehydration)?

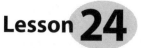

Getting Enough to Drink

 Fitness tip: Drink plenty of water before, during, and after exercising.

Dehydration Means Your Body Has Lost a Lot of Water

- To prevent dehydration, drink plenty of fluids before, during, and after exercise.
- Don't rely on thirst to tell you when to drink. It is not a good indicator because you won't feel thirsty until after your body has lost fluid and most people don't drink enough to replace the fluid they've lost.

Drink Water to Avoid Dehydration

- Water is the best and most economical drink for activities lasting less than an hour.
- Water will help you replace your body's water lost from sweating and will keep you from getting overheated and dehydrated, which can be dangerous.

Sports Drinks Offer an Alternative to Water

- Sports drinks are recommended for exercise that lasts longer than 1 hour and/or is performed in high temperature and humidity.
- They should taste good and contain 6-8% carbohydrate (20 g per 8 oz). Check the label.
- 100% fruit juices can also be used, if they are diluted with water (half juice/half water).

Warning!

Never use salt tablets. You don't need them. They can make you sick to your stomach. Because one salt tablet increases the amount of water you need by one pint (16 oz; 2 cups), taking salt tables can make a dehydration problem worse.

Your Body's Response to Excess Heat

About 60% of your body weight is water, and about 80% of your muscles is water. Sweat is largely made up of water and just a small amount of minerals and electrolytes (sodium, potassium, and magnesium). Sweating is the body's mechanism for getting rid of excess heat. When sweat evaporates, it cools your skin. This helps keep your body from overheating by constantly drawing heat out to the surface of the skin. When you sweat, you lose water. Not drinking enough during exercise may lead to dehydration and will make you feel bad. Dehydration can cause heat injuries like cramps, exhaustion, and heat stroke. Prevention is easy: drink water before, during, and after you exercise!

1·2·3 HOW TO

1. To avoid dehydration, drink 1 to 2 cups of water before exercising.
2. When you work out, start drinking early and at regular intervals (10-15 minutes).
3. Drink cool rapidly absorbed water, sports drinks, or diluted fruit juices.
4. Continue to drink after your workout is over. Flavored drinks may encourage you to drink more during this recovery period.
5. Avoid drinking soda and caffeinated drinks (such as colas, coffee, and iced tea) to replace water loss, because caffeinated drinks will increase water loss through urine, and large amounts of sugar (from soda) slow down stomach emptying and increase the time it takes for the fluid to reach your blood.

QUESTIONS FOR STUDENTS

1. How can you prevent dehydration?
2. What does water do for you when you exercise?
3. What happens if you don't drink enough water?
4. Is thirst a good sign of whether you are drinking enough water while exercising?

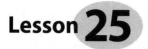

Food and Supplement Myths

Fitness tip: For a healthy, fit body, stay away from drugs and supplements, and concentrate on physical activity and eating well.

Getting Fit

- The best way to get fit is through consistent training and eating well.
- There are no miracle drugs, nutrients, or foods that build fitness or athletic performance.

Stay Away From Drugs and Supplements

- You may have heard that anabolic steroids improve athletic performance, but in fact they are illegal and using them can cause health problems.
- In addition, bee pollen, brewer's yeast, and protein supplements have no proven value in athletics.

Are Anabolic Steroids a Good Way to Build Muscles?

No! Using anabolic steroids to build muscles is dangerous and is against the law! There are many health risks associated with anabolic steroids: stunted growth, acne, liver damage, cancer, and severe behavioral disturbances. Some of the side effects of anabolic steroids can be permanent. While anabolic steroids do build muscles, this effect goes away when you stop taking them.

Are Tea and Coffee Good Drinks Before a Workout?

No. Both tea and coffee contain caffeine, an addictive stimulant. Excessive caffeine intake can cause headaches, nausea, and trembling or "shakes." While caffeine will increase the amount of time you can exercise, it can also increase urine production and this may result in dehydration. For drinks before competition, water and diluted fruit juice are the best choices.

Will Taking Vitamin and Mineral Supplements Improve Strength

No. The vitamin and mineral requirements of an athlete are similar to those of nonathletes. Some vitamins can be toxic if taken in large amounts, while others simply are flushed out in urine when taken in high doses. Vitamins and minerals don't provide any energy. In addition, there is no evidence that special supplements like bee pollen, ginseng, brewer's yeast, DNA, and protein supplements improve strength and endurance.

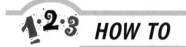

HOW TO

1. Stay away from drugs and supplements.
2. Just work hard every day to improve your fitness the natural way.
3. Have fun and get fit gradually.

QUESTIONS FOR STUDENTS

1. What is the best way to improve performance?
2. Are there any fitness advantages to taking supplements and drugs?
3. Besides the items we discussed, what are some foods or supplements that you have heard of to improve performance?

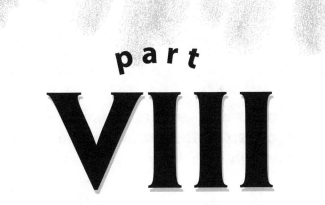

part

VIII

Fitness Can Be Fun!

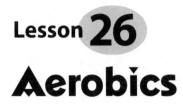

Lesson 26
Aerobics

Fitness tip: Aerobics classes are a fun way to improve strength, flexibility, and cardiovascular endurance while moving to your favorite music.

Aerobics Classes Provide You With a Great Workout!

- Aerobics improve strength, flexibility, and cardiovascular endurance by requiring you to perform many different movements to the beat of music.
- Both boys and girls can do aerobics.

There Are Many Different Types of Aerobics

- Some aerobics classes use special
  - slides,
  - step benches, and
  - small weights.
- Other classes require use of just the arms and legs to create specific steps or moves.
- Some classes may seem like dance classes, but many have easy steps that can be done with little practice.

Where

Provide information on local aerobics classes if possible.

You might try a high school, a YMCA, a Boys & Girls Club, a church, or a fitness club. You can also buy, rent, or borrow an aerobics videotape and do your aerobics at home by yourself or with your family and friends.

Equipment

For aerobics, you will need a good pair of exercise shoes that support your feet well to prevent injury to your ankles, knees, hips, and back. Dress in comfortable clothes that allow you to move your arms and legs freely.

Safety Tips

In order to be safe while doing aerobics, be sure to follow these safety tips:
- Always warm up and cool down.
- If you feel dizzy or light-headed, slow down or walk or jog in place briefly, check your heart rate, drink some water, and take time out! Stop if you are ever in pain.
- Follow your teacher's instructions carefully to avoid joint or muscle injury.

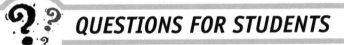

HOW TO

1. Try doing aerobics with your friends.
2. Remember to start out slowly, and gradually build to doing longer and tougher workouts.
3. Finally, always remember to wear proper clothing and follow the safety tips!

QUESTIONS FOR STUDENTS

1. Do you know of any aerobics centers in town? What aerobics classes do they offer?
2. What should you do if you feel dizzy or light-headed when you are doing aerobics?

Lesson 27
Calisthenics

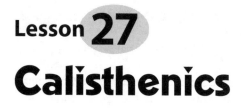 **Fitness tip: Calisthenics are a great way to increase muscular endurance, strength, and flexibility.**

What Are Calisthenics?

- Calisthenics are repetitive body movements that increase muscle strength, endurance, and flexibility using little or no equipment.
- The biggest advantage of this type of exercise is that you do not need any expensive equipment or clothing.

Examples of Calisthenics

- Some examples of calisthenics that work your upper body are
  - chin-ups,
  - dips,
  - push-ups, and
  - pull-ups.
- A variety of abdominal curls (sit-ups) can be done to work your stomach muscles.
- A variety of leg lifts and extensions can be done to work your leg muscles.

Where
You can do calisthenics anywhere!

Equipment
You should wear loose-fitting clothing and comfortable athletic shoes when you are doing calisthenics.

Safety Tip
Warm up and cool down to avoid joint and muscle injury.

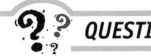

HOW TO

1. Remember to warm up with light flexibility exercises before beginning your calisthenics exercises.
2. To increase your muscular endurance, gradually increase the number of times (repetitions) you do each exercise.
3. To increase your muscular strength, you can gradually add weights to your wrists or ankles.
4. Be sure to include exercises that work all of your major muscle groups: trunk, arms, and legs.
5. Leave time for some stretching exercises at the end of your workout.
6. Try some calisthenics with your family.

QUESTIONS FOR STUDENTS

1. What is one major advantage of doing calisthenics?
2. Which components of fitness will calisthenics help you improve?

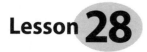

Running, Jogging, and Fitness Walking

 Fitness tip: Distance running, jogging, and fitness walking are good for you and can be done anywhere. Go out and explore your neighborhood!

Running and Jogging

- Running and jogging are excellent forms of exercise that do not require learning any new skills.
- Running and jogging (which is slower and less vigorous running) will improve your cardiovascular (aerobic) fitness and will condition your leg muscles.
- The advantage of running and jogging as a form of fitness exercise is that you can run or jog almost anywhere or anytime—as long as it's not dark!

Fitness Walking

- Brisk walking is also a good form of cardiovascular exercise.
- You can walk practically anywhere. Just remember to walk with a buddy!
- Walking and talking can be a lot of fun!

Where

As long as it is safe, you can do these aerobic activities almost anywhere. Packed dirt and clay surfaces are better for your joints than concrete surfaces. Also, avoid roads with a lot of traffic.

Equipment

Dress for the weather—wear layers if it's cold; dress lightly if it's hot. You need good running or walking shoes; they can be expensive, but shoes are the only thing you have to buy. Have a salesperson at a sporting goods store explain the different shoes to you; do some comparison shopping before you buy. You will need shoes that fit you well, give your foot room to expand, and support and stabilize your heel. Running shoes should be loose in the toes and snug in the heel. Running in the wrong shoes can stress your feet, ankles, knees, hips, and spine.

Safety Tips

When you go running, be sure to follow these safety tips:

1. Run with a buddy.
2. Talk over your running route with your parents before you go.
3. Don't run at night. Even at twilight, be sure to wear reflective gear.

HOW TO

1. Warm up with flexibility exercises before running, jogging, or fitness walking.
2. In the beginning, set a pace slow enough to carry on a conversation. In time your body will figure out the best running pace.
3. Stop or slow down if you experience pain.
4. To avoid injuries, build up distance and speed gradually.
5. Keep your body straight and comfortable, shoulders dropped, elbows comfortably bent, and fingers lightly closed.
6. Cool down with gentle stretching after you finish your workout.

QUESTIONS FOR STUDENTS

1. Why is it better to run on packed dirt and clay surfaces instead of concrete surfaces?
2. What is a good way to warm up before you walk, jog, or run?

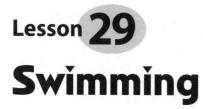

Swimming

 Fitness tip: Swimming is one of the best exercises for cardiovascular endurance and general conditioning.

Swimming Is One of the Best Exercises You Can Do!

- Long-distance swimming improves cardiovascular endurance.
- When you swim, you use almost every major muscle group in your body, promoting flexibility and strength.
- Because your body is supported by water, there is less risk of injury compared to some land sports.

Water Games Are Good Forms of Exercise, Too

- Remember, to keep fit, you need to keep moving.
- Water games like water polo, sharks and minnows, and Marco Polo keep you moving and are fun to play.
- Going swimming with your friends or family can be a lot of fun.

Where

Provide information on local swimming pools if possible—check the Yellow Pages for help in locating swimming pools.

You might try a high school, a YMCA, a Boys & Girls Club, or a municipal pool.

Equipment

You will need goggles, a good swimsuit designed for swimming (for girls this means a one-piece suit with a racing back so your straps stay put), and possibly a bathing cap. Remember, no cutoff shorts!

Safety Tips

In order to be safe when you swim, remember to follow these safety tips:

1. Swim only where there are lifeguards.
2. Swim with a buddy.
3. Never dive into shallow water or in places where you can't see the bottom—you may hit your head on a shallow bottom.
4. Don't push, grab, or jump on others in the pool.
5. If you are tired or get a cramp, float on your back and gently kick to shallow water.
6. Never run on the pool decks.
7. Always check out the pool rules before you go swimming.

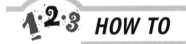 ## HOW TO

1. Learn to swim through a Red Cross or YMCA certified program, with qualified instructors.
2. When you are tired of swimming, try some games like water basketball, water polo, tag, or whatever you can make up.

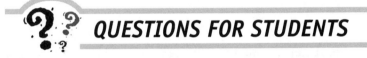 ## QUESTIONS FOR STUDENTS

1. What is one safety tip to remember when you go swimming?
2. Why is swimming one of the best exercises for you?

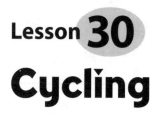

Lesson 30
Cycling

Fitness tip: Bicycling is an excellent cardiovascular exercise that helps build strong leg muscles.

Cycling Is Fun and It's Good for You!

- Cycling is an excellent cardiovascular (aerobic) exercise.
- It builds leg strength and can make small improvements in flexibility in the ankles, knees, and hips.
- It is a fun exercise that you can do either by yourself or with friends.

Choosing the Right Bike

- A great range of bicycles are available, but the important thing is to make sure your bike is the right size for you and that it works well.
- To make sure your bike is the right size, follow these tips. For a racing bike (dropped handlebars):
    - Make sure there is no more than an inch clearance between you and the top tube.
    - Adjust the seat so your leg is just slightly bent at the bottom of your pedal stroke.
    - Adjust the handlebars to a comfortable height and angle.
- For mountain bikes:
    - Make sure there is 2 to 3 inches clearance between you and the top tube.
    - Adjust the seat so your leg is just slightly bent at the bottom of your pedal stroke.
    - Adjust the handlebars so you tilt slightly forward. Make sure your elbows are slightly bent and not locked.

Where

Use maps and guidebooks (sometimes free at bike shops), and ask around to find bike paths and roads with less traffic, or try biking off-road if you have a mountain bike.

Equipment

As with most sports, you can get very technical with bikes and buy all kinds of expensive extras. All you really need is a bike, comfortable clothes, sneakers, and a helmet. In time, when you are riding longer distances, you may consider getting some bike gloves, a bicycle pump, and tools.

Safety Tips

For maximum fun, follow these safety instructions:

- Always wear a helmet. Your helmet should fit comfortably and not move around on your head. Don't tilt your helmet back off of your forehead—this exposes the front of your head to injury. Cyclists without helmets risk serious head injuries if they are hit by cars or fall off their bikes.
- Bike on sidewalks and trails if they are available. Watch for cars backing out of driveways.
- If you bike on the road, pay attention to the traffic. Enter the roadway when there is no traffic. Always ride on the right (not left) side with the traffic. Keep to the edge; ride in a line, not beside your friends.
- Before turning, stop, look, listen, and use hand signals.
- Obey stop signs and traffic lights.
- Don't bike at night.
- Don't remove your bike's reflectors.
- Learn to change and patch a tire, and always carry your tools and a pump with you on long trips.

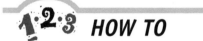 **HOW TO**

1. If your bike has gears, use the easy gears to warm up.
2. Switch gears *before* you start climbing a hill.
3. Try to pedal at an even pace.
4. Shift gears to keep the pace you set.

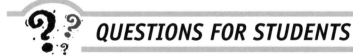 **QUESTIONS FOR STUDENTS**

1. What side of the road should you ride on?
2. How can you tell if a bike fits you properly?

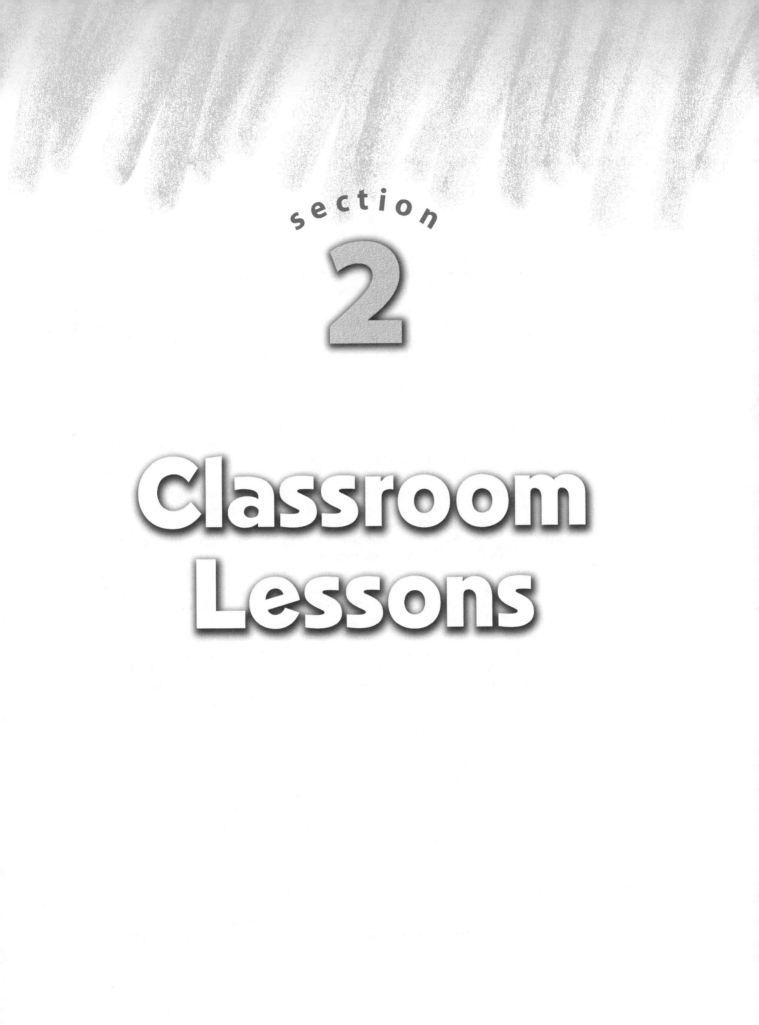

section

2

Classroom Lessons

Introduction to Classroom Lessons

The *Planet Health* classroom curriculum is composed of an introductory lesson and eight lessons in each of the following subject areas: language arts, math, science, and social studies. Read this section before proceeding to the lesson plans; it will provide you with useful information on how to select and teach the lessons and how to incorporate them into your existing curriculum. Because the *Planet Health* curriculum also focuses on developing literacy across the curriculum, this introduction offers teachers helpful suggestions on how to make every lesson literacy-rich.

Components of the Classroom Curriculum

The classroom curriculum contains an introductory lesson (*Do You Make Space for Fitness and Nutrition?*); four units (one each for the subject areas language arts, math, science, and social studies) with eight lessons in each unit; and *Power Down*, a TV reduction campaign.

The introductory lesson, *Do You Make Space for Fitness and Nutrition?*, should be used to introduce students to the *Planet Health* curriculum and health messages. Students will assess their own nutrition and activity behaviors using a short questionnaire and demonstrate their understanding of these concepts by answering an open-ended or key question. The self-assessment can be repeated at the end of the school year to help students and teachers reflect on changes in student knowledge and behavior. This lesson can be taught in any subject area, but is well-suited for health classes and other classes that practice answering open-ended and key questions as part of their curriculum.

The four units address each of the major subject areas of language arts, science, math, and social studies. There are eight lessons in each unit, a total of 32 lessons in all. Each lesson addresses one of the four *Planet Health* themes: eating fat in moderation; eating five fruits and vegetables daily; participating in regular, preferably daily, physical activity; and limiting TV, videos, and computer games to no more than 2 hours per day. At the beginning of each unit, a *Planet Health* At A Glance chart identifies the subject area theme, level of difficulty, subject-specific skills, and materials needed for each lesson.

Power Down is a TV reduction campaign. This lesson is included in appendix D. This two-week exercise is appropriate for use in a math, science, or health education class, and is adaptable as a school-wide campaign. *Power Down* asks students to assess and reflect on their current TV, video, and computer habits and strive to reduce their "screen time." Teachers may choose to teach this in place of one of the other lessons listed under the activity or lifestyle theme.

Resources

Background information on nutrition (appendix A) and physical activity (appendix B), useful in teaching lessons in all major areas, can be found at the back of this book. Appendix C contains resources for the social studies lessons.

Lesson Design

All lesson plans provide

- a summary paragraph,
- behavioral objectives,
- learning objectives,
- materials,
- a teaching procedure,
- teacher resources, and
- student activity sheets.

Some lessons also include

- student resources, and
- overhead transparency masters.

Educational Approach

Each classroom lesson uses subject-specific skills and competencies to convey *Planet Health*'s messages. Innovative, student-centered teaching methods are used to engage students. For example, brainstorming, debates, case studies, classroom demonstrations, games, group projects, and presentations are incorporated into lesson activities. The lessons foster critical thinking and responsible decision making, in addition to offering skill-building exercises.

Planet Health addresses four major concerns in educational practice: achieving learning standards, emphasizing literacy learning across the curriculum, fostering constructivist teaching and learning, and emphasizing discussion and cooperative learning.

Achieving Learning Standards

The *Planet Health* curriculum is aligned with the Massachusetts Department of Education Curriculum Frameworks (learning standards). The lessons address learning standards in health, English language arts, math, science, and social studies.

Emphasizing Literacy Learning Across the Curriculum

In addition to encouraging learning standards from many curriculum areas, *Planet Health* emphasizes literacy learning in each lesson. With the recent nation-wide focus on literacy, teachers seem to regularly ask themselves, "How do I cover subject-area content while at the same time focusing sufficiently on literacy?" A partial answer is that literacy learning should be a component of every lesson, whether the subject area is health, math, science and technology, or history and social science. Learning is accomplished through language, and literacy learning should be a part of all lessons. Every *Planet Health* lesson integrates a range of English language arts curriculum learning standards in a manner that will make classroom implementation easy. To assist teachers with long-term planning, the learning standards covered are outlined at the beginning of each part.

Fostering Constructivist Teaching and Learning

Planet Health also draws upon the constructivist approach to teaching and learning. Constructivist thinking emphasizes the idea that students learn best when they actively construct meaning for themselves. Students come to the classroom lessons with different knowledge and experiences. Constructivism encourages teachers to create learning environments that activate and build on this diversity in a manner that is active, inquiry-based, and student-centered.

Thus, *Planet Health* lessons begin by the activating and assessing of prior knowledge. Lessons proceed to inquiry-based activities in which the students read, write, speak, listen, experiment, and reflect in order to answer health-related questions. *Planet Health* provides a range of teacher and student resources to support this inquiry.

To promote this type of inquiry, multiple student resources are provided. *Planet Health* also points teachers to comprehensive nutrition and physical activity resources so that each teacher can knowledgeably facilitate students' learning experiences.

Emphasizing Discussion and Cooperative Learning

Every *Planet Health* lesson specifies discussion ideas for small and/or large groups to cooperatively learn and solve health-related issues. Higher-level thinking and cognition are encouraged by active discussion, and social development is enhanced by working with peers in groups.

Incorporating Planet Health Into Your Curriculum

Ideally each 6th, 7th, and 8th grade classroom teacher should teach two or three lessons per year. The lessons within each subject area can be taught in any sequence. However, we strongly recommend that clusters or departments coordinate, to ensure that students first complete the introductory self-assessment lesson (lesson 31), followed by language arts lesson 32 on the Food Guide Pyramid. (This lesson is also well-suited for a health or consumer science class.) If this is not possible, spend a few minutes reviewing *Planet Health*'s four health messages and the Food Guide Pyramid before teaching one of the other lessons.

A middle school planner can be found at the end of the introduction to the book (page xviii). It was designed to help you make your implementation plan and coordinate it with other *Planet Health* teachers. We recommend that you talk with other teachers to learn what lessons they are using and when they will be introducing them. This approach will help you to build upon and reinforce lessons taught in each other's classes. You will also need to be aware of which lessons teachers introduced to your students last year.

Selecting Lessons

To help you identify lessons that best fit your curriculum objectives, consult the *Planet Health* At-A-Glance charts located at the beginning of each subject area. The At-A-Glance charts include a list of lesson titles, themes, levels of difficulty, subject-specific skills, and materials needed. You also may wish to review the Massachusetts Curriculum Frameworks for each unit. These tables list the health, language arts, and subject-specific learning standards addressed by each lesson.

Familiarize yourself with the lesson(s) you have selected by reviewing the following sections in the order listed:

- introductory paragraph,
- learning objectives,
- materials,
- student activity sheets,
- teacher procedures, and
- teacher resources.

Many of the lessons offer a choice of activities. Adapt the lesson procedure to fit your teaching style, students' skills, and time constraints.

Resources

A teacher resource section is located at the end of each lesson. This section contains health-related information specific to the lesson. The material in this section is meant to serve as a resource for teachers, not to be presented in its entirety to students. General resources on nutrition and physical activity are described in the appendices. Appendix A contains nutrition resources; appendix B contains physical activity resources; and appendix C contains social studies resources. Appendix E contains a table that outlines how the lessons are aligned with the Massachusetts Curriculum Frameworks. Notes in the teacher resources for each lesson list the items in the appendixes that are most relevant.

Make Every Lesson a Literacy-Rich Experience

The *Planet Health* curriculum provides many opportunities to foster literacy learning. To make the most out of literacy-related activities, a teacher may choose to focus on reading comprehension, pose questions, emphasize key vocabulary prior to reading, refine word-identification strategies, or encourage students to work through steps in the writing process.

Focus on Reading Comprehension

Prepare your students for reading by giving them a framework (or umbrella idea) that helps them more easily understand what they will read. For example, you could say, "We will now read *Carbohydrates: Energy Foods* (lesson 33). This article will help us to understand the role of carbohydrates in a healthy diet and will help us to understand what foods contain carbohydrates."

Pose Questions

A second way to focus on reading comprehension is to help students pose questions that will be answered by reading. A teacher may follow the framework for comprehension used above, requesting, "Students should read *Carbohydrates: Energy Foods* with a mind to answering the questions: What role do carbohydrates play in a healthy diet? And, what foods contain carbohydrates?" Helping students to focus their reading in this manner will enhance their understanding of the specific material. Students can utilize this comprehension strategy with other reading materials.

Emphasize Key Vocabulary Prior to Reading

Some words are more important to understanding text than others and are, at the same time, difficult to figure out using context and other word identification strategies. These words need to be taught prior to reading so that reading comprehension is not unnecessarily hindered. Examples of such words may be "pyramid" (as in "food pyramid") or "balanced" (as in "balanced diet") or "glucose" (as in "blood glucose").

Refine Word-Identification Strategies

When a reader comes upon an unknown word, several strategies can be used to identify the unknown word. Students should be taught (by teacher modeling) to use a combination of these strategies. These strategies are

- read ahead and try to figure out the word from context clues,

- sound out the word or look for "word chunks" and make a guess at how the whole word sounds, and
- put that sound for the word back.

Encourage Students to Work Through Steps in the Writing Process

In all writing activities, encourage students to engage in pre-writing activities (such as brainstorming and webbing), drafting (to get initial ideas down on paper), revising (to refine ideas), and editing/proofreading (to polish writing).

Do You Make Space for Fitness and Nutrition?

Use this lesson in the classroom to introduce students to the Planet Health curriculum and health messages. Students will assess their own nutrition habits and level of physical activity using a short questionnaire and demonstrate their current understanding of these concepts by answering an open-ended or key question. The self-assessment and open-ended question can be repeated at the end of the school year as a way of helping students and teachers reflect on changes in student behavior and knowledge in this area. This lesson can be taught in any subject, but is well-suited for science, math, and health classes or classes that practice answering open-ended or key questions as part of their curriculum. Student portfolios may also be used to document changes in student understanding and knowledge.

▶▶ Behavioral Objective

For students to reflect on their eating habits and level of daily physical activity.

▶▶ Learning Objectives

Students will be able to

1. accurately answer questions about their eating habits and level of daily physical activity,
2. state the *Planet Health* messages,
3. interpret histograms and demonstrate their knowledge and understanding of the benefits of proper nutrition and physical activity by answering open-ended questions that require them to use higher order thinking skills (interpret, analyze, evaluate, apply, connect, generalize, and predict).

▶▶ Materials

- Activity 1 *Student Self-Assessment*
- Activity 2 *Class Summary*
- Activity 3 *Reflecting on Your Habits,* a key question activity, or activity 4 *What Do You Know?,* an open-ended question activity
- Parent letter (page 129)
- Overhead transparency 1: *Planet Health* overview
- Overhead transparency 2: *Planet Health* messages
- Overhead transparency 3: *Class Summary*

▶▶ Procedure

The purpose of this lesson is to introduce students to the *Planet Health* curriculum and health messages and to assess their current knowledge and behaviors related to eating and physical activity. To assess changes in student behavior, the lesson should be repeated at the end of the year.

Overview:

Activity 1

Activity 2

Activity 3 or 4
(choose one)

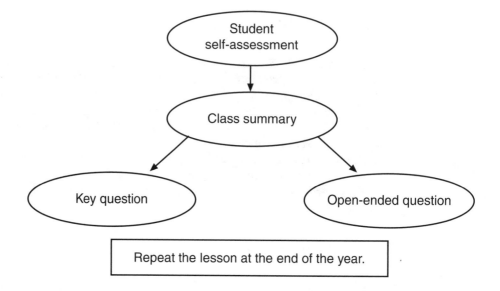

Student self-assessment

Class summary

Key question

Open-ended question

Repeat the lesson at the end of the year.

Day 1

1. (5 minutes) Give a brief overview of the *Planet Health* curriculum. (See the Teacher Resources for help describing *Planet Health*). You may wish to display overhead transparency master 1 *Overview of Planet Health* to help students see the big picture. Do not give much detail or background regarding the health messages at this point as this may impact student assessment responses. Make the following points:

- *Planet Health*'s goal is to encourage students to eat a healthy diet and be physically active.

- Students will be involved with this curriculum in math, science, social studies, language arts, and physical education classes over the next few years.

2. (2-3 minutes) Hand out activity 1 *Student Self-Assessment*. Explain that the purpose of this activity is for students to reflect on their current eating and physical activity patterns.

3. (10 minutes) Have students complete activity 1.

4. (20 minutes) Graph the class data by having each student shade in the appropriate box on the histogram in activity 2 *Class Summary*. We recommend you display an example of a completed histogram and go through a step-by-step explanation of how to graph student responses. For example, let's say your students totaled their fruit consumption and found the following:

- 12 students ate three fruits

- 3 students ate four fruits

- 2 students ate five fruits

- 1 student ate six or more fruits

The graph would look like this:

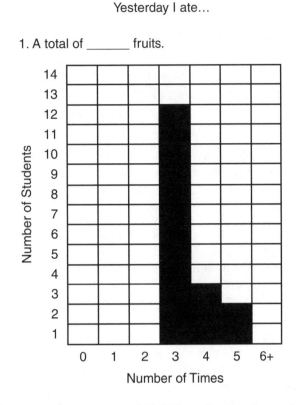

Yesterday I ate...

1. A total of _____ fruits.

Pass around the graphs on pages 120-125 so that students can graph their data anonymously. Each student locates the total number of fruits (or other food or activity) eaten on the *x*-axis, then shades in the blank box closest to the *x*-axis in that column. For example, if the first student ate four fruits, she would shade in the box that corresponds to four fruits (*x*-axis) and one student (*y*-axis). If the second student also ate four fruits, he would shade in the box that corresponds to four fruits (*x*-axis) and two students (*y*-axis). See the graph below.

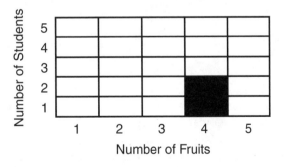

As students take turns shading in their totals, a histogram representing the number of students in each category appears. This provides a method for anonymously tallying the class responses.

Other options for graphing class data:

- Use a show of hands to tally students' responses, then have a volunteer or volunteers graph the information.
- Collect the self-assessments and graphs the data yourself.

5. While the graphs are being passed around, have students work on activity 3 *Reflecting on Your Habits* or activity 4 *What Do You Know?*

Activity 3 has a key question format. This activity requires students to

1. compare their nutrition and physical activity patterns with the *Planet Health* recommendations and goals,
2. point out which goals they meet by providing supporting data from activity 1,
3. conclude whether "good nutrition and fitness" are a part of their lives, and
4. identify issues in their daily habits or environment that make it difficult for them to achieve the goals.

This activity gives students an opportunity to reflect on their own eating and activity patterns and practice answering key questions. Students will probably need to complete this assignment as homework.

Activity 4 *What Do You Know?* consists of a brainstorming activity and an open-ended essay. Your students will likely have very different background knowledge and experiences with nutrition and physical activity. This lesson will help you activate and assess their knowledge and understanding of good nutrition and adequate physical activity. It will also give students an opportunity to practice essay writing. Students will probably need to complete this assignment as homework.

For help grading these activities, see the Teacher's Guides (pages 111-112).

Day 2

1. (10 minutes) Use overhead transparency master 2 *Planet Health Messages* to review the *Planet Health* goals for students. Display an overhead transparency of the class graphs from activity 2. Ask students to compare the class data with the *Planet Health* messages. What conclusions can they draw? What goals can the class set as a whole? Record and save these conclusions and goals on the *Class Summary* sheet.

2. (10 minutes) Discuss the following question: What are the benefits of a healthy diet and regular physical activity? Don't tell students the answer to this question. Use this as a brainstorming session, as well as an opportunity for you to get a feeling for what the class already knows about this subject.

End of the Year

1. Administer activities 1, 2, and 3 or 4 at the end of the year.

2. Discuss the class results. Ask students to compare the year-end graphs with those they made in the fall. Have the class's eating and activity habits changed? Did they reach their goals?

3. Grade activity 3 or 4 and assess whether students' knowledge, behavior, and/or ability to answer open-ended questions have improved during the year.

►► Extension Activities

1. Have students complete activity 3 or 4 as homework.

2. Have each student take home a copy of the parent letter on page 129. Ask them to read it with their parents. You may wish to ask them to get their parents' signatures acknowledging that they have seen the letter.

▶▶ Teacher Resources

General Background Material

In preparing for this lesson, you may want to refer to the following resources:

- *Nutrition and Your Health: Dietary Guidelines for Americans.*
- *Centers for Disease Control and Prevention Fact Sheets on Physical Activity.*
- *Television Viewing as a Cause of Increasing Obesity Among Children in the United States, 1986-1990.*
- *Healthy People 2010.*

See appendixes A and B for information on obtaining these resources.

Specific Background Material

What is Planet Health?

Planet Health is an interdisciplinary health curriculum that provides children with the knowledge and skills they need to choose nutritious diets and be physically active. Research shows that a good diet and adequate physical activity can significantly reduce the risk of obesity and chronic diseases, such as heart disease, high blood pressure, diabetes, and cancer. Yet many children today are not eating the fruits and vegetables nor getting the physical activity they need to be healthy both now and in the future.

Planet Health provides children with the tools to turn this trend around! Through exciting lessons designed to be incorporated into math, science, social studies, language arts, and physical education classes, the curriculum introduces and reinforces four simple health messages/goals:

- Be physically active daily or nearly every day.
- Limit your screen time to no more than 2 hours each day.
- Eat five or more fruits and vegetables (combined) every day.
- Choose a diet low in saturated fat and trans fat and moderate in total fat.

Planet Health is **not** about dieting. Putting these four health messages into practice can help everyone, children and adults, improve their current well-being and decrease their risks for many chronic conditions and diseases. When talking to students about these messages, emphasize the benefits of a healthy lifestyle. Avoid conveying an attitude of restriction. Kids don't need to give up all high-fat and sugar foods or TV. Moderation is the key. The *Planet Health* curriculum will encourage students to think about their choices for nutrition and activity and give them practice developing strategies for achieving these goals.

What are the Benefits of Eating a Healthy Diet and Being Physically Fit?

Some benefits of good nutrition and physical activity are

- Eating well and being active help reduce the risk of obesity, heart disease, cancer, high blood pressure, and diabetes.
- Being physically active helps students feel better.
- Eating well helps children grow, develop, and do well in school.

Why do Children Need Encouragement and Education Around the Planet Health Messages?

Some facts about children's health:

- Children are eating fewer than the recommended number of daily servings of fruits and vegetables.

- Children are eating more fat than experts recommend.

- Only about one-half of young people regularly participate in vigorous physical activity.

- The percentage of young people who are overweight has more than doubled in the last 30 years.

- Many children spend more time watching television than in any other activity besides sleep.

Children are at Risk

Poor diet and physical inactivity are the second leading cause of death in the United States, accounting for at least 300,000 deaths each year. Obesity, coronary heart disease, certain cancers, diabetes, and high blood pressure are affected by a person's diet and physical activity level. In many cases, disorders such as obesity and coronary heart disease begin early in childhood. Yet many children are not eating the food and getting the exercise they need to prevent these chronic diseases and promote lifelong good health.

It is especially troubling that as children age they become progressively less active and choose less healthy diets. Establishing healthy eating habits at a young age is critical because changing poor eating patterns in adulthood can be difficult.

Unfortunately, children do not always have the chance to benefit from a good diet and adequate physical activity. Food industry advertising encourages them to choose high-fat/high-sugar foods. Inadequate safe play spaces may make it difficult for children to be physically active. Unlimited access to TV, videos, and computer games is also likely to make them less active. *Planet Health* encourages children to make healthy food choices, be physically active, and limit their screen time to less than 2 hours per day.

What Background Information Will Students Need to Complete the Planet Health Lessons?

The *Planet Health* curriculum teaches students how to eat a balanced diet based on the Food Guide Pyramid (FGP). Language arts lesson 32 provides teachers and students with an introduction to the FGP principles and practice applying them. (This lesson is also well-suited for a health or consumer science class.) We recommend that all students begin with this lesson as many of the other lessons assume students are familiar with the FGP. However, if it is not possible to fit lesson 32 into your schedule, spend a few minutes reviewing the FGP before teaching one of the other lessons. Other lesson-specific background information is provided as student resource handouts within individual lessons.

The Food Guide Pyramid is an eating guide designed by the United States Department of Agriculture. It helps people understand the five food groups as well as the importance of variety, proportionality, and moderation in the diet. It tells us to choose foods from all of the food groups daily and to choose a variety of foods within each food group. Following the FGP recommendations ensures consuming essential nutrients sufficient to meet the dietary needs of most people.

What are the Four Planet Health Messages?

1. Be physically active daily or nearly every day.

How much activity is needed to obtain health-related benefits?

Moderate amounts of activity are recommended for people of all ages. However, physical activity need not be strenuous to be beneficial. Thirty minutes of moderately intense activity, such as walking, can generate genuine health benefits, such as reducing body weight and lowering the risk of heart attack, hypertension, and death. Some kind of regular vigorous activity however, is the best way to improve cardiovascular fitness.

Physical activity recommendations for adolescents:

- Be moderately active for at least 30 minutes every day or nearly every day as part of play, games, sport, chores, transportation, or planned exercise.
- Aim for at least three sessions per week of vigorous physical activity lasting 20 minutes or more.

What are the benefits of an active lifestyle?

Physical activity

- helps develop cardiovascular fitness, muscle strength, and confidence in physical ability.
- helps in maintaining a healthy body weight and reducing fat.
- reduces stress and brightens a person's mood.
- lowers the risk of diabetes, high blood pressure, and colon cancer, which can lead to premature death.

2. Limit screen time to no more than 2 hours each day.

What are the risks of a sedentary lifestyle?

Activity is required for health. Studies suggest that physically active individuals enjoy lower risks of developing cardiovascular disease, diabetes, colon cancer, osteoporosis, anxiety, and depression relative to sedentary individuals. Sedentary habits increase the risk of death from these diseases. TV viewing is one of the major causes of overweight (obesity) among youth. TV watching has also been associated with elevated cholesterol levels and poor cardiovascular fitness.

How much time do adolescents spend watching TV?

According to Dietz (1991), American children spend more time watching TV than in any other activity except sleeping. In 1988, the average adolescent viewed approximately 22 hours per week. The percentage of youth watching TV or playing computer or video games for 5 or more hours per day has increased greatly, from 13% in the late 1960s to 43% in 1990. Essentially, TV watching for many children has become a full-time job! The American Academy of Pediatrics recommends limiting TV viewing to 2 hours or less per day.

What are some examples of things you can do to increase your activity and decrease your inactivity?

Take the stairs; don't park next to the building; walk around the mall or the neighborhood with friends; only watch your favorite TV shows; remove or unplug the TV in your bedroom; play catch with a sibling, friend, or parent.

3. Eat five or more fruits and vegetables (combined) per day.

What are the main benefits of fruits and vegetables?

- Many are good sources of potassium, fiber, and vitamins C, A, and B.
- They are low in fat.
- They reduce the risk of certain forms of cancer.
- They provide nutrients important for immunity, healing, and healthy skin and eyes, among other functions.

How many fruits and vegetables should we eat daily?

The 5-A-Day campaign promotes consumption of five or more fruits and vegetables everyday. Also, the Food Guide Pyramid recommends consuming 2-3 servings of fruits and 3-5 servings of vegetables every day. Encourage students to eat at least two servings of fruit and three servings of vegetables (including at least one serving of a dark green or orange vegetable) each day.

4. Choose a diet low in saturated fat and trans fat and moderate in total fat.

What are the recommendations for fat intake?

The National Research Council's Dietary Guidelines recommend consuming no more than 30% of calories from total fat (unsaturated, saturated, and trans fat) with no more than 10% of calories from saturated fat. Individual foods can have more or less fat. It's the total that counts. Although the guidelines do not mention an upper limit for trans fat, new scientific evidence points to the harmful effects of trans fat. Therefore, it is important to limit trans fat intake as well. Recommended fat intake:

- for 11–14-year-old girls, about 73 grams per day with 24 or fewer grams saturated fat (based on a 2,200 calorie diet), and
- for 11–14-year-old boys, about 83 grams per day with 28 or fewer grams saturated fat (based on a 2,500 calorie diet).

Should we try to eliminate fat from our diets?

NO! Fat has many important functions in our bodies.

- Fats and oils (also called lipids) add flavor, aroma, and texture to food. Lipids provide a feeling of fullness because they take longer to digest than carbohydrates and proteins and remain in the stomach for a longer time.
- Dietary fat is essential for the absorption of the fat-soluble vitamins A, D, E, and K.
- Fat is a major source of energy.
- Essential fatty acids are needed for normal tissue function throughout the body. Deficiency syndromes can develop if they are missing from the diet.

These are just a few important functions of fat. For a more complete list see lesson 49 (page 327). This lesson discusses the different types of fat and their impact on health.

Facts associated with excess fat intake:

- Habitual fat intake in excess of physiological needs increases risk for chronic disease in adulthood. This risk can begin in the teen years.
- Excess fat intake, especially from animal fat, can cause blocked arteries and the development of heart disease as well as certain cancers in adult years.
- Arteriosclerosis, the process of fatty substances building up in the arteries, can begin early in life.

References

Dietz, W. 1991. Physical activity and childhood obesity. *Nutrition* 7(4):295-296.

Dietz, W.H., and Strasburger, V.C. 1991. Children, adolescents, and television. *Current Problems in Pediatrics* 21(1):8-31.

U.S. Department of Agriculture and U.S. Department of Health and Human Services. 2000. *Nutrition and your health: Dietary guidelines for Americans* 2000, 5th edition. **www.usda.gov/cnpp**

U.S. Department of Health and Human Services. 2000. Healthy People 2010, conference edition, vols. I and II. **www.health.gov/healthypeople**

Whitney, E.N., and Rolfes, S.R. 1993. *Understanding nutrition.* 6th ed. St. Paul, MN: West Publishing Co.

►► Answer Keys

Teacher's Guide to Grading the Key Questions (Activity 3)

You may design your own criteria for grading the key questions. We recommend assessing two criteria:

1. the understanding and thoroughness of students' self-assessments of their eating and physical activity habits, and
2. students' thesis statements.

Tally the number of students who rate themselves as having healthy nutrition and physical activity habits and the numbers who don't think they have healthy habits. This assessment will give you information regarding the students' abilities to answer key questions and their eating and activity behaviors. Repeat these tallies at the end of the year to determine whether there has been any change in your class profile.

Student Understanding and Thoroughness

	Number of students
Thorough understanding	
Basic understanding	
Basic but superficial understanding	
Little understanding	

Student thesis statements

	Number of students
Yes, I have healthy eating and physical activity habits	
No, I don't have healthy eating and physical activity habits	
Other (make other categories as necessary)	

Teacher's Guide to Grading the Open-Ended Essay (Activity 4)

Decide whether you will grade the essay for content and style (grammar, punctuation, spelling, and format) or just content. We suggest that you grade the content as follows: Set the value of the content portion of the essay equal to 12 points. Students should address each of the four *Planet Health* messages in their essay. Give them a point for each correct piece of information. Subtract a point for incorrect information or misconceptions and for neglecting to mention any one of the messages. Only credit a maximum of four points for any one health message; many points are possible.

Why Eat Five Fruits and Vegetables Every Day?

- Many are good sources of potassium, fiber, and vitamins C, A, and B.
- They are low in fat.
- They reduce the risk of certain forms of cancer.
- They provide nutrients important for immunity, healing, and healthy skin and eyes, among other functions.

Why Eat Fat in Moderation?

- The Dietary Guidelines recommend consuming no more than 30% of calories from fat in the total diet with no more than 10% of calories from saturated fat. Future lessons will discuss the different types of fat.
- Fat has many important functions (see the Teacher Resources) in our bodies, so it should not be eliminated from our diets.
- Excess saturated fat can cause blocked arteries and the development of heart disease as well as certain cancers in adult years.
- Arteriosclerosis, the process of fatty substances building up in the arteries, can begin early in life.

Why Be Physically Active Daily or Nearly Every Day?

Physical activity

- helps develop cardiovascular fitness, muscle strength, and confidence in physical ability.
- helps maintain a healthy body weight and reduce fat.
- reduces stress and brightens a person's mood.
- lowers the risk of diabetes, high blood pressure, and colon cancer, which can lead to premature death.
- is fun.

Why Limit Screen Time to No More Than 2 Hours Per Day?

- Activity is required for health. Studies suggest that physically active individuals enjoy lower risks of developing cardiovascular disease, diabetes, colon cancer, osteoporosis, anxiety, and depression relative to sedentary individuals. Sedentary habits increase the risk of death from these diseases.
- TV viewing is one of the major causes of overweight (obesity) among youth.
- TV watching has also been associated with elevated cholesterol levels and poor cardiovascular fitness.

Planet Health Overview

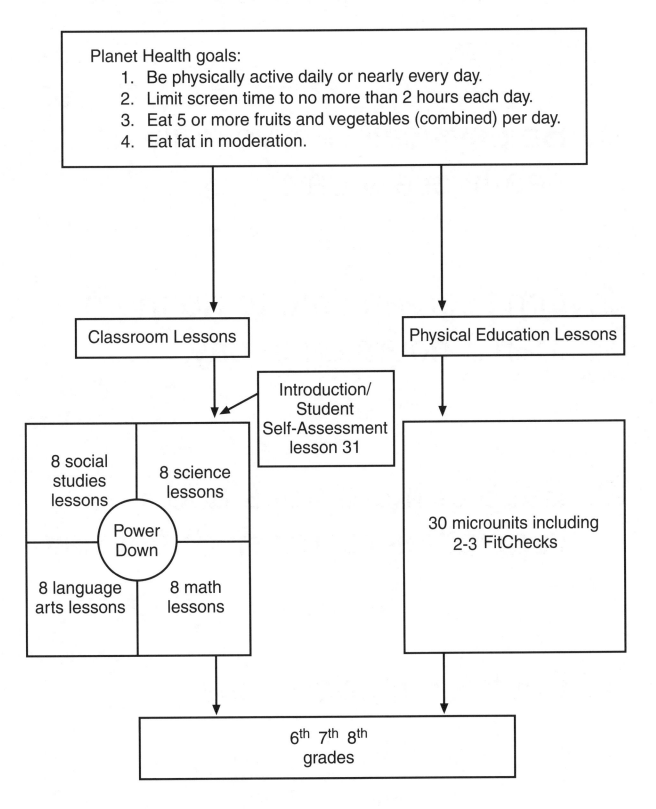

Planet Health goals:
1. Be physically active daily or nearly every day.
2. Limit screen time to no more than 2 hours each day.
3. Eat 5 or more fruits and vegetables (combined) per day.
4. Eat fat in moderation.

Classroom Lessons

Physical Education Lessons

Introduction/
Student
Self-Assessment
lesson 31

8 social
studies
lessons

8 science
lessons

Power
Down

8 language
arts lessons

8 math
lessons

30 microunits including
2-3 FitChecks

6th 7th 8th
grades

Planet Health Messages

1. Be physically active daily or nearly every day.

2. Limit screen time to no more than 2 hours each day.

3. Eat 5 or more fruits and vegetables (combined) per day.

4. Eat fat in moderation.

Yesterday I ate…

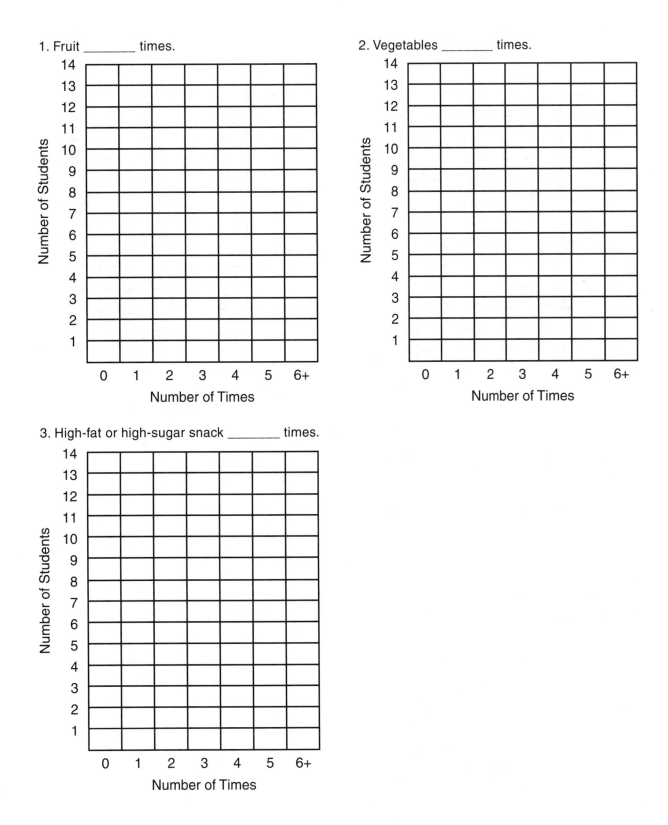

1. Fruit _____ times.

2. Vegetables _____ times.

3. High-fat or high-sugar snack _____ times.

In the past 7 days…

4. I participated in moderate physical activity for at least 30 minutes on _____ days.

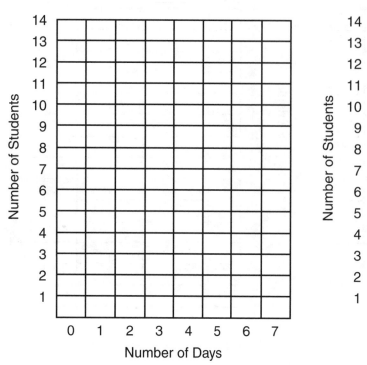

5. I participated in vigorous activity for at least 20 minutes on _____ days.

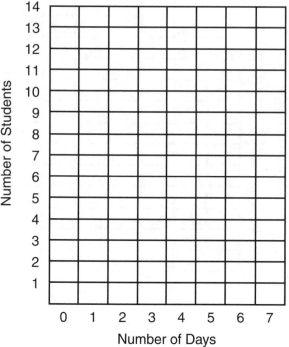

6. I spent *on average* _____ hours each school day watching TV.

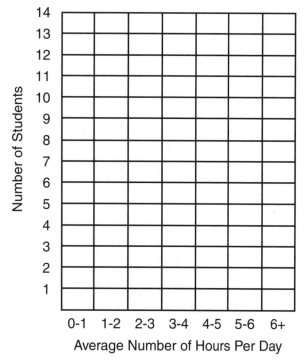

Do You Make Space for Fitness and Nutrition?

Think About Your Nutrition

Think about all the meals and snacks you ate yesterday from the time you got up until you went to bed. Answer the following questions as best you can. Remember, there are no right or wrong answers. Circle your response.

1. Yesterday, how many times did you eat fruit or drink 100% fruit juices such as orange juice, apple juice, or grape juice? (Do not count punch, Kool-Aid, sports drinks, or other fruit-flavored drinks.)

    0

    1

    2

    3

    4

    5

    6 or more

2. Yesterday, how many times did you eat vegetables (e.g., green salad, carrots)?

    0

    1

    2

    3

    4

    5

    6 or more

3. Yesterday, how many times did you eat snacks such as chips, cookies, doughnuts, pie, cake, candy, etc?

    0

    1

    2

    3

    4

    5

    6 or more

All questions in this activity were adapted from the Center for Disease Control's Youth Risk Behavior Surveillance System.

Think About Your Physical Activity

Think about how active you have been during the past 7 days. Think about the games you play, chores, sports, and other exercise or activity both in and out of school. Answer the following questions as best you can, and remember: there are no right or wrong answers. Circle your response.

4. On how many of the past 7 days did you participate in physical activity for at least 30 minutes that did not make you sweat or breathe hard, such as fast walking, slow bicycling, skating, pushing a lawn mower, or mopping floors? (moderate activity)

   0 days

   1 days

   2 days

   3 days

   4 days

   5 days

   6 days

   7 days

5. On how many of the past 7 days did you exercise or participate in physical activity for at least 20 minutes that made you sweat and breathe hard, such as basketball, soccer, running, swimming laps, fast bicycling, fast dancing, or similar aerobic activities? (vigorous activity)

   0 days

   1 days

   2 days

   3 days

   4 days

   5 days

   6 days

   7 days

Think About Your Screen Time

Now think about a typical school day (Monday through Friday). Answer the following question, and remember that there are no right or wrong answers. Circle your response.

6. On an average school day, how many hours do you watch TV?

   None-1 hour per day

   1-2 hours per day

   2-3 hours per day

   3-4 hours per day

   4-5 hours per day

   5-6 hours per day

   6 or more hours per day

Name _____

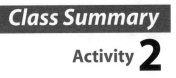

Directions: All class members should shade in one block on each graph. Have students refer to their self-assessments to determine how to respond to each statement. Record the conclusions and goals emerging from the class discussion in the tables below.

	Conclusions
Vegetables	
Fruits	
High-fat and high-sugar snacks	
Daily activity	
Vigorous activity	
TV time	

	Goals
Vegetables	
Fruits	
High-fat and high-sugar snacks	
Daily activity	
Vigorous activity	
TV time	

Yesterday I ate…

1. Fruit _____ times.

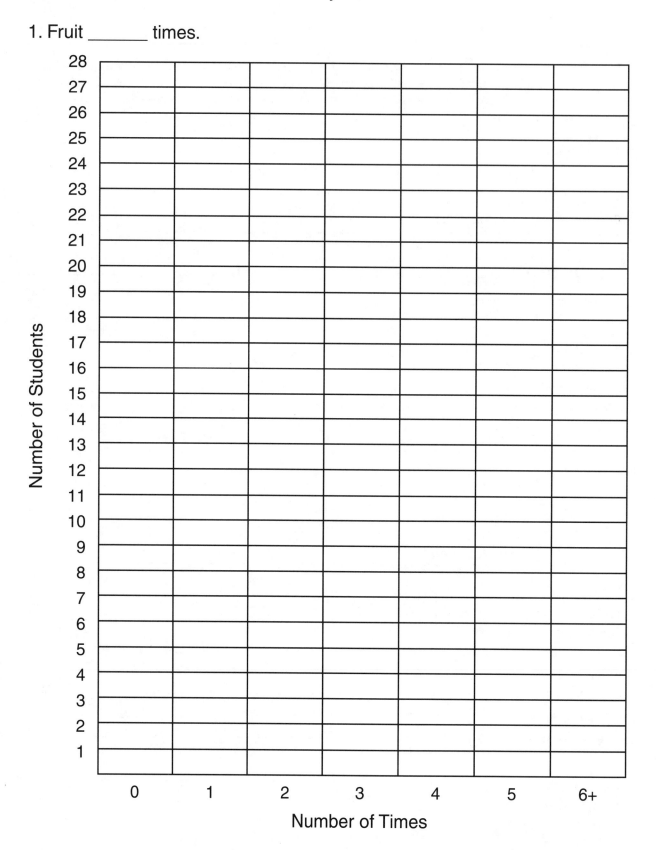

Number of Times

(Y-axis: Number of Students, 1–28; X-axis: Number of Times, 0, 1, 2, 3, 4, 5, 6+)

Yesterday I ate…

2. Vegetables _____ times.

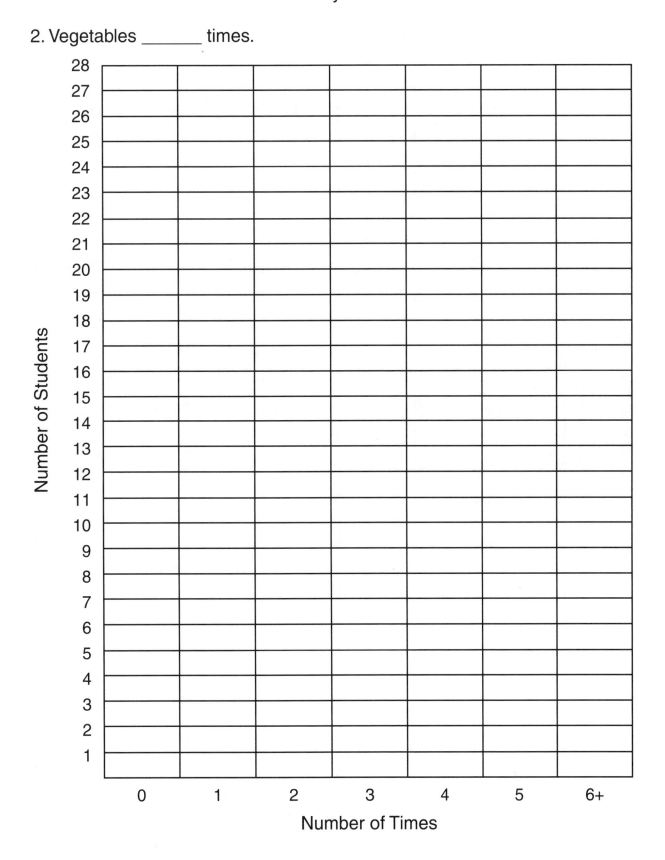

Yesterday I ate…

3. High-fat or high-sugar snacks _____ times.

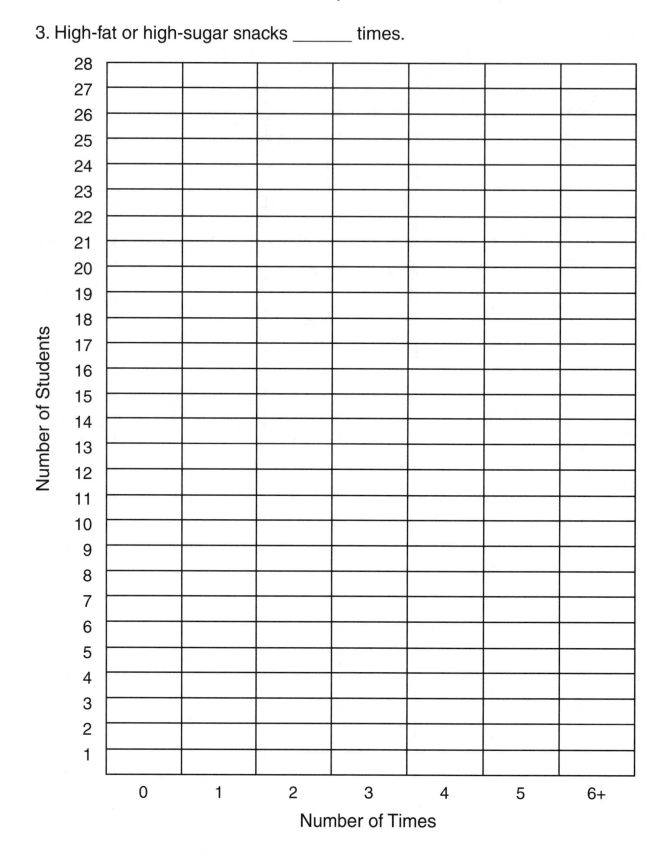

Number of Times

Planet Health: Do You Make Space for Fitness and Nutrition?

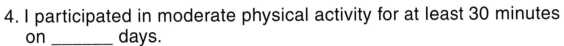

In the past 7 days…

4. I participated in moderate physical activity for at least 30 minutes on _____ days.

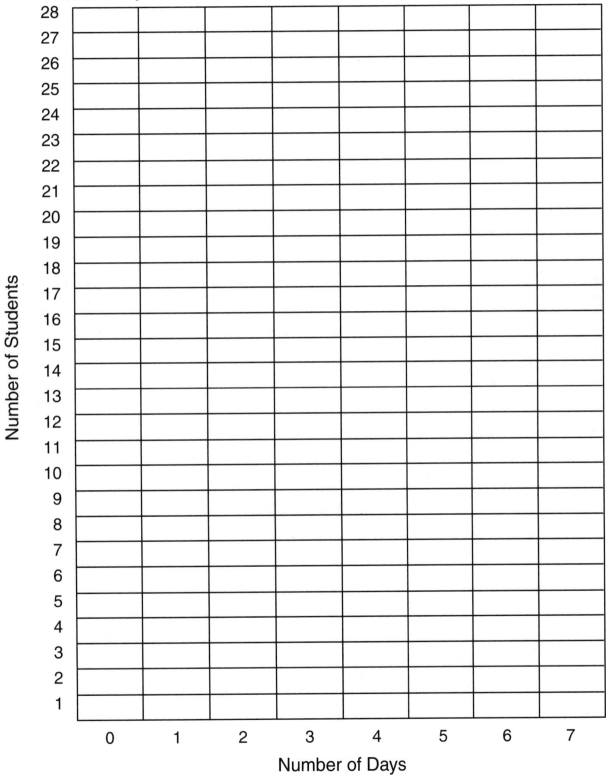

Number of Students

Number of Days

In the past 7 days…

5. I participated in vigorous activity for at least 20 minutes on _____ days.

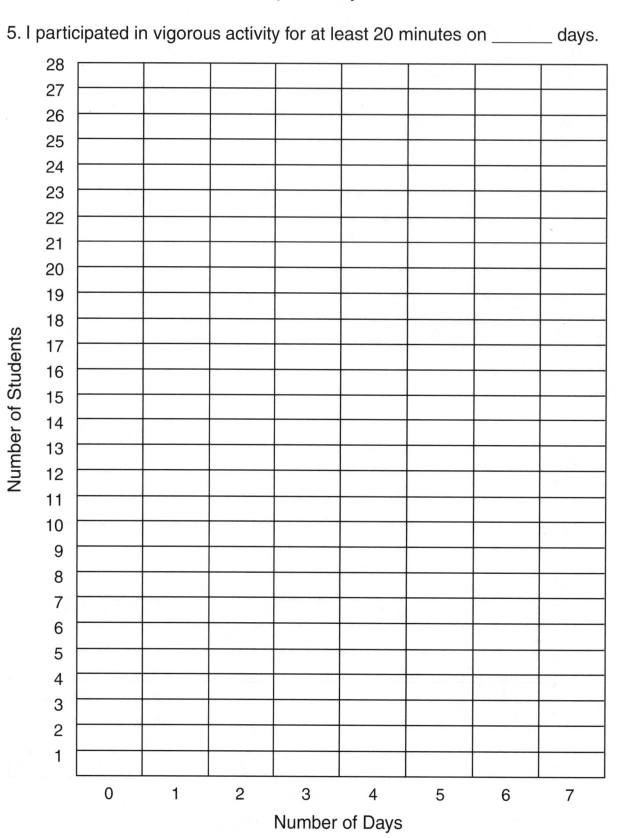

In the past 7 days…

6. I spend *on average* _____ hours each school day watching TV.

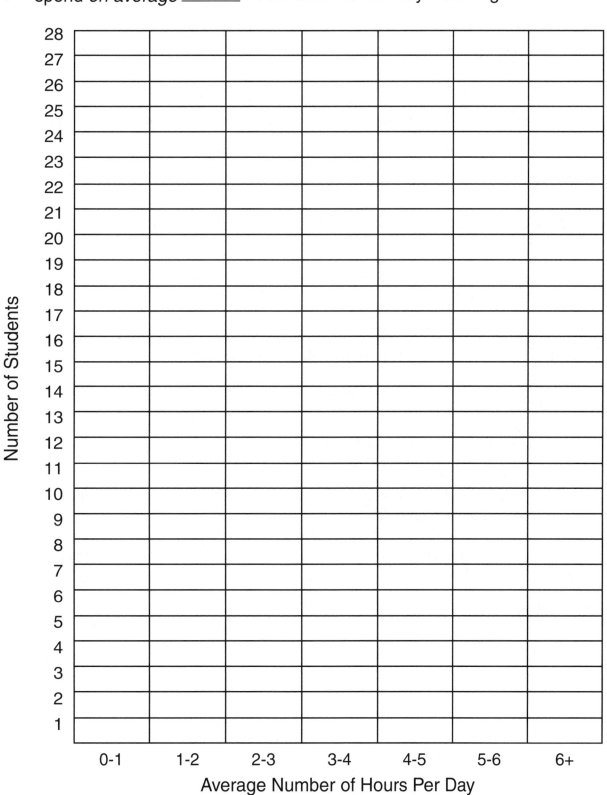

Are You in the Habit of Eating Healthy Foods and Being Physically Active?

To help you answer this question, compare your eating and physical activity patterns in activity 1 _Student Self-Assessment_ with the _Planet Health_ recommendations below. Point out which goals you meet by providing supporting information from activity 1. Conclude whether or not you are in the habit of eating healthy food and being physically active. Finally, if you don't meet one or more of the _Planet Health_ recommendations, why not? Can you identify things in your daily habits or environment that make it difficult for you to reach these goals?

Planet Health Nutrition and Physical Activity Recommendations

1. Eat at least five fruits and vegetables (combined) every day.
2. Choose a diet low in saturated fat and trans fat and moderate in total fat.
3. Be physically active daily or nearly every day.
4. Limit screen time to no more than 2 hours each day.

Student Checklist for Answering Key Questions

Your answers should include the following:

_____ _Thesis statement:_ A direct response to the question that includes your point of view.

_____ _Background:_ A summary of important information related to the question that will help the teacher understand your point of view. This might be knowledge about nutrition and physical activity that you have learned in this class, another class, or at home. The background information should be included at the beginning of a response, before or after the thesis statement.

_____ _Supporting details:_ Evidence from activity 1 or other sources that supports your point of view.

_____ _Conclusion:_ One or more sentences to bring the answer to a close, including a summary of your point of view and the most important details.

_____ _Correct format:_ Use paragraphs, complete sentences, proper punctuation, spelling and grammar, and clear penmanship.

Directions: Complete the first chart by writing what you **know** about good nutrition in the "K" column, what you **think** you know in the "T" column, and what you **want** to know about this topic in the "W" column. Brainstorm what you know, think you know, and want to know about being physically active throughout your life in the second chart.

Topic: Good Nutrition		
K: I Know	T: I Think I Know	W: I Want to Know

Topic: Being Physically Active Throughout Your Life		
K: I Know	T: I Think I Know	W: I Want to Know

An Open-Ended Essay

Examine the *Planet Health* recommendations for nutrition and physical activity. Based on what you know, explain why youth are encouraged to follow each of these recommendations.

Planet Health nutrition and physical activity recommendations

1. Eat at least five fruits and vegetables (combined) every day.
2. Choose a diet low in saturated fat and trans fat and moderate in total fat.
3. Be physically active daily or nearly every day.
4. Limit screen time to no more than 2 hours each day.

INFORMATION ABOUT PLANET HEALTH

Dear Parents,

Your children will be participating in an exciting health curriculum called *Planet Health*. *Planet Health* equips children with the knowledge and skills they need to choose nutritious diets and be physically active. Research shows that a good diet and adequate physical activity can significantly reduce the risk of obesity and chronic diseases, such as heart disease, high blood pressure, diabetes, and cancer. Yet children today are not eating the fruits and vegetables or getting the physical activity they need to be healthy both now and in the future.

Planet Health provides children with the tools to turn this trend around! Through exciting lessons designed to be incorporated into math, science, social studies, language arts, and physical education classes, the curriculum introduces and reinforces simple health messages.

- Eat five or more fruits and vegetables (combined) every day.
- Choose a diet low in saturated fat and trans fat and moderate in total fat.
- Be physically active daily or nearly every day.
- Limit screen time to no more than 2 hours each day.

Your child will receive up to 12 *Planet Health* lessons each year in grades 6, 7, and 8 as part of the math, science, social studies, and language arts curriculum. The concepts will also be taught in physical education classes. These lessons give students the opportunity to read, write, speak, listen, experiment, work cooperatively, and think for themselves to answer health-related questions.

Planet Health was developed and evaluated by the Harvard Prevention Research Center on Nutrition and Physical Activity. Over 100 teachers and 1,200 students in four school districts tested the materials. The curriculum improved student knowledge and helped students adopt more healthy behaviors.

Please reinforce the *Planet Health* messages at home. Encourage your children to make healthy food choices, help them identify safe opportunities to be physically active, and limit screen time to no more than two hours per day.

Sincerely,

part

IX

Language Arts

This unit contains eight lessons. Use the At A Glance chart below to help you select the lessons that best fit your curriculum objectives. Some of the lessons offer a choice of activities. Adapt the lesson procedures to fit your teaching style, students' skills, and time constraints.

Lessons in this unit meet many Massachusetts learning standards that may be similar to standards in your state. Refer to appendix E (page 508) to see which of the 1996-1999 Massachusetts Curriculum Frameworks (MCFW) each lesson incorporates.

Language Arts At A Glance

Theme	Lesson	Level of difficulty (grade) *			Subject specific skills	Materials needed
		6th	7th	8th		
Balanced diet	32 Pyramid Power	M	M	L	Persuasive writing	Posterboard
Balanced diet	33 Carbohydrates: Energy Food	H	M	M	Reading comprehension, analyzing and interpreting nonfiction, concept mapping	None
Fruits and vegetables	34 The Language of Food	M	M	L	Writing and analyzing poetry	Dr. Seuss's *Green Eggs and Ham* (optional)
Fruits and vegetables	35 Keep it Local	H	M	M	Persuasive writing	Overhead transparency
Activity	36 Write a Fable: Important Messages About Activity	H	M	M	Reading comprehension, writing, critiquing, and revising fables	None
Activity	37 Go for the Goal	M	M	L	Writing goals	None
Lifestyle	38 Lifetime Physical Activities: Research One, Describe One, Try One!	H	M	M	Research, writing nonfiction	Books on sports and leisure activities
Lifestyle	39 Choosing Healthy Foods	M	M	M	Persuasive writing	Advertisements

* Level of difficulty: L = low, M = medium, H = high

Lesson 32

Pyramid Power

In this lesson, students will learn about the importance of eating a balanced diet based on the Food Guide Pyramid (FGP). They will participate in a group activity where they will plan a balanced meal for a special event and write promotional materials for the event.

▶▶ Behavioral Objective

For students to eat a balanced diet based on the Food Guide Pyramid.

▶▶ Learning Objectives

Students will be able to

1. organize their ideas,
2. write clearly and persuasively, and
3. choose from each food group and within each food group in the Food Guide Pyramid.

▶▶ Materials

- Activity 1 *Balancing Meals*
- Activity 2 *Global Foods Puzzle* or activity 3 *Food Guide Pyramid Fun*
- Student resource 1 *Global Foods in the Food Guide Pyramid*
- Posterboard

▶▶ Procedure

1. (15 minutes) Explain the rationale for the shape of the pyramid, and the three principles of the Food Guide Pyramid (variety, moderation, and proportionality). Discuss the importance of all the food groups. Explain the importance of a balanced diet. (Different foods contain different nutrients. Eating a balanced diet provides us with energy and nutrients to do work and to play.) Discuss recommended number of servings and serving sizes. Finally, encourage students to follow the U.S. dietary guidelines.

- Make grains (especially whole grains), fruits, and vegetables the foundations of your meals.
- Be flexible and adventurous. Try new choices from these three groups in place of some of the less nutritious foods you eat.

2. (5 minutes) Define *mnemonic* (a device or formula to assist the memory.) Have students or class as a whole develop a mnemonic. Think of a five-word sentence whose

words start with the same letters of the five food groups, e.g., *My Mother Voted for Greg* (meats, milk, vegetables, fruit, and grains). The words can be in any order. Share the mnemonics with the class.

3. (25 minutes) Have students count off by five, so that they are randomly dispersed into groups of four or five, or use cooperative groups. Hand out one copy of activity 1 *Balancing Meals* per group. Groups will meet, plan a meal, and then present their ideas to the class. (Hand out posterboard to each group for making presentations.) Encourage groups to divide the workload. Please note, presentations may have to be part of the following day's class due to time constraint.

4. *Optional activity*: Discuss the fact that the FGP is meaningful internationally by using the student resource *Global Foods in the Food Guide Pyramid*. You will find two exercises: activity 2 *Global Foods Puzzle* and activity 3 *Food Guide Pyramid Fun*. You can use either exercise with your students. The first sheet has a "global" focus, while the second concentrates on foods more frequently consumed in the United States. The student resource *Global Foods in the Food Guide Pyramid* is included to accompany the "globally focused" word exercise.

▶▶ Extension Activities

Ask students to write a few paragraphs answering the following questions:

- Are you eating a balanced diet?
- Are you eating the same foods each day?
- In which group do you get the most variety?
- In which group is it hardest to get variety?
- What are some other foods you might eat to add variety to your diet?

▶▶ Teacher Resources

General Background Material

In preparing for this lesson, you may want to refer to the following resources:

- *Nutrition and Your Health: Dietary Guidelines for Americans* (appendix A)
- *Fat: Where It's At* (p. 252)
- *Guide to Good Eating* (appendix A)

Specific Background Material

The following will provide the background information necessary to teach this lesson.

Highlights of the Food Guide Pyramid

The Food Guide Pyramid (FGP) was designed by the U.S. Department of Agriculture (USDA) and released in 1992. The FGP is an eating guide that helps people understand the five food groups as well as the importance of variety, proportionality, and moderation in the diet. Following the FGP recommendations ensures consuming essential nutrients sufficient to meet the dietary needs of most people.

The Food Guide Pyramid
A Guide to Daily Food Choices

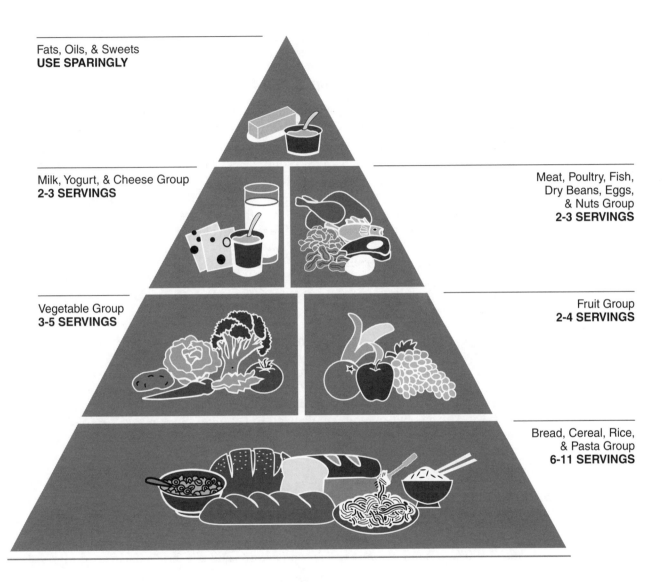

Fats, Oils, & Sweets
USE SPARINGLY

Milk, Yogurt, & Cheese Group
2-3 SERVINGS

Meat, Poultry, Fish,
Dry Beans, Eggs,
& Nuts Group
2-3 SERVINGS

Vegetable Group
3-5 SERVINGS

Fruit Group
2-4 SERVINGS

Bread, Cereal, Rice,
& Pasta Group
6-11 SERVINGS

Looking at the Pieces of the Pyramid

The Food Guide Pyramid emphasizes foods from the five major food groups shown in the three lower tiers of the Pyramid. Each of these food groups provides some, but not all, of the nutrients you need. Foods in one group can't replace those in another. No one of these major food groups is more important than another—for good health, you need them all (USDA and DHHS).

The position of the food groups in the FGP reflects the number of servings people should eat from each food group *every day*. The pyramid has a wide base and a small tip, showing that the food group requiring the most daily servings is at the bottom, and the group requiring the least is at the top. Specifically, the grain group forms the pyramid's base, indicating we should eat more servings of grain products, especially whole grains, than of any other food group. The tip includes foods such as fats, oils, and sweets. These foods should be consumed in small amounts.

The FGP tells us that foods from all food groups are important. It also tells us

- to choose foods from all of the food groups daily;
- to choose a variety of foods within each food group;
- to choose a diet that is moderate in total fat and low in saturated fat and cholesterol; and
- to choose a diet that is low in sweet, salty, and high-fat foods.

The Three Principles of the Food Guide Pyramid

1. *Proportionality (or balance)*: Eat the recommended number of servings from each group (see *Recommended Number of Servings for Girls and Boys Aged 11–14*).

2. *Variety*: Select a variety of foods within each of the five food groups. For example, while selecting from the grains food group, select bread, rice, pasta, tortillas, and cereals. Choose whole grain varieties when possible.

3. *Moderation*: Eat the appropriate number of servings from each food group, using the FGP serving sizes as a guide. Eat foods in the tip of the pyramid sparingly. These foods are low in essential vitamins and minerals and high in calories from fat or sugar. Eating fats, especially animal fats, and sweets in moderation can lower the risk of developing many health problems in adulthood.

The FGP applies to diets around the world. For example, 1/2 cup of mango juice from Brazil is a serving of juice. (See the student resource *Global Foods in the Food Guide Pyramid.*)

Number of Servings From Each Food Group

The FGP suggests a range for number of servings from each group. It provides a chart that explains how many servings you will need from each group based on your age and sex. The FGP can be used by anyone—girls, boys, men, or women—regardless of their age. The amount of food people need to eat differs by age and sex. Most boys and men need more food than most girls and women. Also, growing, active teenagers need more food than many sedentary adults. Review *Recommended Number of Servings for Girls and Boys Aged 11-14.*

Serving Size

To understand how easy it is to eat the recommended number of servings from each group, review the foods included in each food group and review what equals one serving (see *What Counts as One Serving?* on page 138 and pages 488-490 in appendix A).

Combination Foods

These are foods made from ingredients that fit into more than one food group. One example is pizza, which can provide grain, dairy, and vegetable servings. Learning the constituents of combination foods can help with comparing intake to the FGP.

Whole Grain Options

Whole grain products are made from intact kernels of grain. The germ and bran from the kernels make these foods naturally high in nutrients and higher in fiber than refined breads, cereals, pasta, and rice. Eating these foods can reduce the risk of developing diabetes and heart disease. Encourage students to try whole grain foods: whole wheat bread, whole grain ready-to-eat cereal, oatmeal, corn tortillas, whole wheat pasta, tabouli salad, whole barley soup, popcorn, and brown rice. Check food labels. Don't be fooled by foods made from wheat flour, enriched flour, or degerminated corn meal. These are not whole grains.

References

National Dairy Council. 1994. *Guide to good eating.* Rosemont, IL: National Dairy Council.

National Dairy Council. 1997. *The daily food guide pyramid.* Rosemont, IL: National Dairy Council.

U.S. Department of Agriculture and U.S. Department of Health and Human Services. Food Guide Pyramid.

▶▶ Answer Keys

Activity 2 Global Foods Puzzle

1. Fruit
2. Fats, oils, and sweets
3. Lalo
4. Dairy
5. Grain
6. Tofu
7. Fish
8. Candy
9. Vegetable
10. Pasta
11. Variety
12. Moderation
13. Cassava
14. Mango
15. Milk
16. Noodles

Activity 3 Food Guide Pyramid Fun

1. Fruit
2. Fats, oils, and sweets
3. Broccoli
4. Dairy
5. Grains
6. Nut
7. Fish
8. Candy
9. Vegetable
10. Pasta
11. Variety
12. Moderation
13. Carrot
14. Melon
15. Milk
16. Noodles

Recommended Number of Servings for Girls and Boys Aged 11–14

Food group	Girls (2,200 calories/day)	Boys (2,500 calories/day)
Bread, cereal, rice, and pasta	9	11
Vegetable	4	5
Fruit	3	4
Milk, yogurt, and cheese	2.5	2.5
Meat, poultry, fish, dry beans, eggs, and nuts	2.5	2.5

What Counts as One Serving?

Food group	One serving
Bread, cereal, rice, and pasta	1 slice of bread 1 tortilla, roll, muffin 1/2 bagel, English muffin, hamburger bun 1/2 cup cooked cereal, grits, rice, pasta 1 oz. (about 1 cup) ready-to-eat breakfast cereal
Vegetable	1 cup raw leafy vegetables 1/2 cup other chopped vegetables 1/2 cup other cooked vegetables 3/4 cup vegetable juice
Fruit	1 medium apple, banana, orange, pear 1/2 grapefruit 1/4 cantaloupe 1/2 cup of raw, canned, cooked, frozen fruit 1/4 cup raisins, dried fruit 3/4 cup of fruit juice
Milk, yogurt, and cheese	1 cup milk or yogurt 1.5 oz. natural cheese (like cheddar) 2 oz. processed cheese (like American)
Meat, poultry, fish, dry beans, eggs, and nuts	2.5 oz. of cooked, lean meat, poultry, or fish 1/2 cup cooked dry beans, peas 1 egg 2 tablespoon peanut butter 1/3 cup nuts, seeds

Food name	Food group	Some countries where food is consumed regularly
Rice There are many different varieties, white, brown, etc. All can be eaten.	Bread, cereal, rice, and pasta	Brazil, Cambodia, Haiti, Puerto Rico, U.S., Japan, China, Greece, Ethiopia, Korea, India, Mexico
Millet Cultivated for the white seed and used as a food grain. It is high in protein.	Bread, cereal, rice, and pasta	Brazil, Cambodia, China, Iran, Iraq, Jordan, Haiti, Puerto Rico, and U.S. among some populations.
Cassava Also known as manioc, it is a starchy root. There are two varieties, sweet and bitter. The sweet cassava is consumed as a vegetable, and the bitter variety is used to thicken soups and puddings.	Vegetable	Brazil is the world's largest grower of cassava. Also, West Africa, Spain, Phillipines.
Lalo A green leafy vegetable that is high in iron.	Vegetable	Haiti
Plantain It looks like a large banana, but it is much starchier (harder). They grow 1 to 2 feet long and are green, yellow, or black. When they are boiled, roasted, fried, or baked, their taste is similar to a potato.	Fruit	Brazil, Columbia, Cambodia, Haiti, Puerto Rico, Venezuela. It originated in southeastern Asia.
Mango A tropical fruit that is sweet, aromatic, and juicy. It is peeled before consumption.	Fruit	Africa, Brazil, Cambodia, Haiti, India, Puerto Rico. The original home of the mango is Southeastern Asia, and it is imported to U.S.
Papaya Looks like a melon and is often called a "tree melon." Weight ranges from 1 to 20 pounds.	Fruit	Brazil, Cambodia, Haiti, Puerto Rico. The original home of the papaya was Mexico or the West Indies.
Dried fish Like codfish, it is a fish that has been dried and often salted.	Meat, poultry, fish, dry beans, eggs, and nuts	Africa, Brazil, Cambodia, Haiti, India, Korea, Puerto Rico
Tofu Bean curd, a by-product of the soybean.	Meat, poultry, fish, dry beans, eggs, and nuts	Cambodia, China, Korea, Japan, U.S. among some populations, Vietnam.

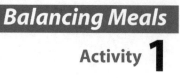

The Student Council needs help in planning a series of great events this year at your school. There are five events where meals will be served, and the student council needs students with expertise in the Food Guide Pyramid to plan nutritious meals that include a food from each of the five food groups. The events are: a breakfast before the pep rally, a Saturday lunch for the fund-raiser for the field trip into Boston, a special dinner before the school talent show, a day's snacks for the car wash, and a lunch for Earth Day.

You have been asked to help plan one of these meals. As a group, decide which meal and then begin the balancing act! Be prepared to present your ideas to the class.

As you plan your meal, think about the following:

• Who will be attending this event (teachers, students, parents, etc.)?

• What extra incentive would encourage people to come to the event?

1. Write your meal plan.

2. Describe how the meal fits into the theme of the event.

3. How many food groups are represented? How many foods in each food group are represented?

4. Why is it important to eat foods from every food group each day?

5. Make a poster advertising the event and promoting the healthy food that will be available.

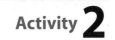

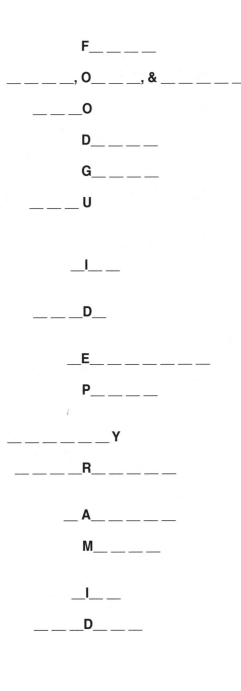

F __ __ __

__ __ __ __ , O __ __ __ , & __ __ __ __ __ __ __

__ __ __ O

D __ __ __ __

G __ __ __ __

__ __ __ U

__ I __ __

__ __ __ D __ __

__ E __ __ __ __ __ __ __

P __ __ __ __

__ __ __ __ __ __ __ Y

__ __ __ __ R __ __ __ __

__ A __ __ __ __ __

M __ __ __ __

__ I __ __

__ __ __ D __ __

1. Mangoes belong in this group.

2. The group at the tip of the pyramid.

3. A Haitian green vegetable high in iron.

4. Milk, yogurt, and cheese are ____ products.

5. Cereal and rice are types of _____.

6. A common source of protein in parts of Asia. It falls in the meats, poultry, ____, dry beans, eggs, and nuts group.

7. The meat, poultry, ____, dry beans, eggs, and nuts group.

8. Something for one's sweet tooth that falls in the fats, oils, and sweets group.

9. Carrots belong in this group.

10. A type of grain product that comes in many shapes and sizes.

11. Eat a ____ of foods (lots of different kinds).

12. This principle explains that we need to make sure our diet does not contain too much of certain foods.

13. A starchy tuber (root vegetable) eaten in tropical areas.

14. A juicy tropical fruit eaten in many different countries, but not grown in the US.

15. A beverage often consumed with cereal.

16. A product in the grain group eaten around the world. These are long and skinny.

F_ _ _ _

1. Mangoes belong in this group.

_ _ _ _ , O_ _ _ , & _ _ _ _ _ _ _

2. The group at the tip of the pyramid.

_ _O_ _ _ _ _

3. This green vegetable is high in Vitamin C.

D_ _ _ _

4. Milk, yogurt, and cheese are ____ products.

G_ _ _ _ _

5. Cereal and rice are types of _____.

_U_

6. Cashews are a type of ____. They are high in protein and fat.

_I_ _

7. The meat, poultry, ____, dry beans, eggs, and nuts group.

_ _ _D_

8. Something for one's sweet tooth that falls in the fats, oils, and sweets group.

_E_ _ _ _ _ _ _

9. Spinach belongs in this group.

P_ _ _ _

10. A type of grain product that comes in many shapes and sizes.

_ _ _ _ _ _ _Y

11. Eat a ____ of foods (lots of different kinds).

_ _ _ _R_ _ _ _

12. This principle explains that we need to make sure our diet does not contain too much of certain foods.

_A_ _ _ _

13. An orange vegetable with a green top (high in Vitamin A).

M_ _ _ _

14. Cantaloupe is from the ____ family.

_I_ _

15. A beverage high in Vitamin D often consumed with cereal.

_ _ _D_ _ _

16. A product in the grain group eaten around the world. These are long and skinny.

Carbohydrates: Energy Foods

Students will read a passage that describes the importance of carbohydrates in a healthy diet. The reading will be preceded and followed by activities designed to improve reading comprehension and retention. Then, you choose whether to have students build their vocabulary (crossword puzzle), make connections (concept mapping), or apply the information (discussion/skits) presented in the reading to make recommendations about healthy eating choices. The final activity offers students the opportunity to practice their critical thinking skills.

▶▶ Behavioral Objective

For students to make healthy food choices based on the Food Guide Pyramid.

▶▶ Learning Objectives

Students will be able to

1. comprehend and identify basic facts and ideas introduced in a nonfiction essay (activities 1 and 2),

2. use vocabulary introduced in a reading assignment to complete a crossword puzzle (activity 3),

3. complete a concept map to illustrate the connections among major ideas presented in a reading assignment (activity 4),

4. apply information obtained from reading to make recommendations for healthy food choices (activity 5),

5. discuss their thoughts and opinions and persuade others to follow their recommendations (activity 5),

6. explain why it's important to include complex carbohydrates in their diet, and

7. use their new understanding of carbohydrates to explain why grains make up the base of the Food Guide Pyramid (activity 6).

▶▶ Materials

- Activity 1 *Word Splash* (overhead transparency, or handout, or use chalkboard)
- Activity 2 *Reading Comprehension*
- Activity 3 *Crossword Puzzle* or activity 4 *Concept Map* or activity 5 *What Would You Say?* (discussion or skits)
- Activity 6 *Critical Thinking*
- *Optional:* Overhead transparency *Good and Poor Sources of Carbohydrates*

▶▶ **Procedure**

Overview (modify this to fit your needs):

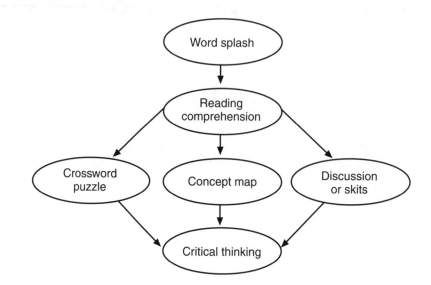

1. Point out the goals of this lesson:
   - To improve reading comprehension
   - To learn about the importance of carbohydrates
   - To make healthy food choices in the future
2. Post an itinerary of the activities. This helps students who need to see the big picture of what's going to happen in order to be able to focus on the details.

Activity 1 Word Splash

This activity is designed to help students access their prior knowledge of carbohydrates, get them to make predictions about concepts they will read about, and develop a purpose for reading the new information. This type of activity facilitates comprehension of expository text (Stern 1996). It is a good idea to tell students why this type of activity is useful. This will help them reflect on the learning process, as well as on the specific material they are learning.

1. Display an overhead transparency of the Word Splash (activity 1).
2. Ask students to predict connections among at least five of the words in the splash and the topic in the center (carbohydrates). They should write down their predictions. For example: "Pasta is a food that contains a lot of carbohydrates."

Activity 2 Reading Comprehension

Activity 2 *Reading Comprehension* will provide your students with practice reading nonfiction materials. Combining this activity with activity 3 *Crossword Puzzle* will help their vocabulary development.

1. Have students read the passage to check the accuracy of their predictions from activity 1. As they read, they revise their statements as needed.

2. Discuss the reading by asking students some of the following questions. This discussion may take place after students complete activity 3 or 4, but should take place before activity 5.

- What was the main idea?
- What's the difference between simple and complex carbohydrates?
- What types of foods are high in simple carbohydrates? complex carbohydrates?
- How many servings of grain products should you eat daily?
- Why do experts say whole grains should comprise at least half of the grain products you eat each day?

You also may wish to give students some examples of good and poor sources of carbohydrates. To do this, you may display the overhead transparency *Good and Poor Sources of Carbohydrates* (or use the chalkboard).

Choose activity 3, 4, or 5 to help reinforce (activity 3), make connections (activity 4), or apply (activity 5) information about carbohydrates.

Activity 3 Crossword Puzzle

Activity 3 *Crossword Puzzle* requires students to reread parts of the passage on carbohydrates. It emphasizes the important points in the reading by asking students to recall vocabulary. This would make a good homework assignment.

1. Have students complete the crossword puzzle.
2. If you haven't already discussed the reading passage of activity 2, please do so now. Then proceed to activity 6 *Critical Thinking*.

Activity 4 Concept Map

Activity 4 *Concept Map* will be most successful if your students are familiar with concept mapping or webbing. If they are not, you should precede the activity with the following explanation.

1. Explain the following:
    - *Why should I do concept maps?*
        - They are important study tools that help you store information in your long-term memory.
        - They help you figure out the main ideas in a piece of reading material.
        - They help you organize new material and establish relationships between ideas.
    - *How do you make a concept map? What are the rules?*
        - A feature of concept maps is that main ideas are placed at the top of the map. Smaller, more specific concepts and examples go below the main ideas.
        - Concept words go in the circles or boxes. These are labels for ideas or concepts. All of these words are concepts because they cause a picture to form in your mind. Examples: *car, dog, thinking, bread, carbohydrates.*
        - Concepts should never contain more than three words.
        - Linkage words connect, or link, concept words. They go on a line connecting the circles or boxes. Examples: *are, the, when, is, to.*
        - Concepts should not be repeated. Instead, extend the linkage line to where that concept first appeared.
2. Have students complete the concept map. (The answer key follows the references.)

3. If you haven't already discussed the reading passage of activity 2, please do so now. Then proceed to activity 6 *Critical Thinking*.

Activity 5 What Would You Say?

Activity 5 *What Would You Say?* requires students to apply the information they read in the passage on carbohydrates. They must read the situations listed on the activity sheet and make recommendations about appropriate food choices.

1. If you haven't already discussed the reading passage of activity 2, please do so now. Then you may proceed with this activity.
2. Divide the class into groups of three or four students. Assign each group one of the situations listed on the activity sheet. Ask each group to discuss the situation and come up with a recommendation. You may wish to have each group present their recommendation in the form of a short skit. Proceed to activity 6 *Critical Thinking*.

Activity 6 Critical Thinking

The following activity provides students the opportunity to interpret and apply what they have learned about carbohydrates in the other activities.

1. Use the chalkboard or an overhead transparency to present the Food Guide Pyramid.
2. Ask students the following question:
   • Based on what you know about carbohydrates, why do grains form the base of the Food Guide Pyramid?
3. Write their responses on the board. (Be sure to clarify any misconceptions. See the Teacher Resources for an answer to this question.)

►► Extension Activities

Ask students to write a few paragraphs answering the following:

• Why do grains form the base of the Food Guide Pyramid?
• How many servings of grain products do you usually eat each day? What proportion are whole grain?
• Are you consuming an appropriate amount of carbohydrates in your diet?

►► Teacher Resources

General Background Material

In preparing for this lesson, you may want to refer to *Nutrition and Your Health: Dietary Guidelines for Americans*. See appendix A for information on obtaining this resource.

Specific Background Material

For an overview of the types of carbohydrates, their function in the body, dietary recommendations, and examples of foods high in carbohydrates, see activity 2 *Reading Comprehension*.

Dietary Recommendations for Carbohydrates, Fat, and Protein

Carbohydrates (carbos) provide 4 calories per gram. Carbos are our major source of energy and include sugars (simple carbohydrates) and starches (complex carbohydrates). The rationale for the recommendation that 55-60% of daily calories come from carbohydrates is not based on a physiological requirement. Rather, it is derived from the need to provide an upper limit on fat and protein intake! Thus, if fat and protein intake combined account for 40-45% of intake, the rest should be from carbohydrates. Fruits, vegetables, and grain products (whole grain breads, cereals, pasta, and rice) are excellent sources of carbohydrates.

For an adolescent boy eating 2,500 calories per day, carbohydrate intake would be as much as 375 grams. Grams of total carbohydrate per serving are listed on food labels.

Fat provides 9 calories per gram. It's important for cell structure, transporting fat-soluble vitamins (A, D, E, and K), and insulating our bodies. Body fat also functions as an energy store. However, it's important to note that calories from any source—protein, carbohydrate, fat, or alcohol—are stored as fat when energy intake exceeds expenditure. Weight gain occurs when this imbalance persists over time.

Not all fats are created equal. The U.S. Dietary Guidelines recommend a diet that is low in saturated fat (no more than 10% of calories), low in cholesterol, and moderate in total fat (no more than 30% of calories). Foods high in saturated fat (for example, butter or lard) tend to be solid at room temperature and come from animal sources. Foods high in dietary cholesterol, such as meat and dairy products, also come from animal sources. Foods high in saturated fat and dietary cholesterol raise blood cholesterol. Consequently, eating a diet high in these foods increases the risk of heart disease.

In contrast unsaturated fats, such as olive, peanut, and vegetable oils, tend to be liquid at room temperature. Unsaturated fats help keep blood cholesterol low and substituting them for saturated fats has been shown to decrease the risk of heart disease. However, through a commercial process called hydrogenation these healthy liquid fats can be converted into solids called *trans fats;* this is how some margarines are made. On food labels for products such as commercially-made cookies and crackers, trans fats are often referred to as partially hydrogenated vegetable oil. Not surprisingly foods high in trans fats have been found to increase the risk of heart disease. Americans typically get about 33% of their total calories from fat, 11% from saturated fat and 2.6% from trans fat.

An adolescent girl whose total calorie requirement is 2,200 calories can get about 660 calories from fat each day, which is 73 grams. No more than 24 grams of this should come from saturated fat. Food labels list total fat, saturated fat, and unsaturated fat grams per serving. The FDA has recently proposed including trans fats on food labels as well.

Protein provides 4 calories per gram. Proteins are essential to growth, building and repairing cells, making enzymes and hormones, and other processes. Proteins are produced by cells. Dietary protein needs vary over the life span. Generally expressed in terms of grams needed per kilogram of body weight, protein needs are highest during infancy, at about 2.2 g/kg, and decline to 0.8 g/kg in adulthood. Adolescents need to consume about 1 g/kg/day.

Experts recommend that 10-15% of daily calories come from protein. During a growth spurt, adolescents may require more calories from protein. However, they should consult with their pediatricians before increasing their protein consumption. American diets usually exceed protein requirements and are rarely deficient in this nutrient. Lean red meat, chicken, fish, nuts, and legumes are excellent sources of protein. Dairy products like cheese and milk are also good sources of protein. To avoid consuming excess amounts of saturated fats and cholesterol, eat red meat in moderation and choose low-fat dairy products.

An adolescent boy who needs 2,500 calories per day needs about 250 calories from protein each day, which is 63 grams. Food labels list protein grams per serving.

Alcohol

Alcohol provides 7 calories per gram. There is no dietary requirement for alcohol. Evidence suggests that moderate consumption by healthy adult men and healthy, nonpregnant, nonlactating adult women (equivalent to one glass of wine per day for women, two for men) may lower the risk of heart disease in some individuals. Higher levels of alcohol consumption increase the risk of high blood pressure, stroke, heart disease, liver disease, certain cancers, accidents, violence, suicide, birth defects, and death. Even moderate consumption may increase the risk of certain cancers. Children and youth should not consume alcohol.

Grains Form the Base of the Food Guide Pyramid

Experts recommend that 55-60% of our daily energy intake come from carbohydrates. Grains contain large amounts of carbohydrates, the energy foods. They are usually low in fat and provide protein, fiber, some vitamins (riboflavin, thiamin, and niacin), and some minerals (iron and magnesium). The Dietary Guidelines for Americans as depicted in the Food Guide Pyramid recommend consuming 6-11 servings of grain per day depending on calorie needs, with about half of the servings coming from whole grain food products. The guidelines also recommend that grain products be prepared with little to no fats or sugars.

Whole Grain Options

Whole grain products are made from intact kernels of grain. The germ and bran from the kernels make these foods naturally high in nutrients and higher in fiber than refined breads, cereals, pasta, and rice. Eating whole grain, high-fiber foods reduces the risk of developing diabetes and heart disease. According to *Healthy People 2010,* some clinical evidence suggests that eating food with water-soluble fiber decreases blood glucose and blood lipid levels. Currently only about 7% of Americans two years old and older eat three or more servings of whole grain each day.

Try eating whole grain foods such as whole wheat bread, whole grain ready-to-eat cereal, long cooking oatmeal, corn tortillas, whole wheat pasta, whole grain tabouli salad, whole barley soup, popcorn, and brown rice. Check food labels. Don't be fooled by foods made from wheat flour, enriched flour, or degerminated corn meal. These are not whole grains.

Some Common Grain Foods

Bread usually contains flour, water, yeast, salt, and some sugar. Although breads are generally good sources of carbohydrates, vitamins, and protein, whole grain bread contains about four times as much fiber as white bread. One slice of bread counts as one serving of grain, and breads are usually low in fat. Check the ingredient list on bread packages.

For whole wheat bread, the label must specify that the product is made from whole wheat flour. Many commercial wheat breads use enriched white flour and brown syrup, so that they have the brown appearance of wheat bread. Other whole grain breads include rye and oat, among others.

White bread is made from bleached white flour, which loses 70% of its nutrients in the milling process. Although some nutrients are added back in a process called fortification, enriched white bread contains less fiber and nutrients than whole grain breads.

Pasta means "paste" in Italian and is very nutritious. It is rich in carbohydrates, high in protein, and low in fat and sodium. The fat content of pasta dishes depends upon the toppings selected. Meat, cheese, and tomato sauce are often used but can be high in sodium and fat. Check the labels of sauces to determine the percentage of calories from fat per serving. Adding vegetables to pasta dishes adds taste and nutritional value.

Rice is the cereal of choice in most damp tropical climates. In this country, white rice is usually enriched with iron and other nutrients. Brown rice, a whole grain, is unpolished, which means it retains the bran and germ that contains much of the fiber in rice. Brown rice also takes longer to cook than white rice (40-50 minutes). Processed rice usually has no bran or germ and is available in the form of rice flakes and rice puffs, often eaten as snacks.

Breakfast cereals vary greatly in their nutritional value. While grains are naturally high in fiber and low in fat, sodium, or sugar, the final product on the supermarket shelf may not have these characteristics. Breakfast cereals may be made from rice, wheat, corn, or oats, or a combination of these. The grains are often exploded into puffs, pressed into flakes, shredded and spun into biscuits, or baked into various shapes. They are commonly toasted, and sweeteners, nuts, raisins, salt, fat, and preservatives are often added. Hot cereals are usually made from unrefined grains (e.g., oats and wheat), which are high in fiber, vitamins, and minerals, and low in fat. Instant varieties of hot cereals, however, may have various sweeteners and other ingredients added to them.

For all cereal products, check the label for the following items:

- the ingredient list,
- how much fiber (this varies widely),
- how much fat (e.g., granola products are often high in fat because of added coconut oil),
- how much sodium, and
- how much sugar.

Many breakfast cereals are fortified with vitamins and minerals.

See the table for examples of good and poor sources of carbohydrates.

Good and Poor Sources of Carbohydrates

Good sources		Poor sources
Baked potato	Mango	Beef
Banana	Mashed potatoes	Celery
Black beans	Oatmeal	Cheese
Blackberries	Oranges	Chicken
Black-eyed peas	Pancakes	Cucumbers
Bread	Pasta	Eggs
Cereal	Pinto beans	Fish
Corn	Plums	Hot dogs
Garbanzo beans	Polenta	Lettuce
Grapes	Rice	Nuts
Green beans	Squash	Pork

Good sources		Poor sources
Lima beans	Strawberries	
Low-fat milk	Sweet potatoes	
Low-fat yogurt	Waffles	

References

Bierer, L.A., Warner, L., Lawson, S., and Cohen, T. 1991. *Life science: The challenge of discovery.* Lexington, MA: Heath. (For ideas on concept mapping)

Cheung, L., Gortmaker, S., and Dart, H. 2001. *Eat well & keep moving.* Champaign, IL: Human Kinetics.

Hu, F.B., Stampfer, M.J., Manson, J.E., Rimm, E., Colditz, G.A., Rosner, B.A., Hennekens, C.H., and Willett, W.C. 1997. Dietary fat intake and the risk of coronary heart disease in women. *New England Journal of Medicine* 337(21): 1491-1499.

McArdle, W.P., Katch, F.I., and Katch, V.L. 1991. *Exercise physiology: Energy, nutrition, and human performance.* Philadelphia: Lea & Febiger.

National Dairy Council. 1994. *Guide to good eating.* Rosemont, IL: National Dairy Council.

National Dairy Council. 1997. *The daily food guide pyramid.* Rosemont, IL: National Dairy Council.

National Research Council. 1989. *Recommended dietary allowances.* 10th ed. Washington, D.C.: National Academy Press.

Stern, A. 1996. Instructional strategies and techniques to enhance motivation and achievement. Workshop, Weston, MA.

U.S. Department of Agriculture and U.S. Department of Health and Human Services. 2000. *Nutrition and your health: Dietary guidelines for Americans 2000,* 5th edition. **www.usda.gov/cnpp**

U.S. Department of Health and Human Services. 2000. Healthy People 2010, conference edition, vols. I and II. **www.health.gov/healthypeople**

Willett, W. 2000. Got fat? Exploding nutrition myths. *World Health News.* **www.worldhealthnews.harvard.edu**

▶▶ Answer Keys

Activity 3 Crossword Puzzle

Solution to the crossword puzzle

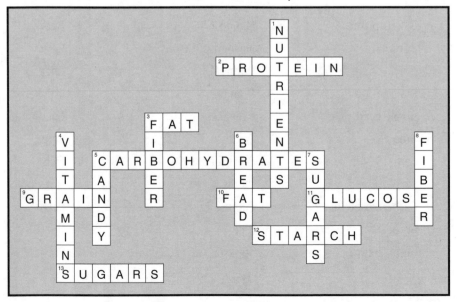

Activity 4 Concept Map

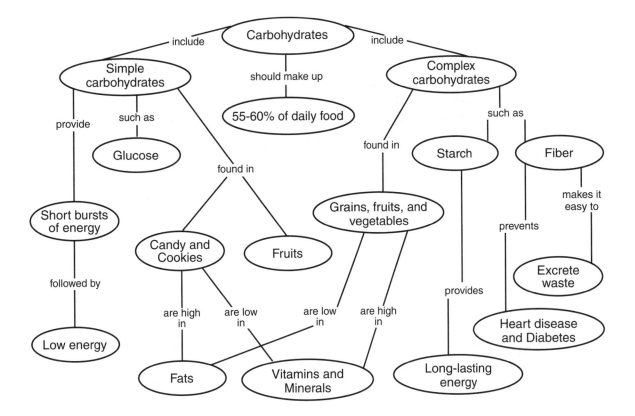

Activity 5 What Would You Say?

Situation 1

Carbohydrates should be the largest part of each day's total energy intake in a healthy diet. They provide us with an excellent energy source. Since we are going to be hiking all day, we need to make sure we will have enough energy. Bringing fruit is a good snack idea. Fruit has carbohydrates, vitamins, minerals, and fiber, but we need to eat more than just fruit. We should bring some sandwiches on whole grain bread for lunch and unsweetened dry cereal and rice cakes for snacks. Bread and cereals are members of the grain group. They contain a large amount of complex carbohydrates, vitamins, minerals, and fiber, and are low in fat. According to the Food Guide Pyramid, we should eat 6-11 servings of grains per day and about half from whole grains. As for protein, we need some protein, but not lots. If the sandwiches had peanut butter or some type of meat, we'd be okay. We also should bring some raw veggies and lots of water.

Situation 2

Carbohydrates should be the largest part of each day's total energy intake in a healthy diet. Experts recommend 55-60% of your total day's calories should come from carbohydrates, 10-15% from protein, and no more than 30% from fat. I recommend that you eat a balanced diet by following the Food Guide Pyramid recommendations and make sure you are doing physical activity every day. Eat sweets and high-fat foods in moderation. Stay away from "diets"! You don't need to starve yourself.

Situation 3

Eating foods that are high in sugar causes a sharp increase in blood glucose, followed by a sharp decrease. Eating sweets prior to participating in sporting events *may* result in a feeling of low energy in some people. Athletes should be encouraged to eat foods that are high in complex carbohydrates during daily meals. This will ensure they have plenty of carbohydrates (glycogen) stored to get them through their sporting event. A pre-game meal should be eaten 2 to 3 hours prior to the event, and it should be high in carbohydrates and relatively low in fat and protein (no steak-and-egg pre-game meals).

whole grain foods

pasta   proteins

grains

fats   starch

balanced diet   candy

Carbohydrates

sugar   rice

bread   energy source

low in fat   55-60%

complex carbohydrates   vitamins

Good sources of carbohydrates

Baked potato	Lima beans	Polenta
Banana	Low-fat milk	Popcorn
Barley	Low-fat yogurt	Rice
Black beans	Mango	Squash
Blackberries	Oatmeal	Strawberries
Black-eyed peas	Oranges	Sweet potatoes
Bread	Pancakes	Tortillas
Brown rice	Pasta	Waffles
Cereal	Pinto beans	Whole grain:
Corn	Plums	• cereal
Garbanzo beans		• bread
Grapes		• pasta

Poor sources of carbohydrates

Beef	Fish
Celery	Hot dogs
Cheese	Lettuce
Chicken	Nuts
Cucumbers	Pork
Eggs	

Planet Health: Carbohydrates: Energy Foods

Carbohydrates: Energy Foods in the Pyramid

The foods we eat contain many kinds of nutrients. Nutrients are the chemical substances in food that our bodies use to keep us healthy. Macronutrients (carbohydrates, fats, and proteins) are the major food components. Micronutrients (vitamins and minerals) are the nutrients that we need in very small amounts and are present in many foods. Both groups of nutrients are important for a healthy body.

All foods are made up of one, two, or all three of the macronutrients. **Protein** provides the body with the building blocks for making and repairing tissue (like muscle and skin). **Fat** helps keep the body warm, helps protect the internal organs (like the heart and liver), helps the body transport certain vitamins, and is a rich source of energy. **Carbohydrates** provide the body with energy. Protein and fat can also provide energy, but carbohydrates are the quickest source of energy and the only nutrient that can be used for energy in every single cell in the body. Carbohydrates should make up the largest part (55-60%) of each day's total calorie intake in a healthy diet. Only 10-15% of daily calories should come from protein and no more than 30% from fat.

There are two kinds of carbohydrates: simple and complex. Simple carbohydrates are composed of one or two small molecules and are also called sugars. Glucose, fructose, maltose, and sucrose are examples of sugars commonly found in the foods we eat. They are found in especially large quantities in sweet foods like soda, cookies, and candy. However, they are also found naturally in fruits and other foods made from plants. Sugars are easily absorbed into the blood from the digestive system. Eating a meal high in simple carbohydrates gives us a short burst of energy. Unfortunately, this is sometimes followed by a feeling of drowsiness or low energy.

Complex carbohydrates, like starch, are made up of long chains of simple sugars that are linked together. These large molecules provide us with a longer-lasting source of energy. Breads, cereals, pasta, rice, and other grain products are high in complex carbohydrates; so are many fruits and vegetables. Foods that are high in complex carbohydrates are usually low in fat and provide us with protein, some vitamins (folic acid, riboflavin, thiamin, and niacin), and some minerals (iron and magnesium).

The starches found in foods made from whole grains, like whole wheat bread, raisin bran, popcorn, and brown rice, are surrounded by intact kernels of grain. They are broken down more slowly than the starches found in foods made from refined grains, such as white bread and white rice. Whole grain foods and some fruits and vegetables are high in fiber, a complex carbohydrate that helps the digestive system function properly. Fiber can't be broken down by our digestive juices, so it passes through our intestines, soaking up water and making it easier for waste to pass from our bodies. Eating plenty of fiber may help prevent heart disease and diabetes.

Carbohydrates are found in many foods and in all groups of the Food Guide Pyramid. However, the grain, fruit, and vegetable groups contain the greatest amount of carbohydrates and are the foundation of a healthy diet. Eat six or more servings of grain products daily, and include at least three whole grain varieties. Eat five or more servings of fruits and vegetables daily. Be sure to choose a variety of foods within these groups. This will help you get the nutrients and fiber you need. Go easy on sweet foods like soda, cookies, and candy. Although these foods provide carbohydrates, they are usually low in vitamins and minerals and can be high in saturated and trans fat.

Adapted from the classroom lesson of L. Cheung, S. Gortmaker, and H. Dart, *Eat Well & Keep Moving*, 2001.

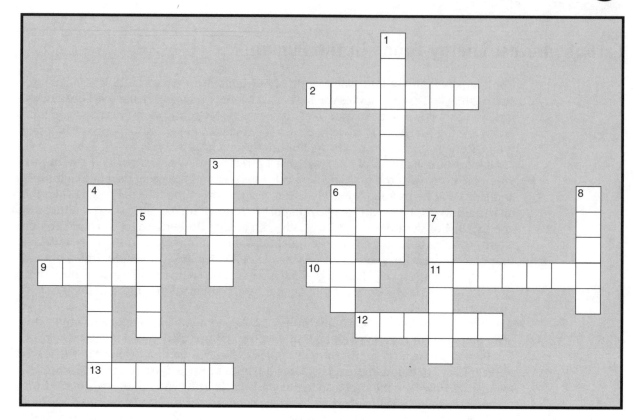

Across

2. Provides the body with building blocks for repairing tissue.

3. Helps keep the body warm.

5. The macronutrient that should make up the largest part of each day's total food intake.

9. A food group that contains foods high in complex carbohydrates.

10. Foods that are high in complex carbohydrates are usually low in _____.

11. Blood sugar; a simple carbohydrate.

12. Provides us with long-lasting energy.

13. Carbohydrates that are easily absorbed into the blood.

Down

1. Chemical substances in food that our bodies need to stay healthy.

3. May lower your risk for heart disease and some cancers.

4. Grains usually contain these micronutrients.

5. Foods that contain large amounts of simple sugars.

6. An example of a food high in complex carbohydrates.

7. Provide short bursts of energy.

8. Absorbs water and makes it easy for waste to pass from our bodies.

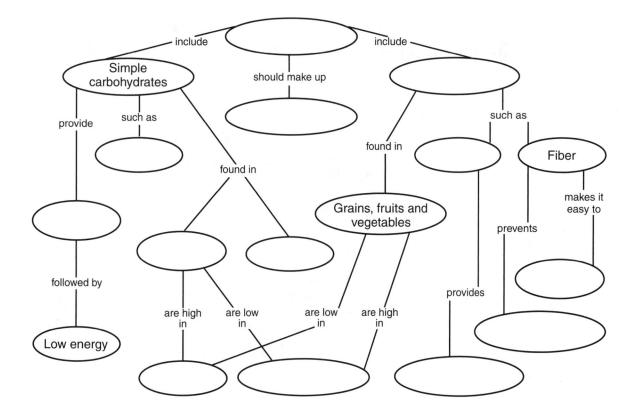

What would you say or do if you were presented with the following situations?

Situation 1

You and a group of your friends are planning a day hike into the White Mountains. Everyone is trying to decide what to bring for lunch and snacks. One of your friends thinks you should bring food high in protein. Another friend says she just wants to bring fruit. What would you recommend? What would you say to convince your friends they should follow your suggestions?

Situation 2

Your sister tells you she is interested in going on the "Zone Diet." She explains that the diet is a high-protein, low-carbohydrate diet. The diet recommends that 40 percent of daily calories come from protein, 30 percent from carbohydrates, and 30 percent fat. She asks you whether you think this is a good idea. What would you recommend and why?

Situation 3

Your soccer game begins in 30 minutes. Your friend offers you a candy bar. He says it will give you a quick burst of energy for the game. Would you accept his offer? Why or why not?

Lesson **34**

The Language of Food

This lesson will teach students about the importance of eating fruits and vegetables and will encourage them to taste new and different varieties of these foods. It is designed to be integrated into a poetry unit. Students will read and interpret poems that describe the feelings associated with trying new foods. They will taste a fruit or vegetable that they have never eaten before and write a poem which describes the fruit or vegetable and their experience tasting it.

▶▶ Behavioral Objectives

- For students to eat five or more fruits and vegetables per day.
- For students to try a variety of fruits and vegetables.

▶▶ Learning Objectives

Students will be able to

1. read and analyze poems to determine common themes,
2. observe foods critically and list adjectives to describe their characteristics,
3. write poems that depict emotions and experiences associated with trying new foods,
4. explain why it's important to eat fruits and vegetables, and
5. cite the 5-A-Day recommendation for fruits and vegetables.

▶▶ Materials

- Activity 1 *Poetry Writing*
- Poems (included): "The Sad Tale of Jonathan Who Wouldn't Eat His Vegetables," "Something Green for Dinner," "Celery," "Stuart McGroo," "I'd Never Eat a Beet," "Taste of Purple," **OR**
- *Green Eggs and Ham* by Dr. Seuss (not included)

▶▶ Procedure

Day 1

1. (5-10 minutes) We recommend you read aloud Dr. Seuss's *Green Eggs and Ham* or two of the poems included in the lesson.
2. (5 minutes) Discuss the main points of the selected poems and/or *Green Eggs and Ham*.

159

Themes From Selected Poems

When discussing the selected poems, ask students what themes are common to these reading selections.

How will you identify these as possible answers? Here are four answers to elicit.

- Children often don't like to eat vegetables or green things.
- Children often don't like to try new foods.
- Sometimes it's hard to try unfamiliar foods or foods that look different.
- Try it, you might like it.

Green Eggs and Ham

When discussing *Green Eggs and Ham*, ask students to respond to some of the following questions:

- Why did Dr. Seuss choose the color green for the new food the main character is asked to try?
- Does the green food symbolize vegetables?
- Which is more difficult: trying foods that look different from those we usually eat or trying foods that look similar to those we usually eat?
- Who does Sam represent?
- Have you ever had a similar experience when someone tried to get you to taste a new food?

3. Then, ask students to point out the sensory imagery used in the poem(s).

4. Point out the lesson goals:

- Discuss the importance of eating fruits and vegetables.
- Try a new fruit or vegetable.
- Write a poem that describes the appearance, smell, feel, and taste of the fruit or vegetable they tried.

5. (5 minutes) Ask students the following:

- Why is it important to eat fruits and vegetables? (See the Teacher Resources.)
- How many fruits and vegetables do you eat on a typical day?
- How many fruits and vegetables should you eat daily? (See the Teacher Resources.)

6. (5 minutes) Discuss the correct answers to the questions. To get students thinking about the kinds of vegetables and fruits they eat, have students complete part I of activity 1.

7. For homework, ask students to try one fruit or vegetable that they have never tasted before. (If you are worried students might not be able to buy one of these foods, you can bring in several unusual fruits or vegetables to class. Before sharing what you bring in, wash foods and ask if anyone has relevant food allergies.) Ask students to list at least three to five adjectives that describe the appearance, taste, feel or texture, and smell of their food choice, and bring this list to class.

Day 2

8. (Time will vary: at least 20 minutes) Ask students to write a poem that describes the fruit or vegetable they tried and their feelings associated with the experience. Did they like the food? Were they surprised by its taste? You may wish to make certain

style or length requirements that fit your students' skills or previous experiences with poetry writing. (Possible poetic forms: free verse, rhymes, shape poems; possible literary elements to include: alliteration, onomatopoeia, or metaphors.) *Optional:* To give students more time to work on their poems or reduce class time spent on this activity, you may wish to have students complete their poem for homework.

9. (5 minutes) To give students an example of what you're asking them to do, read one or two of the poems included in the lesson.

10. (Time will vary: at least 5 minutes) Have some of the students share their poems with the class.

11. (5 minutes) To help students realize that their food preferences will change as they get older, ask students some of these questions:

- If you didn't like the fruit or vegetable you tried, does that mean you will never like it?
- Are there any foods or drinks that you like now that you used to dislike?
- Can you think of any foods or drinks that adults like that you might like when you get older?

Suggest that they continue to try new foods and foods that they haven't liked in the past. They may change their opinions. Who knows, maybe someday they'll even like spinach!

▶▶ Extension Activities

Ask students to do one of the following:

1. Use a scoring rubric to evaluate their own and others' poems.
2. Make an illustration that complements the poems they wrote.
3. List 10 fruits and vegetables and write down three adjectives for each.
4. Make a poster telling people about the benefits of eating fruits and vegetables. (See Teacher Resources.) Use persuasive writing and appealing graphics.

▶▶ Teacher Resources

General Background Material

In preparing for this lesson, you may want to refer to *Time to Take Five*. See appendix A.

Specific Background Material

What are the main benefits of fruits and vegetables?

- Many are good sources of vitamin C: oranges, lemons, grapefruits, cantaloupe, raspberries, strawberries, tomatoes, cabbage, potatoes, spinach, cauliflower, peppers, radishes, and green leafy vegetables such as spinach and kale.
- Many are good sources of vitamin A: bright orange vegetables like carrots, sweet potatoes, and pumpkin; dark green leafy vegetables such as spinach, collards, and turnip greens; and bright orange fruits like mango, cantaloupe, and apricots.

- Many fruits and vegetables are important sources of the B vitamins: leafy vegetables, cooked dried beans and peas, and oranges.
- They are an important source of potassium and fiber.
- They are low in fat.
- They reduce the risk of certain forms of cancer.
- They provide nutrients important for immunity, healing, and healthy skin and eyes, among other functions.

How many fruits and vegetables should we eat daily?

The 5-A-Day campaign promotes consumption of five fruits and vegetables every day. The Food Guide Pyramid recommends consuming 2-4 servings of fruits and 3-5 servings of vegetables every day.

How should we select fruits and vegetables?

- The U.S. Dietary Guidelines advise that in many cases "the brighter the color, the higher the content of vitamins and minerals." However, no one food supplies all the necessary nutrients, so try many colors and kinds.
- Choose fresh, frozen, or canned fruits and vegetables, fruit and vegetable juices, or dried fruits. All provide vitamins and minerals.
- Canned fruits in fruit juice or light syrups are more nutritious than canned fruits in heavy syrups.
- Choose whole or cut up fruits and vegetables most often since they are higher in fiber than juices.
- Fruit punch and fruit sodas contain little fruit juice and plenty of added sugars. They don't count as a serving of fruit juice.

How can we include plenty of different fruits and vegetables in our meals and snacks?

The U.S Dietary Guidelines provide this advice:

- Keep ready-to-eat raw vegetables handy in clear containers in the front of your refrigerator for snacks or meals on the go.
- Keep a day's supply of fresh or dried fruit handy on the table or counter.
- Enjoy fruits as a naturally sweet end to a meal.
- When eating out, choose a variety of vegetables at a salad bar.
- Serve raw vegetables with dip.
- Mix fruits or vegetables with other foods in salads, casseroles, soups, and sauces (for example, add shredded vegetables to pasta sauces).

References

U.S. Department of Agriculture and U.S. Department of Health and Human Services. 2000. *Nutrition and your health: Dietary guidelines for Americans* 2000, 5th edition. **www.usda.gov/cnpp**

Sample Poems

The Sad Tale of Jonathan Who Wouldn't Eat His Vegetables

Jonathan hated vegetables,
I mean he HATED vegetables!
"I'll NEVER eat a vegetable,"
He said, "of any kind!"
"You won't grow up," our mother sighed.
She served them boiled and stewed and fried,
But Jonathan said, "I won't! I won't!
And you can't make me mind!"
Every day our sister, Sue,
Said, "Vegetables are good for you!
You won't grow up without them."
But he said, "I'd rather die!"
"Try some, Jonathan," begged our dad,
"These vegetables are not so bad."
But Jonathan cried, "I hate them!
You'll never make me try!"
"You won't grow up," our brother said,
But nothing got through Jonathan's head.
He kicked and screamed and pitched a fit
And drove the family wild.
And so it grieves me to report
That Jonathan met the saddest sort
Of fate because he wouldn't eat
His veggies as a child.
Our friends all gobbled vegetables,
They slurped and swallowed vegetables,
And that's the reason, I suppose,
They grew up one and all.
While Jonathan, as I'm sure you know,
Never did begin to grow,
And now he's ninety-seven,
But he's only two feet tall.

David L. Harrison

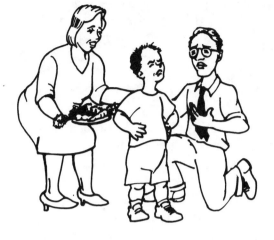

Something Green for Dinner

They served something green for dinner
And we wondered what it was.
Kenny whispered that it looked like
Someone's old lawn-mower fuzz.
Dad said, "Try a bite, you'll like it!"
We said, "Tell us, please, what is it?"
Dad said, "Ground up alien fern-tips
From the Martian spaceship's visit."
(They tasted great with the burgers.)

Jeff Moss

Celery

Celery, raw,
Develops the jaw,
But celery, stewed,
Is more quietly chewed.

Ogden Nash

Stuart McGroo

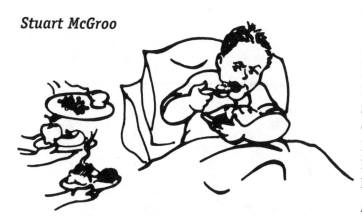

Let me tell you the story of Stuart McGroo,
A person who never tried anything new.
As a boy he ate nothing but gooseberry pie,
Not one bit of any new food would he try,
Not one pea or donut, not one brussels sprout,
And that's what young Stuart McGroo was about.
He would make no new friends so you couldn't invite
Stuart over to your house to stay for the night.
"I like my own bed!" cried young Stuart McGroo.
"I'm a person who never tries anything new!
I will stay safe at home! I will never go out!"
And that's what young Stuart McGroo was about.
Well, Stuart grew up but his heart did not throb
To raise a nice family or have a good job.
He just stayed in bed with his gooseberry pie
Saying, "Families and jobs are just new things to try
And I *never* try new things, there can be no doubt!"
And that is what Stuart McGroo was about.
The years hurried by, Stuart grew old alone
But he wondered about things that he'd never known.
And one day an old man with beard and a cane
Was seen strolling slowly down Tea Garden Lane.
He smiled at the people, they smiled at him, too,
And he made some new friends, did old Stuart McGroo.
Then a family he met asked him home for a meal.
For the first time he tasted spaghetti and veal
And pudding and milk and he loved every bite.
And Stuart dreamed happy dreams all through the night
Till he woke with a start and let out a shout,
"Now I finally see what the world's all about!"

Jeff Moss

Taste of Purple

Grapes hang purple
In their bunches,
Ready for
September lunches.
Gather them, no
Minutes wasting.
Purple is
Delicious tasting.

Leland B. Jacobs

I'd Never Eat a Beet

I'd never eat a beet, because
I could not stand the taste,
I'd rather nibble drinking straws,
or fountain pens, or paste,
I'd eat a window curtain
and perhaps a roller skate,
but a beet, you may be certain
would be wasted on my plate.
I would sooner chew on candles
or the laces from my shoes,
or a dozen suitcase handles
were I ever forced to choose,
I would eat a Ping-Pong paddle,
I would eat a Ping-Pong ball,
I might even eat a saddle,
but a beet? No! Not at all.
I would swallow talcum powder
and my little rubber duck,
I'd have doorknobs in my chowder,
I would eat a hockey puck,
I would eat my model rocket
and the socks right off my feet,
I would even eat my pocket,
but I'd never eat a beet!

Jack Prelutsky

Name _____

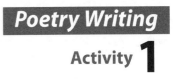

Part I

1. Put a check next to the fruits and vegetables listed below that you have tried.
2. Circle the ones that you like.

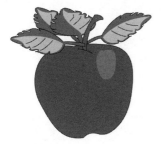

- ☐ apple
- ☐ apricot
- ☐ artichoke
- ☐ asparagus
- ☐ avocado
- ☐ bamboo shoots
- ☐ banana
- ☐ beets
- ☐ black-eyed peas
- ☐ blueberry
- ☐ broccoli
- ☐ brussels sprouts
- ☐ cabbage
- ☐ carrots
- ☐ cassava
- ☐ cauliflower
- ☐ celery
- ☐ cherries
- ☐ chiles

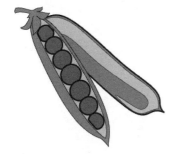

- ☐ collard greens
- ☐ corn
- ☐ cucumber
- ☐ currant
- ☐ date
- ☐ eggplant
- ☐ endive
- ☐ fig
- ☐ garbanzo beans
- ☐ gooseberry
- ☐ goya beans

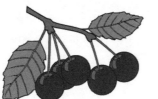

- ☐ grapefruit
- ☐ grapes
- ☐ green beans
- ☐ huckleberry
- ☐ jalapeno
- ☐ jicama
- ☐ kidney beans
- ☐ kiwifruit
- ☐ kohlrabi
- ☐ kumquat
- ☐ leek
- ☐ lemon
- ☐ lettuce
- ☐ lima beans
- ☐ lime

- ☐ mango
- ☐ melon
- ☐ mushrooms
- ☐ nectarine
- ☐ okra
- ☐ onion
- ☐ orange
- ☐ papaya
- ☐ parsnip
- ☐ patchoi
- ☐ pea
- ☐ peach
- ☐ pear
- ☐ pepper
- ☐ persimmon
- ☐ pineapple
- ☐ plantain
- ☐ plum
- ☐ pomegranate
- ☐ potato
- ☐ pumpkin
- ☐ radicchio
- ☐ radish
- ☐ raspberry
- ☐ red chili
- ☐ rhubarb
- ☐ rutabaga
- ☐ scallions
- ☐ snow peas
- ☐ spinach
- ☐ squash
- ☐ star fruit

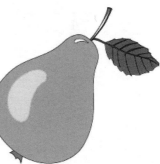

- ☐ strawberry
- ☐ sweet potatoes
- ☐ Swiss chard
- ☐ tangerine
- ☐ tomato
- ☐ turnip
- ☐ ugli fruit
- ☐ water chestnuts
- ☐ watercress
- ☐ watermelon
- ☐ wax beans
- ☐ xigua
- ☐ yam
- ☐ yuca
- ☐ zucchini

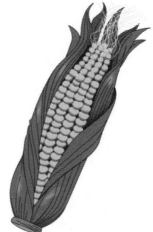

Part II

1. Choose one of the foods above that you HAVE NOT TASTED and try it. If you have tried them all or if you can't find one that you haven't tried in your local store, pick one that you don't like and try it again!

2. List as many adjectives as you can think of to describe the food's taste, smell, appearance, and texture.

	Adjectives that describe _____
Taste	
Smell	
Appearance	
Texture	

Part III

Write a poem that describes the food you tried. Include your feelings about the experience. Did you like it?

Part IV Extension Activity

Draw a picture that illustrates your poem.

Keep It Local

Students will write public service announcements to promote the 5-A-Day theme of eating five fruits and vegetables every day, with a focus on produce grown in Massachusetts (or your home state). This lesson is designed to infuse information about choosing healthy foods into a classroom unit on writing promotional messages.

▶▶ Behavioral Objective

For students to eat five or more fruits and vegetables per day.

▶▶ Learning Objectives

Students will be able to

1. list some locally grown fruits and vegetables,
2. organize their ideas and write them clearly and persuasively,
3. as a group, write a public service announcement, and
4. explain the 5-A-Day fruit and vegetable recommendation.

▶▶ Materials

- Student resource 1 *Massachusetts Grown . . . and Fresher!*
- Student resource 2 *What's a PSA?*
- Activity 1 *Writing a PSA*
- *Optional:* Overhead transparency of Teacher Resources

▶▶ Procedure

To make this more relevant to your students, contact your state department of agriculture to obtain information about foods grown in your state. You can modify the procedure to substitute information on your state for the Massachusetts resources we provide.

1. (8 minutes) Review the 5-A-Day recommendation with students, making sure they understand that "five a day" refers to eating fruits and vegetables combined, not to eating five a day each of fruits and vegetables. Discuss the Massachusetts Agriculture Facts and the Fruit and Vegetable Facts (see Teacher Resources) and relate them to the 5-A-Day theme. If possible, provide students with copies of the Teacher Resources or display them on an overhead.

2. (5 minutes) Pass out student resource 1 *Massachusetts Grown . . . and Fresher!*, which details the months when you can buy fresh Massachusetts-grown produce. Highlight the variety and diversity of fruits and vegetables grown in Massachusetts using discussion questions A through E below (some of these questions could be used for homework):

A. What produce is available locally in each of the seasons? Why are fruits and vegetables available locally at certain times and seasons? (Make sure students know that nutritious produce is available year-round via imports from other sources.)

B. What are your favorite fruits and vegetables that are grown in Massachusetts?

C. What fruits and vegetables do you consume that aren't from Massachusetts?

D. If you are not originally from the United States, what other fruits and vegetables did you grow up eating that you can't buy here?

E. Which locally grown fruits and vegetables have you tried for the first time in the past two years?

3. (15-20 minutes) Distribute student resource 2 *What's a PSA?* and discuss the sample PSA. Have students analyze the sample PSA and how it incorporates the Tips for Developing PSAs (in *What's a PSA?*). (See the Teacher Resources for additional examples of PSAs.)

4. Hand out activity 1 *Writing a PSA*.

- Have students form groups of four to five and as a group write a PSA for the radio promoting eating five a day with Massachusetts-grown fruits and vegetables.

- Allow 15 minutes for students to brainstorm and write their PSAs. Each group then will present their PSA to the class.

- Students can record messages on audiotapes and replay them.

▶▶ Extension Activities

Videotape or audiotape student presentations. You might involve the art and/or music teachers in a project where students would produce a visual representation or select or create music to go along with their PSAs.

▶▶ Teacher Resources

General Background Material

In preparing for this lesson, you may want to refer to *Time to Take Five*. See appendix A.

Specific Background Material

Massachusetts Agriculture Facts

Massachusetts ranks

- #1 in the United States for production of cranberries,
- #9 for production of sweet corn,
- #15 for production of apples, and
- #17 for production of tomatoes.

Massachusetts farms average 100 acres in size (1 acre is about the size of a football field). There are about 6,000 farms and 600,000 acres of farmland in the state of Massachusetts. There are more than 400 roadside farm stands in Massachusetts as well as 95 farmers' markets.

The 5 A Day Recommendation

The 5 A Day campaign promotes eating five servings of fruits and vegetables every day.

Fruit and Vegetable Facts

- Massachusetts-grown fruits and vegetables that are good sources of vitamin C include cantaloupe, raspberries, strawberries, tomatoes, cabbage, potatoes, cauliflower, peppers, radishes, and green leafy vegetables such as spinach and mustard greens.
- Some Massachusetts-grown fruits and vegetables that are good sources of vitamin A include cantaloupe, carrots, asparagus, red pepper, tomato, and green leafy vegetables such as spinach and kale.
- Most fruits and vegetables contain large amounts of fiber and are low in fat.
- Eating at least five fruits and vegetables a day may reduce the risk of certain forms of cancer.
- Fruits and vegetables provide nutrients important for immunity, healing, healthy skin and eyes, and other functions.

Selecting Fruits and Vegetables

- According to the U.S. Dietary Guidelines, in many cases "the brighter the color, the higher the content of vitamins and minerals." However, no one food supplies all the necessary nutrients, so try many colors and kinds.
- Choose fresh, frozen, or canned fruits and vegetables, fruit and vegetable juices, or dried fruits. All provide vitamins and minerals.
- Canned fruits in fruit juice or light syrups are more nutritious than canned fruits in heavy syrups.
- Choose whole or chunked fruits and vegetables most often, since they are higher in fiber than juices.
- Fruit punch and fruit sodas contain little fruit juice and plenty of added sugars. They don't count as a serving of fruit juice.

Including Different Fruits and Vegetables in Meals and Snacks

Here are some tips from the U.S. Dietary Guidelines:

- Keep ready-to-eat raw vegetables handy in a clear container in the front of your refrigerator for snacks or meals on the go.
- Keep a day's supply of fresh or dried fruit handy on the table or counter.
- Enjoy fruits as a naturally sweet end to a meal.
- When eating out, choose a variety of vegetables at a salad bar.
- Serve raw vegetables with dip.
- Mix fruits or vegetables with other foods in salads, casseroles, soups, and sauces. (For example, add shredded vegetables to pasta sauces.)

Sample Public Service Announcements

- CBS TV 7-9 P.M.: *And now some helpful hints on recycling from Danny DeVito and Rhea Pearlman . . . DO IT!*
- NBC TV 8-10 P.M.: "The More You Know," Courtney Cox says: *"What if I told you that you could save a friend's life with these?" (car keys). "Be a designated driver."*

References

Massachusetts Department of Food and Agriculture and Massachusetts Office of Business Development. 1994. *New England agricultural statistics.* Concord, NH: New England Agricultural Statistics Services.

U.S. Department of Agriculture and U.S. Department of Health and Human Services. 2000. *Nutrition and your health: Dietary guidelines for Americans 2000,* 5th edition. **www.usda.gov/cnpp**

U.S. Department of Agriculture and National Agricultural Statistics Service. 1992. *U.S. census of agriculture.* Washington, D.C.

U.S. Department of Health and Human Services. 1989. *Making health communication programs work.* Baltimore, MD: National Cancer Institute.

Massachusetts grown...and fresher!

Buying Guide

	May	June	July	August	September	October
Fruits						
Apples			■	■	■	■
Blueberries			■	■		
Cantaloupes				■	■	
Cranberries					■	■
Grapes				■	■	
Peaches			■	■	■	
Raspberries			■	■	■	
Strawberries		■	■			
Vegetables						
Asparagus	■	■				
Beans			■	■	■	
Beets		■	■	■	■	■
Cabbage		■	■	■	■	■
Carrots			■	■	■	■
Cauliflower		■	■	■	■	■
Celery				■	■	■
Chinese cabbage		■	■	■	■	■
Corn			■	■	■	■
Cucumbers		■	■	■	■	
Eggplant			■	■	■	■
Escarole - endive			■	■	■	■
Lettuce, greens	■	■	■	■	■	■
Onion			■	■	■	■
Parsnips					■	■
Peas (green and snap)		■	■	■	■	■
Peppers			■	■	■	■
Potatoes			■	■	■	■
Pumpkins					■	■
Radishes		■	■	■	■	■
Scallions	■	■	■	■	■	■
Spinach	■	■	■	■	■	■
Summer squash		■	■	■	■	
Winter squash					■	■
Tomatoes			■	■	■	■
Turnips				■	■	■

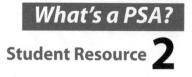

Public Service Announcements (PSAs) are usually 30- or 60-second radio or TV advertisements that create awareness around a health problem or issue. Nonprofit and government agencies often sponsor PSAs to provide new information, to reinforce prevailing knowledge or attitudes, or to promote programs, services, activities, or issues of community interest. Commercial advertisements, on the other hand, try to sell an actual product. Radio and TV stations and networks donate the broadcast air time for PSAs. In recent years, public service campaigns have been used frequently by health promotion and disease prevention programs. Some campaigns you might be familiar with promote NOT smoking and drinking more milk. For example, the message "milk, it does a body good" is probably familiar to you. What other PSAs do you recall?

Tips for developing PSAs

1. Keep messages short and simple—just one or two key points.
2. Identify the main issue (health problem) in the first 10 seconds in an attention-getting way and summarize or repeat the main point or message at the close.
3. Use a memorable slogan, theme, music, or sound effects to aid recall.
4. Present the solution as well as the problem.

Sample Public Service Announcement

From the New England Dairy and Food Council

Is a Vegetarian Diet a Healthy Way to Eat? (60-Second PSA)

Is a vegetarian diet a healthy way to eat? This is Sue Barton of the New England Dairy and Food Council with the September Nutrition Report.

According to the new U.S. Dietary Guidelines released in January 1995, vegetarian diets can be a healthy way to eat. However, the guidelines said people who eat only vegetarian foods need to make sure that they are consuming enough calcium, protein, and B vitamins. This can easily be done by choosing foods from the Food Guide Pyramid. Beans and eggs help to provide protein. At least two daily servings of milk, yogurt, or cheese (four servings for teenagers) supplies the recommended amount of calcium. Fortified breads and cereals can help meet B vitamin requirements. If you decide to go vegetarian, keep nutrition in mind and the Food Guide Pyramid by your side.

Directions

1. Break into groups of about four to five students.

2. Your assignment for the next 10 minutes is to address the need for middle school children to eat more fruits and vegetables by writing a 60-second Public Service Announcement (PSA) for a local radio station. Your PSA should target middle school students and promote eating five a day with MA grown fruits and vegetables. (One group of local middle school students reported eating 3.3 servings instead of 5 servings of fruits and vegetables a day.)

3. Create a humorous advertisement if you like. Each group will present their final PSA draft to the class. Everyone must have a part in the presentation.

4. Choose a local radio station where you will broadcast this PSA. _____
   Why did you choose this station?

5. Create a 30–40 second ad (five to seven short sentences) that will promote the 5-A-Day theme and write below. Include information highlighted under "Fruit and Vegetable Facts" as well as any other helpful information that you would like to add.

Write a Fable: Important Messages About Activity

In this lesson, students will learn about what it means to be "physically fit" and why an active lifestyle is important. They will read a short essay about the topic and use their knowledge to write three important lessons or "morals" about physical fitness. Finally, they will write a fable that illustrates one important lesson. An alternative activity is included for teachers who just want to work on reading comprehension.

▶▶ Behavioral Objective

For students to be more active.

▶▶ Learning Objectives

Students will be able to

1. comprehend and identify basic facts and ideas introduced in a nonfiction essay (activities 1 and 2),

2. write a fable that illustrates the importance of physical fitness and an active lifestyle (activity 3),

3. critique and edit one another's work (activity 4),

4. revise their writing to improve organization, diction, sentence structure, mechanics, and spelling,

5. list the four components of physical fitness, and

6. suggest ways to improve their own physical fitness.

▶▶ Materials

- Activity 1 *Reading Comprehension*
- Activity 2 *Reading Review* or activity 3 *Writing a Fable*
- *Optional:* Activity 4 *Guidelines for Critiquing Fables*

▶▶ Procedure

Overview: Modify this to fit your time constraints and students' skill levels. If you are short on time, you may wish to do only activity 1 and activity 2.

Activity 1

Activity 2 OR 3
(choose 1)

Activity 4 (optional)

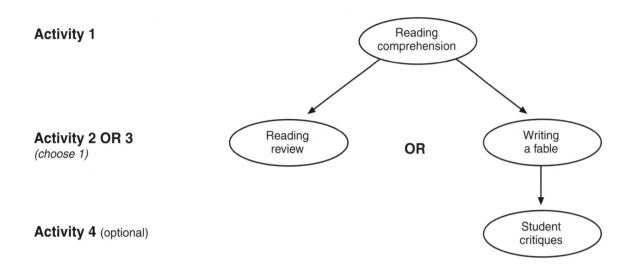

1. Decide which activities best fit your curriculum and students' abilities.

2. Point out the goals of the activity:

   • Discuss the importance of physical fitness and an active lifestyle.

   • Comprehend and identify basic facts and ideas introduced in a nonfiction essay (activities 1 and 2).

   • Write a fable that illustrates the importance of physical fitness and an active lifestyle (activity 3).

Activity 1 Reading Comprehension

1. (10–15 minutes) Hand out activity 1 *Reading Comprehension*. Have students read this silently and underline statements they think convey an important message. (*Optional:* You could assign this for homework to be done the night before you planned on doing this lesson.)

Activity 2 Reading Review

2. (10–15 minutes) Hand out activity 2 *Reading Review*. Have students work in pairs or groups to complete these questions.

3. Discuss answers to the questions. See Teacher Resources for answers.

Activity 3 Writing a Fable

4. (5–10 minutes) This lesson is designed to be incorporated into a unit on fables. However, if your students are not familiar with fables, read a short fable aloud (for example, *The Tortoise and the Hare,* an Aesop fable). Discuss this literary style. Remind students that fables are fictitious, short stories designed to teach an important lesson or "moral" and impart some wisdom. The moral of the story is usually clearly stated at the end of the story. Frequently, the characters in these stories are animals that speak and act like humans.

5. (10 minutes) Hand out activity 3 *Writing a Fable*. Have students work in pairs to develop three important lessons, or "morals to the story," based on the statements they underlined in activity 1.

6. (10-15 minutes) Have each student choose one of the three morals to write a fable about. Partners should work together to brainstorm plots and characters they might use in writing their individual fables. Each student should write an outline of their story.

7. Ask students to write a first draft of their fable for homework. (*Optional:* You may choose to give students an opportunity to do the writing in class.)

Activity 4 Guidelines for Critiquing Fables

If you want to shorten this lesson, you could choose to have students hand in their drafts to you and skip the peer review activity.

8. (15 minutes) Hand out activity 4 *Guidelines for Critiquing Fables.* Have students exchange fables with their partners and make comments and suggestions for revision based on the specified criteria.

9. Have students revise their stories during class or for homework.

10. *Optional:* Ask a few students to read their stories to the class.

▶▶ Extension Activities

1. Have students write their fables in a storybook format with illustrations.

2. Choose one of the fables to have students act out in class.

3. Take a field trip to a local elementary school or preschool. Have students read their fables to the younger children.

4. Ask students to write a reflective essay about the amount of physical activity they participate in regularly. What types of physical activities do they do? How can they increase the amount of physical activity in their lives? Have them make a plan for the next five days.

▶▶ Teacher Resources

General Background Material

In preparing for this lesson, you may want to refer to the following resources:

- *Centers for Disease Control and Prevention Fact Sheets on Physical Activity*
- *Television Viewing as a Cause of Increasing Obesity Among Children in the United States, 1986-1990*
- *Healthy People 2010*

See appendix B for information on how to obtain these resources.

Specific Background Material

What is physical fitness? Why is it important?

See activity 1 *Reading Comprehension.*

How much activity is needed to obtain health-related benefits?

Moderate amounts of activity are recommended for people of all ages. However, physical activity need not be strenuous to be beneficial. Just a small increase in physical activity can generate genuine health benefits, such as reduction of body weight and the risk of heart attack, hypertension, and death. Thirty minutes or more of moderately intense activity, such as walking, is beneficial for your health when performed regularly. Some kind of regular vigorous activity, however, is the best way to improve cardiovascular fitness.

How much activity is needed for fitness?

See activity 1 *Reading Comprehension*.

What are some examples of things you can do to increase your activity and decrease your inactivity?

Take the stairs; don't park next to the building; walk or ride your bike to school if there is a safe route; walk around the mall or the neighborhood with friends; watch only your favorite TV shows; remove or unplug the TV in your bedroom; play catch with a sibling, a friend, or parent.

What are the benefits of a more active lifestyle?

See activity 1 *Reading Comprehension*.

What changes in society have brought about a decrease in daily physical activity?

In the latter part of the 20th century, there was a dramatic reduction in the amount of physical activity performed in daily life. An increase in the number of sedentary white-collar jobs and a decrease in blue-collar and farming jobs that required physical work has occurred. Modern appliances, machinery, and motorized transportation have decreased the amount of activity required to complete household chores and work-related tasks. The growth of technology and inactive leisure activities has also been enormous, with computers, video, and TV being the major factors. The Internet, CD-ROM, and continued expansion of the TV channel market will help these trends continue.

How much time do adolescents spend watching TV?

According to Dietz (1991), American children spend more time watching TV than they do engaging in any other activity except sleeping. In 1988, the average adolescent viewed approximately 22 hours per week. The percentage of youth watching TV and playing computer or video games for 5 or more hours per day has increased greatly, from 13% in the late 1960s to 43% in 1990. Essentially, TV watching for many children has become a full-time job! On average, adolescents spend more time watching television than they spend in school. The American Academy of Pediatrics recommends limiting TV viewing to 2 hours or less per day.

What are the risks of a sedentary lifestyle?

Activity is required for health. Studies suggest that physically active individuals enjoy lower risks of developing cardiovascular disease, diabetes, colon cancer, osteoporosis, anxiety, and depression relative to sedentary individuals. Sedentary habits increase the risk of death from these diseases. Television viewing is one of the major causes of overweight (obese) youth. TV watching has also been associated with elevated cholesterol levels and poor cardiovascular fitness.

What are the alternatives to TV viewing?

Anything that involves movement! Limiting TV time can ensure children do other activities that involve more physical activity. Also, you don't have to sit still while you watch TV—you can be dancing, cleaning, cooking, and so on. One easy way to cut down on TV time is to take the TV out of the room where you sleep. If you don't want to physically remove it, just unplug it. Watch TV only if your favorite show is on.

References

Blair, S. 1993. C.H. McCloy research lecture: Physical activity, physical fitness, and health. *Research Quarterly for Exercise and Sport* 64(4): 365-376.

Dietz, W.H., and Strasburger, V. 1991. Children, adolescents, and television. *Current Problems in Pediatrics,* January, pp. 8-30.

Gortmaker, S.L. 1990. National health examination survey, 1967-70. Unpublished data.

Gortmaker, S.L. 1990. National longitudinal survey of youth. Unpublished data.

Park, R. 1992. Human energy expenditure from *Australopithecus afarensis* to 4-minute mile: Exemplars and case studies. *Exercise and Sport Sciences Reviews* 20: 185-220.

Sallis, J.F., and Patrick, K. 1994. Physical activity guidelines for adolescents: Consensus statement. *Pediatric Exercise Science* 6:302-314.

U.S. Department of Health and Human Services. 2000. Healthy People 2010, conference edition, vols. I and II.. **www.health.gov/healthypeople**

▶▶ Answer Key

Activity 2 Reading Review

1. _F_ To improve your physical fitness, you must exercise every day for 60 minutes. *Experts recommend that people of all ages be moderately active for 30 minutes or more every day or nearly every day. How long, how hard, and how often you are active will determine how fit you are! You can improve fitness by increasing the frequency (if you are not exercising regularly), increasing the intensity (doing something faster, doing more repetitions), or increasing the time you spend on each exercise.*

2. _T_ To be physically fit, you must work on aerobic fitness, muscle strength and endurance, and flexibility.

3. _T_ Walking to school, climbing stairs, chasing after younger brothers and sisters, and walking the dog are all physical activities that provide the health benefits of exercise.

5. _F_ To strengthen your heart, lungs, and circulatory system, you need to do at least *five* sessions per week of vigorous physical activity lasting for 20 minutes or more. *Three sessions of vigorous activity are recommended to improve cardiovascular fitness. However, moderately intense activity can also improve cardiovascular fitness. It should be done nearly every day and for a longer duration (30 minutes or more).*

6. _T_ Physical activity helps relieve stress.

7. _T_ Regular physical activity NOW will help you develop an active lifestyle, something that will help prevent heart disease later in life.

8. _F_ Flexibility is the ability of the heart, lungs, and circulatory system to deliver oxygen and nutrients to all areas of your body. *Aerobic fitness is the ability of the heart, lungs, and circulatory system to deliver oxygen and nutrients to all areas of your body.*

What exactly is physical fitness? Being fit means you have more energy to do daily tasks, can be more active, and do not tire as easily during the day. Being fit also helps you build a positive self-image and feel better about yourself.

You can gain the health benefits of physical activity without spending hours in a gym. Every time you throw a softball, swim a lap, or climb up a flight of stairs, you improve your health and fitness level. How long, how hard, and how often you are active will determine how fit you are!

Benefits of Physical Activity

Physical activity has many proven benefits. Physical activity can help

- prevent high blood pressure;
- strengthen your bones;
- ward off heart disease, some cancers, and diabetes;
- relieve stress;
- make you feel and look better;
- keep you active as an adult; and
- maintain or achieve an appropriate weight for your height and body build.

Regular physical activity can help you be more self-confident, organize your time better, learn new skills, and meet people with similar interests. It also helps reduce stress. Learning to cope with stress is an important part of healthy living. Family problems, conflicts with friends, and school pressures can cause stress. Major changes in your life, such as moving to a new home or school, are also sources of stress. Exercise helps you relax by causing physical changes inside your body that help it react to and handle stress.

Overeating, not exercising enough, or both, often lead to more body fat. Being overweight increases your risk of diabetes, high blood pressure, and heart attack. Physical activity can help you maintain or achieve an appropriate weight for your height and body type.

Physical activity also helps ward off heart disease, the leading cause of death in the United States. You might say, "I don't need to worry about having a heart attack. That only happens to people when they get old." But research has shown that risk factors for developing heart disease as an adult start during childhood. A lack of physical activity is one of the major risk factors influencing heart disease. So being active now will help you develop an active lifestyle that you can maintain throughout your life, something that will help prevent heart disease later.

Physical Fitness is a Balance of Many Areas

To be physically fit, you must work on all aspects of fitness, including the following:

- **Aerobic fitness**: This is the ability of the heart, lungs, and circulatory system to deliver oxygen and nutrients to all areas of your body. When you are active, you breathe harder and your heart beats faster so that your body is able to get the oxygen it needs. If you are not fit, your heart and lungs have to work extra hard during physical activity.

• **Muscle strength and endurance:** This is the amount of work and the amount of time that your muscles are able to do a certain activity before they get tired, such as lifting heavy objects or in-line skating.

• **Flexibility:** Flexibility is the ability of joints and muscles to move and stretch through a full range of motion. For example, people who are very flexible can bend over and touch the floor easily. A person with poor flexibility is more likely to get hurt during physical activity.

What Can I Do to Become More Fit?

First, you have to make the commitment to become **more** physically active. Try to do some physical activity every day, whether it is through physical education classes in school or an activity on your own. Choose an activity you like. You are more apt to stay in the habit of doing it if it's one you enjoy. Anything that involves movement qualifies as physical activity. You do not have to be on a sports team, have expensive athletic clothes or shoes, or be good at sports to become more fit. Any type of regular, physical activity is good for your body. Household chores, such as mowing the lawn, vacuuming, or scrubbing, involve exercise and may have fitness benefits, depending on how vigorously you do the chores. The most important thing is that you keep moving. Walking is better than riding in a car, and using the stairs is better than taking the elevator. Making small changes like these in your everyday life can make you more fit.

It may help to plan a physical activity with a friend. Many people find that it is more fun to exercise with someone else.

You should incorporate moderate and vigorous aerobic exercise into your regular activity plans. Aerobic activity is continuous. It makes you sweat, causes you to breathe harder, and increases your heart rate. Examples of aerobic activities are brisk walking, basketball, bicycling, swimming, in-line or ice skating, jogging, dancing, and taking an aerobics class. Baseball and football do not involve as much continuous exercise because you are not active the whole time.

To make more time for physical activity, limit the amount of time you watch TV or play computer or video games.

How Often Should I Exercise?

Make physical activity a part of your lifestyle. Your goal should be to do some type of moderately intense activity for at least 30 minutes every day or nearly every day and aim for at least three sessions per week of vigorous physical activity lasting 20 minutes or more. If you are not exercising now, increase your level of activity gradually.

Include stretching exercises in your daily routine. Stretching before you exercise warms up your muscles, helps protect against injury, and makes your muscles and joints more flexible. It is also important to stretch out after you exercise to cool down your muscles.

Muscular strength increases when you do all types of regular physical activity. However, you may want to include strength training as part of your exercise regimen. Strength Training, also called "weight training" and "resistance training," is where you use free weights and/or weight machines to increase muscle strength and muscle endurance. You should always have a trained adult supervise you.

You can improve fitness by increasing the frequency (if you are not exercising regularly), increasing the intensity (doing something faster, doing more repetitions), or increasing the time you spend on each exercise. You might choose more types of exercise to do.

Physical activity is an important part of keeping your body healthy. It should be part of your daily lifestyle. Exercise for a better today and a healthier tomorrow.

Like all things, exercise can be overdone. You may be exercising too much if

- your weight falls below what is normal for your age, height, and build;
- exercise starts to interfere with your normal school and other activities; or,
- your muscles become so sore that you risk injuring yourself.

If you notice any of these signs, talk with your parents or pediatrician before health problems occur.

Adapted from the American Academy of Pediatrics' brochure *Better Health and Fitness Through Physical Activity* © 1996.

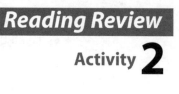

Fact or Fiction?

Read through each of the statements below. Put a "T" in front of the true statements. Put an "F" in front of the false statements and rewrite the statements so that they are correct.

1. ____ To improve your physical fitness, you must exercise every day for 60 minutes.

2. ____ To be physically fit, you must work on aerobic fitness, muscle strength and endurance, and flexibility.

3. ____ Walking to school, climbing stairs, chasing after younger brothers and sisters, and walking the dog are all physical activities that provide the health benefits of exercise.

4. ____ To strengthen your heart, lungs, and circulatory system, you need to do at least *five* sessions per week of vigorous physical activity lasting for 20 minutes or more.

5. ____ Physical activity helps relieve stress.

6. ____ Regular physical activity NOW will help you develop an active lifestyle, something that will help prevent heart disease later in life.

7. ____ Flexibility is the ability of the heart, lungs, and circulatory system to deliver oxygen and nutrients to all areas of your body.

Name _____

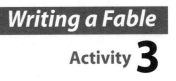
Fables are fictitious, short stories that teach an important lesson or "moral" and share some wisdom. The moral of the story is usually clearly stated at the end of the story. Frequently, the characters in these stories are animals that speak and act like humans. For example, in the fable _The Tortoise and the Hare_, an Aesop fable, the important lesson is, "Hard work and perseverance bring reward."

Step 1

1. Read activity 1 _Reading Comprehension_ and underline statements that you think convey important messages about physical fitness.
2. Work with a partner to write three important lessons about physical fitness.

Important Lessons

1.

2.

3.

Step 2

Choose one of the important lessons above. Brainstorm plots and characters you could use to tell a story that teaches this lesson. Each individual must write his or her own fable.

Step 3

Make an outline of the fable you plan to write.

Help your partner revise his or her fable. As you read the fable, keep the following guidelines in mind.

1. Read the fable at least twice.

2. Remember that when you critique someone else's work, it's a good idea to share your positive reactions first, and then discuss your constructive criticisms.

3. Write down what you like about the story below.

4. The first time you read the story think about what message the story is trying to get across. Does the story clearly portray the wisdom stated in the important lesson? Is the story easy to follow or does it need to be reorganized? Make your suggestions for improving the story.

5. The second time you read the story examine the details of how the story is told.

   • Make any suggestions for changes in vocabulary.

   • Are there any run-on or incomplete sentences?

   • Check for correct usage of punctuation (commas, apostrophes, periods, quotation marks).

   • Check for correct spelling.

Write your suggestions on the story itself, but be sensitive to the way you make your comments. Write legibly, and do not cross out words so that they are no longer readable. Choose words that are not hurtful.

Lesson 37

Go for the Goal

This lesson examines setting fitness goals using activities that complement the goal setting students may be doing in their PE classes. While this lesson may stand alone, consider checking with the PE teachers to verify that they are using Planet Health. You may be able to coordinate timing this lesson for maximum impact in language arts and PE. This lesson is designed to infuse information about increasing physical activity into a language arts class. Students will read several case studies and write physical activity goals aimed at increasing the activity of the individuals discussed in the case studies.

▶▶ Behavioral Objectives

For students to increase their physical activity by

- learning how to set realistic goals, and
- trading inactive time for time to participate in some physical activity.

▶▶ Learning Objectives

Students will be able to

1. read and comprehend case studies,
2. understand the concept of goal setting and its components, including planning, setting, and evaluating progress toward a goal, and
3. write clear and realistic physical activity goals.

▶▶ Materials

- Activity 1 *Making Time to Stay Fit*
- Activity 2 *Choosing a Lifestyle That Helps You Stay Fit* (case studies)
- Copy of the Goal-Setting section of FitCheck (see part II beginning on page 18 for more information about FitCheck)

▶▶ Procedure

Planning: Because this lesson asks students to set a goal over a 24-hour period, it is best not to teach it on a Friday.

1. (Up to 5 minutes) Write "goal" on the board and have students brainstorm what the word means to them. Write each response on the board.

2. (5 minutes) Give examples of a few simple goals, especially goals related to physical activity. Ask students to give examples of goals that they've set in the past

FitCheck # __

Planet Health

Name _____

Date _____

Grade _____

My FitScore was _____

I need to (circle one)	Score
keep it up!	5-7
be more active.	0-4

My Fit ★Score was _____

I need to (circle one)	Score
keep it up!	3 or more
add more vigorous activities.	0-2

My SitScore was _____

I need to (circle one)	Score
keep it up!	5-7
trade screen time for active time.	0-4

You could:
- trade some screen time for active time, like riding your bike instead of watching TV.
- do more of what you're already doing, like in-line skating for 30 minutes instead of 15.
- work harder at what you're already doing.
- add new activities. Check to see if you can walk to school instead of getting a ride.

Set a goal to improve your fitness

For example:
I will _____ *ride my bike instead of watching TV* _____
(for how long?) _____ *for 30 minutes* _____
(when?) _____ *after school on Tuesdays and Fridays* _____

I will _____
(for how long?)_____
(when?)_____

Date: [   ]

Reflect on your progress

Did you meet your goal?   O Yes   O No
Why/why not? Explain how you reached your goal, or why you did not reach your goal.

_____
_____
_____

and why they've been successful. What motivated them to achieve their goals in those cases? Ask students to also think of goals that have failed and why they've failed.

3. (5 minutes) Review the GoAL (*Go* for an *Activity* you *Like!*) and the concept of "trading time."

4. (7 minutes) Distribute activity 1 *Making Time to Stay Fit* and a copy of the Goal Setting section of the *Planet Health* FitCheck sheet. Have the class complete activity 1. Tell them to wait to fill in the FitCheck sheet.

5. (7–10 minutes) Have students fill in the section of the FitCheck sheet on page 186 titled *Set a goal to improve your fitness,* creating goals for themselves that they can complete by class the next day. Make sure students understand that their homework is to pursue their goals over the next 24 hours. These goals can be similar to the goals they set in PE class, but they need to be reached in a day. PE goals are for four to six weeks. Make sure students don't fill in the section titled *Reflect on your progress.* Collect the FitCheck sheets for class tomorrow.

6. (7–10 minutes) Distribute activity 2 *Choosing a Lifestyle That Helps You Stay Fit.* Have the class review each case study. Have students write solutions to the problems individually or, as a group, develop and discuss solutions for the problems presented.

7. (7 minutes) During the next class period, pass out the FitCheck sheets and have students fill in the section *Reflect on your progress.* Discuss the goals and evaluation with the class. Were the goals realistic, or would they like to change them?

▶▶ Extension Activities

Have students interview a member of their family to find out whether they have any goals for themselves (e.g., to be more physically active, to go to college, to get an "A" on the next math test, to get a promotion, to better their time in the 100-yard dash).

▶▶ Teacher Resources

General Background Material

In preparing for this lesson, you may want to refer to the following resources:

• *Planet Health FitCheck Sheets* (see section I, part II).
• *Healthy People 2010.*

See appendix B for information on obtaining the *Healthy People 2010.* You also may want to refer to lessons 4-7 in section I, part II.

Specific Background Material

Planet Health's Activity Message

Physical activity promotes health and well-being, and offers opportunities to socialize and have fun. Adolescents should be moderately active for at least 30 minutes every day or nearly every day as part of play, games, sports, chores, transportation, or planned exercise, AND they should participate in at least three sessions per week of vigorous physical activity lasting 20 minutes or more. Adolescents should aim for a total of 60 minutes or more of activity on five to seven days a week.

Goal Setting

- The *American Heritage Dictionary* defines a goal as "the purpose to which an endeavor is directed."
- A goal is something you are trying to achieve, and the strategy is the plan for how to get there. People set goals and carry out plans all the time. You can remind students that friends, parents, teachers, and other adults all set goals, too.
- Some examples of goals are getting to school on time or reaching the top of Mount Monadnock on a hike.
- It feels good to achieve a goal.
- Students may find it difficult to set realistic goals. Setting goals involves a process of refining and defining. A goal that initially seems realistic may later need adjustment. For example, you may think that you will be able to run a mile three times a week by the end of the month, and come to realize that you need more time in order to reach that goal. You might need to change your goal to half a mile three times a week.
- Difficult goals can be achieved with patience and diligence. Focusing on and achieving goals takes mental discipline.
- Students are also practicing goal setting in PE as part of *Planet Health*. This lesson helps reinforce the PE component.
- The most important part of a goal: *Go* for an *Activity* you *Like!* (GoAL).

Inactivity and Trading Time

- Strive to decrease inactivity. The percentage of youth watching TV and playing computer or video games for 5 or more hours per day has increased greatly, from 13% to 43% during the 1980s.
- Some amount of activity is required for health. Children need activity to develop and retain cardiovascular fitness, muscle strength, flexibility, and confidence in their physical ability.
- Physical activity builds fitness, is fun, and helps release energy! Just a small increase in physical activity can generate genuine health benefits.
- To prevent disease, it is important for students to create lifestyle patterns now that they will carry into adulthood.
- Encourage students to think about *trading* some time they currently spend on activities like TV, computer games, and video games for some moderately intense or vigorous activity. *This is one way to help set achievable fitness goals and to make space for fitness.* Physical activity is a cure for boredom.

References

The American heritage dictionary. 1985. 2d College Ed. Boston: Houghton Mifflin.

Dairy Council of California. 1998. Exercise your options: A food choice and activity program for middle school students. **www.dairycouncilofca.org**

Gortmaker, S.L. 1990. National health examination survey, 1967-70. Unpublished data.

Gortmaker, S.L. 1990. National longitudinal survey of youth. Unpublished data.

Sallis, J.F., and Patrick, K. 1994. Physical activity guidelines for adolescents: Consensus statement. *Pediatric Exercise Science* 6:302-314.

U.S. Department of Health and Human Services. 2000. Healthy People 2010, conference edition, vols. I and II. **www.health.gov/healthypeople**

Physical activity builds fitness! It's good for your health, and it's fun! To improve your physical fitness, you need to be more active. There are many ways to do this. You could:

- trade some screen time for active time, like riding your bike instead of watching TV;
- do more of what you're already doing, like in-line skating for 30 minutes instead of 15;
- work harder at what you're already doing; or
- add new activities, like walking to school instead of getting a ride.

A. Using the strategies above, come up with four ways you could be more active. Write them below. Remember to choose activities you like!

For example: My goal is to be more active.

I could   *ride my bike instead of watching TV*
(for how long?)   *for 30 minutes*
(when?)   *after school on Mondays, Wednesday, and Fridays*

My goal is to be more active. Here are some of my options:

1. I could _____
   (for how long? _____
   (when?)_____

2. I could _____
   (for how long? _____
   (when?)_____

3. I could _____
   (for how long? _____
   (when?)_____

4. I could _____
   (for how long? _____
   (when?)_____

B. Which of your options do you think you would actually do? Why?

Now that you know your options, write a physical activity goal for yourself.
C. *My goal is to be more active.*

I will _____
(for how long? _____
(when?)_____

Example of physical activities:

- Chores: shoveling snow, raking leaves, cleaning, vacuuming
- Conditioning: running, sit-ups, jumping rope, weightlifting
- Recreation: tag, skiing, sledding, skate boarding
- Sports: soccer, swimming, hockey, basketball
- Transportation: walking, biking, in-line skating, climbing stairs

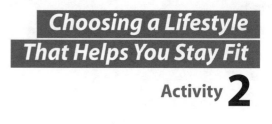

Case Studies

Case Study #1

Julie spends her weekends hanging out with her friends. Her favorite activities include going to movies, shopping at the mall, and watching her little brothers play baseball. When she is at home, she does not watch very much TV. She prefers to read mystery books instead. Julie often feels tired and does not have much energy.

List at least one activity goal for Julie.

Case Study #2

John is in the eighth grade. Every day at school he plays cards with his friends after lunch. After school he comes home and turns on the TV. His parents let him eat in front of the TV, and he has also convinced them that he can do a good job on his homework if he does it while watching TV. John's father has recently asked him to keep track of the number of hours he spends in front of the TV each day. On weekdays, John watches TV from 3:30 until 10:00 P.M., and on the weekends, when he is not playing computer games, John spends about six hours per day in front of the TV.

List at least one activity goal for John.

Case Study #3

David lives three blocks from school. His mother has offered to drive him to school, but David prefers to walk, even in the rain. David participates in after-school sports such as soccer and basketball every day except Friday. He relaxes each night by watching about 1-1/2 to 2 hours of TV. On the weekends, David plays in a basketball league. Do you have any suggestions for David regarding his level of physical activity?

List at least one activity goal for David.

Lifetime Physical Activities: Research One, Describe One, Try One!

Students will discuss the benefits of being physically active throughout life. They will research one type of "lifetime" physical activity and write an article describing the activity for a health fitness newsletter. (An extension activity suggests publishing a health fitness newsletter as a way of displaying the students' Planet Health work and passing on what students have learned about Planet Health concepts to the school community.)

▶▶ Behavioral Objective

For students to be involved in a lifetime physical activity that will help them maintain an active lifestyle.

▶▶ Learning Objectives

Students will be able to

1. obtain information that draws from a variety of sources (experts, observations, experiments, libraries, on-line databases),
2. take notes and summarize information gleaned from reference works and experts,
3. write a coherent composition about a lifetime physical activity,
4. be independent learners, and
5. discuss the importance of being physically active throughout their lives.

▶▶ Materials

- Activity 1 *Lifetime Physical Activities*
- Access to encyclopedias or books that discuss various physical activities
- *Optional:* access to the Internet or other electronic research tools

▶▶ Procedure

1. Point out the goals of this activity:
   - Discuss the benefits of being physically active throughout your life.

- Practice being independent learners: Research a lifetime physical activity of your choosing.
- Write a coherent composition describing the lifetime physical activity you researched.

2. (5–7 minutes) Conduct the following brainstorming activity. Display a model of the "K-T-W chart"* shown. Ask the class what they know, think they know, or want to know about this topic.

The student who offers his/her idea should identify the column in which the idea is to be placed. After eliciting a number of responses, validate or correct the "I Know" and "I Think I Know" responses. The materials listed in the Teacher Resources will help

Topic: The Benefits of Being Physically Active Throughout Your Life

K: I Know	T: I Think I Know	W: I Want to Know

you with this task. If you are unsure of the accuracy of some of their comments, you may wish to ask students to research their questions or verify their statements as part of the research/writing activity. If possible, save a copy of the chart to review at the end of the lesson.

3. (5 minutes) Hand out activity 1 and describe the assignment as outlined on the sheet.

4. (Time will vary) Allow students to begin their research in the library, computer room, or classroom. Assign a deadline for when their research must be completed. You also may wish to require students to record and report their sources of information to you in a standard format of your choosing. (See the Teacher Resources for a list of reference works you may wish to borrow from local libraries.)

5. (Time will vary) Give students time to write their compositions in class or assign it as homework.

6. (5-10 minutes) Review the K-T-W chart. What new information can you add to the "I Know" column?

▶▶ Extension Activities

1. Publish a *Planet Health* newsletter. Include student compositions from this lesson, student poems from lesson 34, public service announcements from lesson 35, fables from lesson 36, and activity goals from lesson 37. Send copies home to parents.

---

*Stern, A. *Instructional strategies and techniques to enhance motivation and achievement.* Workshop, Weston, MA, 1996.

2. Have students make a poster that visually reports the findings of their research on lifetime activity.

3. Have students give oral reports to share their findings.

▶▶ Teacher Resources

General Background Materials

In preparing for this lesson, you may want to refer to the following resources:

- *Centers for Disease Control and Prevention Fact Sheets on Physical Activity*
- *Television Viewing as a Cause of Increasing Obesity Among Children in the United States, 1986-1990*
- *Healthy People 2010*

See appendix B for information on how to obtain these resources.

Specific Background Material

What are lifetime physical activities?

Unlike many competitive team sports, lifetime activities can be done throughout your life. Examples of lifetime activities are running, walking, dancing, hiking, bicycling, swimming, skiing, gardening, and canoeing (see activity 1 for more examples). Team sports require facilities and a number of people, both of which may be difficult to find. Many lifelong activities can be done alone or with a small group of people. You can walk right out your door to participate in many lifetime activities, such as jogging, hiking, bicycling, and swimming. Individuals at various levels of fitness can participate in these types of physical activities by varying the intensity of the activity. Finding a lifetime activity that you enjoy will help you maintain an active lifestyle.

What changes in society have brought about a decrease in daily physical activity?

In the latter part of the 20th century, there was a dramatic reduction in the amount of physical activity performed in daily life. An increase in the number of white-collar jobs has occurred, whereas blue-collar and farming jobs, which require physical work, have decreased. Modern appliances, machinery, and motorized transportation have reduced the amount of activity required to complete household chores and work-related tasks. The growth of technology and inactive leisure activities has also been enormous, with computers, video, and TV being the major factors. The Internet, CD-ROM, and continued expansion of the TV channel market will help these trends continue.

How much time do adolescents spend watching TV?

According to Dietz (1991), American children spend more time watching TV than in any other activity except sleeping. In 1988, the average adolescent viewed approximately 22 hours per week. The percentage of youth watching TV and playing computer or video games for 5 or more hours per day has increased greatly, from 13% in the late 1960s to 43% in 1990. Essentially, TV watching for many children has become a full-time job! On average, adolescents spend more time watching TV than they spend in school. The American Academy of Pediatrics recommends limiting TV viewing to 2 hours or less per day.

What are the benefits of a more active lifestyle?

Activity helps children develop and retain cardiovascular fitness, muscle strength, and confidence in their physical ability. Regular activity helps individuals maintain a healthy weight, build lean muscle, and reduce fat. It can reduce stress and brighten a person's mood. Regular exercise helps build and maintain dense bones, which helps prevent osteoporosis. Active adults have a lower risk of dying prematurely and developing diabetes, high blood pressure, and colon cancer.

What are the risks of a sedentary lifestyle?

Activity is required for health. Studies suggest that physically active individuals enjoy lower risks of developing cardiovascular disease, diabetes, colon cancer, osteoporosis, anxiety, and depression relative to sedentary individuals. Sedentary habits increase the risk of premature death. TV viewing is one of the major causes of overweight youth. TV watching has also been associated with elevated cholesterol levels and poor cardiovascular fitness.

What are the alternatives to TV viewing?

Anything that involves movement! Participate in lifetime physical activities that you enjoy (dancing, bicycling, walking, hiking, gardening, swimming). Limiting TV time ensures that you'll do other activities that involve more physical activity. Also, you don't have to sit still while you watch TV—you can be dancing, cleaning, cooking, and so on.

How much activity is needed to obtain health-related benefits?

Moderate amounts of activity are recommended for people of all ages. However, physical activity need not be strenuous to be beneficial. Just a small increase in physical activity can generate genuine health benefits, such as reduction of body weight and the risk of heart attack, hypertension, and death. Thirty minutes or more of moderately intense activity, such as walking, is beneficial for your health when performed regularly. Some kind of regular vigorous activity, however, is the best way to improve cardiovascular fitness.

How much activity is needed for fitness?

How long, how hard, and how often you are active will determine how fit you are! To be fit, you must work on your cardiovascular (aerobic) endurance, muscular strength (anaerobic fitness), and flexibility. Do strength training two to three times per week. Stretch and do cardiovascular training three to four times per week for at least 20 minutes. You can improve fitness by increasing the frequency (if you are not already exercising regularly), increasing the intensity (doing something faster, doing more repetitions or sets, or using heavier weights), or increasing the time you spend on each exercise. You might choose more types of exercise to do!

What are some examples of things you can do to increase your activity and decrease your inactivity?

Try a new physical activity; take the stairs; don't park next to the building; walk around the mall or the neighborhood with friends; watch only your favorite TV shows; remove or unplug the TV in your bedroom; play catch with a sibling, friend, or parent.

Student Research Activity: Bibliography

These reference books are available at many town libraries.

- *The everything you want to know about sports encyclopedia.* 1994. New York: Bantam Books.

- Mood, D. 1991. *Sports and recreational activities for men and women.* 10th ed. St. Louis: Mosby.
- *Sports encyclopedia.* 1976. New York: Praeger.
- *Sports Illustrated for kids: The everything you want to know about sports encyclopedia* [interactive multimedia]. 1994. Windows CD-ROM. Portland, OR: Creative Multimedia. 2173-01-02.
- Sullivan, G. 1979. *The complete sports dictionary.* New York: Scholastic.
- *Webster's sports dictionary.* 1976. Springfield, MA: Merriam.

References

Blair, S. 1993. C.H. McCloy research lecture: Physical activity, physical fitness, and health. *Research Quarterly for Exercise and Sport* 64(4): 365-376.

Corbin, C., and Lindsey, R. 1979. *Fitness for life.* Glenview, IL: Scott, Foresman.

Dietz, W.H., and Strasburger, V.C. 1991. Children, adolescents, and television. *Current Problems in Pediatrics* 21(1):8-31.

Gortmaker, S.L. 1990. National health examination survey, 1967-70. Unpublished data.

Gortmaker, S.L. 1990. National longitudinal survey of youth. Unpublished data.

Park, R. 1992. Human energy expenditure from *Australopithecus afarensis* to 4-minute mile: Exemplars and case studies. *Exercise and Sport Sciences Reviews* 20: 185-220.

What Are Lifetime Physical Activities?

Unlike many competitive team sports, lifetime activities can be done throughout your life. Examples of lifetime activities are running, walking, dancing, hiking, bicycling, swimming, skiing, gardening, and canoeing. Team sports require facilities and a number of people, both of which may be difficult to find. Many lifelong activities can be done alone or with a small group of people. You can walk right out your door to participate in many lifetime activities like jogging, in-line skating, and bicycling. Individuals at various levels of fitness can participate in these types of physical activities by varying the intensity of the activity. Finding a lifetime activity that you enjoy will help you maintain an active lifestyle and keep physically fit.

Directions

1. Examine the list of lifetime activities below. Choose one of the activities that you enjoy or one that you would like to know more about.

   handball, racquetball, squash

   table tennis

   skating: in-line, ice, roller

   jogging

   judo, karate, tae kwon do

   fencing

   tennis

   swimming

   canoeing, kayaking, rowing

   golf

   snorkeling

   archery

   scuba diving

   gardening

   horseback riding

   mountain climbing

   walking

   orienteering

   hiking

   downhill or cross-country skiing

   dancing: aerobic, ballroom, jazz, line, etc.

2. Research the lifetime activity to determine answers to part A and **one** of the other topics of your choosing.

   A. **Describe the activity**: Where is it done? When is it done? Are there any rules? What equipment or facilities are required?

   B. **History of the activity**: When did people begin doing this activity? In what country did it originate? Where is it currently popular?

C. **Interview someone who does the activity**: Why did they choose to do the activity? Why is it fun? How long have they been doing it? How much does the equipment cost?

D. **Try the activity yourself**: Describe your experience. Where did you do it? Who did you do it with? Did you like it? Would you like to do it regularly?

3. Pretend you are a columnist for a health fitness magazine. Based on your research, write an article that:

A. Informs people about the activity. Be sure to add personal quotes if you researched part C or D in section 2.

B. Encourages people to participate in lifetime activities by pointing out the benefits of maintaining an active lifestyle throughout life.

Lesson 39

Choosing Healthy Foods

In this lesson, students will invent a healthy fast-food product along with an advertising campaign that incorporates the theme of adopting a healthy lifestyle. Students will learn that TV can be a potentially poor dietary influence and can keep children from being active. This lesson is designed to infuse information about choosing healthy foods into a writing activity in a language arts class.

►► Behavioral Objectives

- Students will consume foods high in saturated fat and trans fat less often and in smaller quantities.
- Students will recognize how TV viewing can affect food choices.

►► Learning Objectives

Students will be able to

1. discuss the importance of moderating fat intake,
2. discuss how to incorporate fast-food meals into a healthy diet that includes a variety of foods,
3. organize ideas, collaborate on projects, and write clearly and persuasively, and
4. discuss the media's influence on their diets.

►► Materials

- Student resource 1 *Fast Food Menus*
- Activity 1 *Invent a Food*
- *Optional:* Bring in magazine ads, products, taped TV commercials, or other advertising examples to show students.

►► Procedure

1. (8–10 minutes) Using the following questions (and optional sample advertisements), discuss the overview of the fast-food industry as well as the marketing strategies used by the fast-food industry to reach potential customers.
   - How do you think TV shows and ads affect your choice of foods to eat?
   - If you watched less TV, how might your diet change?
2. (8–10 minutes) Use student resource 1 to review fast-food menus and see how they can be incorporated into a varied diet when eaten in moderation.

3. (20 minutes) Put students into groups of four or five and ask them to invent a healthy fast-food product using student resource 1 *Fast Food Menus* and the activity 1 worksheet *Invent a Food.*

4. (20 minutes) In the next class period, the groups present the food they invented to the class.

▶▶ Extension Activities

Answer the following questions:

- Do you think TV affects the amount of activity you engage in? If so, how? Does it affect what you eat? How?
- Besides TV, what other parts of your life influence your food choices? *(Examples: family, friends, lifestyle, chores, activity schedule.)*
- Can you think of two ways that TV affects your health? *(Keeps us from being active and encourages poor food choices. Some amount of activity is required for health. TV watching has been associated with elevated cholesterol levels and poor cardiovascular fitness among other things.)*

▶▶ Teacher Resources

General Background Material

In preparing for this lesson, you may want to refer to the following resources:

- *Fat: Where It's At*, page 252
- *Television Viewing as a Cause of Increasing Obesity Among Children in the United States, 1986-1990.* See appendix B for information on how to obtain this resource

Specific Background Material

Planet Health endorses the recommendation of the American Academy of Pediatrics to limit TV viewing to 2 hours or less per day.

Planet Health also encourages adolescents to be moderately active for at least 30 minutes every day or nearly every day as part of play, games, sports, chores, transportation, or planned exercise, AND they should participate in at least three sessions per week of vigorous physical activity lasting 20 minutes or more. Adolescents should aim for a total of 60 minutes of activity on five to seven days a week. Physical activity promotes health and well-being, and offers opportunities to socialize and have fun.

Fast Food Facts

- McDonald's opened its first restaurant in 1955 in Des Plaines, Illinois. The company now has over 26,000 restaurants in more than 119 countries.
- 1 in 5 Americans eat at a fast-food restaurant on any given day.
- Eighty-three percent of the time that children under 17 eat out, they eat at fast-food restaurants.

Fast Food Marketing Strategies Targeting the General Population

- *Customizing menus and service to suit local tastes.* McDonald's serves teriyaki burgers and corn soup in Japan, pasta salads in Rome, and has live piano music in Paris and cappuccino and espresso machines in the financial district in New York City.

- *Famous people in TV ads.* For example, basketball players Michael Jordan and Larry Bird have done TV ads for McDonald's.

- *Discount coupons.* In newspapers, magazines, and stores.

- *Flashy billboards.* Colorful logos displaying attractive foods, often with sports heroes (e.g., Drew Bledsoe) prominently displayed along roadways and in front of the restaurants.

- *Sponsorship.* McDonald's runs TV ads during the Olympic Games to promote the fact that it is a proud sponsor of the Olympics.

Fast Food Marketing Strategies Targeting Children

- *Toys.* Fast-food restaurants often offer toys in connection with popular movies or TV shows, for example, Pokemon, Furbys, Teletubbies, Beanie Babies, Inspector Gadget figures.

- *Images.* Ronald McDonald is known by schoolchildren everywhere.

- *Special meals for children.* McDonald's sells "Happy Meals"® for children. Likewise, the other fast-food chains offer similar meal deals for children.

- *TV ads during prime viewing time.* In 1998, McDonald's spent just over a billion dollars in advertising. Fast-food restaurants spend millions of dollars on Saturday morning TV ads aimed at children.

References

Center for Science in the Public Interest. 1991. *The completely revised and updated fast-food guide.* 2d ed. New York: Workman Publishing.

Nestle, M., and Jacobson, M.F. 2000. Halting the obesity epidemic: A public health policy approach. *Public Health Reports* 115:12-24.

Perl, L. 1980. *Junk food, fast food, health food: What America eats and why.* New York: Houghton Mifflin.

Sallis, J.F., and Patrick, K. 1994. Physical activity guidelines for adolescents: Consensus statement. *Pediatric Exercise Science* 6:302-314.

U.S. Department of Agriculture and U.S. Department of Health and Human Services. 2000. *Nutrition and your health: Dietary guidelines for Americans* 2000, 5th edition. **www.usda.gov/cnpp**

U.S. Department of Health and Human Services. 2000. Healthy People 2010, conference edition, vols. I and II. **www.health.gov/healthypeople**

Fast Food Menus: Can Fast Food Contribute to Good Nutrition?

Meals at fast food restaurants can contribute to good nutrition if they are chosen carefully and not eaten too often. When you go, eat in moderation; avoid "supersizing" your menu selections. If you choose foods that are high in fat or sugar, balance them with other foods low in fat and high in nutrients. Order low-fat milk instead of soda.

Strengths of Fast Foods

They have some nutrients in them, are cheap and tasty, and are often served in clean, safe environments. Choose wisely! Examples of nutrient-rich foods include McDonald's Chunky Chicken Salad which is high in vitamin A and protein. Wendy's Baked Potato is high in vitamin C. In addition, some fast food restaurants have salad bars with fruits and vegetables that can provide fiber as well as vitamins A and C.

Weaknesses of Fast Foods

They are typically high in calories, saturated fat, and trans fat (especially the deep-fried items) and sodium, and therefore should be consumed infrequently. In addition, fast foods often have chemical additives and artificial colorings.

Recommended Fat Intake

There is no reason to eliminate fat from your diet. In fact, some fat in your diet is desirable. The total amount of fat you eat is not as important as the type of fat you eat. Choose a diet that is low in saturated fat and low in trans fat (found in margarine and shortening and many bakery goods, packaged snack foods, and fried fast food), since eating too much of these fats can increase your chances of developing heart disease. Substituting unsaturated fats (found in most vegetable oils, most nuts, olives, avocados, and some fish) for saturated and trans fats can decrease your risk of developing heart disease. Of course, eating too much of any type of fat (or other nutrient for that matter) will give you more energy than you need, so choose a diet moderate in total fat.

- Adults should limit fat intake to 15 teaspoons per day, or 65 grams/day (30% of 2,000 calories).
- 11–14-year-old girls should shoot for about 17 teaspoons or 73 grams/day (30% of 2,200 calories). Saturated fat should be limited to no more than 24 grams of the 73 total.
- 11–14-year-old boys should shoot for about 19 teaspoons or 83 grams/day (30% of 2,500 calories). Saturated fat should be limited to no more than 28 grams of the total 83.

Fast Foods to Cut Back on and Avoid

Eat a high-fat food once in a while and choose a lower fat alternative most of the time.

Company/product	Fat (teaspoons)	Fat (grams)
Jack in the Box Ultimate Cheeseburger	16	69
Burger King Double Whopper with Cheese	14	61
KFC Extra Tasty Crispy Thigh and Wing	11	48
McDonald's Thousand Island Dressing, 2.5 oz	9	40
Dunkin' Donuts Chocolate Croissant	9	29

Fast Foods That Can Be Selected Most of the Time

Not all fast foods are high in fat. Become a "fast food sleuth."

Company/product	Fat (teaspoons)	Fat (grams)
Dunkin' Donuts Cinnamon and Raisin Bagel	<1	2
McDonald's Lite Vinaigrette, 2 fl. oz	<1	2
Arby's Light Roast Chicken Deluxe, Garden Salad, and Orange Juice	2	10
KFC Chicken Littles Sandwich	2	10
Jack in the Box Hamburger	2.5	11
McDonald's Hamburger, Carrot Sticks, and Lowfat Milk	2.5	11
Burger King Hamburger	2.5	11

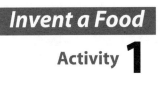

As a team of experts, your task is to invent a healthy, low fat fast food product. Draw up a sample design of your food product and plan your own advertising campaign. Remember to think about who you would like to buy this product. Use additional paper if necessary. Have fun! Be creative! Be ready to report back to the class.

Names of consultants:	

Use the questions below to help you guide your thinking:

1. Name and describe your product.

2. Why is your product healthy? What ingredients does it have? How will it fit into a healthful diet?

3. Why is your product unique? What strategies will you use to get potential customers to buy your product?

4. Where will you advertise?

5. Draw a picture of your product on the other side of this sheet.

6. Think about a logo that will go with your product

7. Write a rap song, TV or radio commercial, or print advertisement for your product.

8. How much will your product cost?

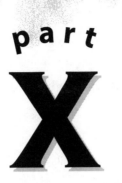

part

X

Math

This unit contains eight lessons. Use the At A Glance chart below to help you select the lessons that best fit your curriculum objectives. Some of the lessons offer a choice of activities. Adapt the lesson procedures to fit your teaching style, students' skills, and time constraints.

Lessons in this unit meet many Massachusetts learning standards that may be similar to standards in your state. Refer to appendix E (page 508) to see which of the 1996-1999 Massachusetts Curriculum Frameworks (MCFW) each lesson incorporates.

Math At A Glance

Theme	Lesson	Level of difficulty (grade)*			Subject-specific skills	Materials needed
		6th	7th	8th		
Balanced diet	40 Problem Solving: Making Healthy Choices 　　Activity 1 　　Activity 2 　　Extension activity	H H M	M H L	M M L	Five-step problem approach; addition, subtraction, and multiplication of integers; the concept of proportionality	None
Balanced diet	41 Figuring Out Fat	H	M	L	Percentages, graphing	Calculators
Balanced diet	42 Looking for Patterns: What's for Lunch? 　　Case study 1 　　　Inequalities 　　　Statistics 　　Case study 2	M H M	M M-H M	L M M	Analyze real-world data from tables and histograms, use inequalities, calculate range, average, difference, and percentage	Calculators
Fruits and vegetables	43 Apples, Oranges, and Zucchini: An Algebra Party	H	H	M	Two-variable equations	Calculators (optional)
Activity	44 Plotting Coordinate Graphs: What Does Your Day Look Like?	H	M	M	Contruct a coordinate system; graphing	Graph paper, ruler, overhead transparencies
Activity	45 Survey the Class	H	M	M	Basic statistical analysis: means, percents, range, ranking	None
Lifestyle	46 Circle Graphs: Where Did the Day Go? 　　Activity 1 　　Activity 2	H M-H	H M	M L-M	Constructing circle graphs; fractions, percentages, decimals, and interconversions	Five pieces of large paper or overhead transparencies, calculator, compass, protractor, plain paper, colored pencils or crayons
Lifestyle	47 Energy Equations	H	M	M	Calculate averages; graphing	

* Level of difficulty: L = low, M = medium, H = high

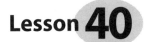

Lesson 40

Problem Solving: Making Healthy Choices

This lesson reinforces the importance of eating a balanced diet based on the Food Guide Pyramid (FGP), a concept introduced in lesson 32. It also introduces the concept of proportionality in the diet. Students will work cooperatively to solve a problem that requires them to use their previous knowledge of the FGP and the five-step problem-solving strategy. Students will apply mathematical thinking and calculations (adding and multiplying whole numbers and fractions) to make healthier menu choices at a fast-food restaurant. This activity requires students to interpret information, plan a problem-solving strategy, draw conclusions, and defend their conclusions. We recommend activity 1 for grades 6 and 7 and activity 2 for grade 8. Extension activity 1 Daily Food Log is appropriate for all grades.

▶▶ Behavioral Objective

For students to make healthy food choices that contribute to a well-balanced diet.

▶▶ Learning Objectives

Students will be able to

1. use the five-step problem-solving approach to make a thoughtful decision,
2. use their knowledge of the Food Guide Pyramid (FGP) to select healthier meals at fast-food restaurants,
3. defend their decisions by calculating differences to compare their food selections with those recommended by the FGP,
4. read and interpret word problems and data tables,
5. explain the concept of proportionality,
6. utilize basic math skills (addition and multiplication of whole numbers) (activity 1) and fractions (activity 2) to solve a word problem, and
7. work cooperatively to solve problems.

▶▶ Materials

- One copy of student resource 1 *Daily Servings* and student resource 2 *Servings of Fast Foods* per group of three
- Activity 1 *Making Healthy Choices* (requires students to add and subtract integers) OR activity 2 *Making Healthy Choices* (requires students to add and multiply fractions)

- Overhead transparency of the Food Guide Pyramid (see Teacher Resources)
- *Optional:* extension activity 1 *Daily Food Log*

▶▶ Procedure

Decide whether problem-solving activity 1 or activity 2 is more appropriate for the skill level of your students. Activity 1 requires students to add and subtract integers. Activity 2 requires students to add and multiply fractions. Extension activity 1 requires students to make comparisons using inequalities.

1. (3 minutes) Remind students of their previous knowledge and experience with the FGP. (Refer to lesson 32.) Explain that today they will be participating in a problem-solving session that requires them to use their previous knowledge of the FGP and previous experience with problem-solving strategies. Ask them, "Why is it important to eat a well-balanced diet?" (See Teacher Resources for possible answers.)

2. (10 minutes) To help students understand the concept of eating a "well-balanced" or "proportional" diet, explain the concept of proportionality as follows (this step is borrowed from the National Dairy Council's *Leader Guide to the Guide to Good Eating and Daily Food Guide Pyramid,* 1994):

    A. Introduce the concept of proportionality with sketches of three houses.

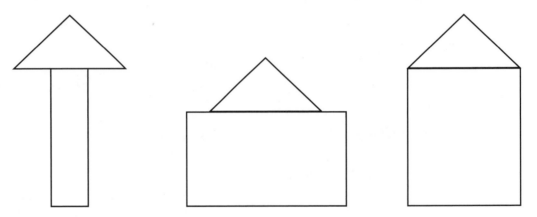

    B. Have students explain the potential problems with houses 1 and 2. Explain that the roof and walls of house 3 are in proportion; those of houses 1 and 2 are not.

    C. Write the word *proportional* on the board and ask for a definition. Help students understand that things are in proportion when they are in their proper dimension as compared with the whole. They are in balance.

    D. Make the following points regarding proportionality in the diet (refer to the overhead transparency of the FGP):

- To get the nutrients you need to stay healthy, you need to eat from all five food groups in the pyramid each day.
- You need more servings from some food groups than others.
- When you eat the recommended number of foods from each food group, you are eating a "proportional" diet.

    E. To check for understanding, ask students to give you an example of a diet that would be unbalanced or disproportional.

3. (3 minutes) Review the steps involved in problem solving.

- *Explore:* Read carefully. What do you know? What do you need to know?

- *Plan:* Design a strategy. Arrange information in tables. Draw pictures. Make an estimate of the answer.
- *Solve:* Test your strategy.
- *Check solutions:* Have you answered the question? Does your answer make sense?
- *Extend:* What have you learned? How can you apply what you've learned?

4. Divide class into groups of three. Hand out student resource sheets 1 and 2 and either activity 1 or activity 2. Give each group only one copy of the problem to increase their need to work cooperatively. You may wish to review the student resource sheets with the class.

5. Point out the goals of the activity:

- To work cooperatively to design a strategy that makes efficient use of class time and all team members. The processes of planning and evaluating choices are the most important parts of the problem.
- To apply their knowledge of the FGP to select a healthy, proportional dinner at a fast-food restaurant.
- To use their math skills to determine their food needs and evaluate their menu options.

6. (30 minutes) Have students work in their groups to solve the problem. The *Menu Analysis* section of the activity will help them summarize their meal selections and can be posted on a bulletin board for other students to look at. (See selected answers in Teacher Resources.)

7. (Time: depends on size of the class) Have students write their group's meal selection on the chalkboard. Choose a reporter from each group to defend the group's selections. (This step can be eliminated to save time. Groups can hand in their worksheets instead.)

8. (5 minutes) Discuss student responses to the questions asked in step 5 *Extend*.

- What was the most difficult part of making this decision in your group? How could you have improved your approach to solving this problem?
- Is it possible to eat at fast-food restaurants and still have a healthy diet overall?
- Why is it important to eat a balanced diet? (See Teacher Resources.)

9. (5 minutes) Help students understand that fast foods generally are high in total fat, saturated fat, trans fat, and calories. (See Teacher Resources for a discussion of the different kinds of fat.) They should limit their visits to fast-food restaurants. However, occasional visits are okay, especially if they choose carefully when eating out and eat a balanced diet most of the time.

▶▶ Extension Activities

1. Hand out the extension activity and student resource sheets. Have students keep a log of their food consumption for one day and analyze its completeness by comparing it to the recommendations made by the FGP. The *Guide to Good Eating* (see appendix A) is an excellent resource for determining which food groups combination foods like pizza fall into.

2. Ask students to go to the local shopping center or mall and

- record the names of fast-food restaurants,
- record the menu items that include vegetables and fruits at each restaurant,
- record the menu items that are labeled low fat or no fat,
- determine which restaurants offer the largest number of healthy eating options, and

• determine which restaurants are the least and most expensive to eat at. This would work best if students worked in teams.

►► Teacher Resources

General Background Material

In preparing for this lesson, you may want to refer to the following resources:

• *Fat: Where It's At,* page 252
• *Daily Food Guide Pyramid,* appendix A
• *Nutrition and Your Health: Dietary Guidelines for Americans, 2000.* See appendix A for information on how to obtain this resource

Specific Background Material

Highlights of the Food Guide Pyramid

• The Food Guide Pyramid was designed by the U.S. Department of Agriculture (USDA) and released in 1992. The FGP is an eating guide that helps people to understand the five food groups as well as the importance of variety, proportionality, and moderation in the diet. Following the FGP recommendations ensures consuming essential nutrients sufficient to meet the dietary needs of most people.

• The position of the food groups in the FGP reflects the number of servings people should eat from each food group daily. The pyramid has a wide base and a small tip, showing that the food group requiring the most daily servings is at the bottom, and the group requiring the least is at the top. Specifically, the grain group is the largest size food group and forms the pyramid's base, indicating we should eat more servings of grain products, especially whole grains, than of any other food group. The tip includes foods such as fats, oils, and sweets. These foods should be consumed in small amounts.

• The FGP tells us that foods from all food groups are important. It also tells us

1. to choose foods from all of the food groups daily, and

2. to choose a variety of foods within each food group.

• The recommended serving numbers are broad dietary goals. An individual's sex, age, weight, activity level, and genetic makeup determine the number and type of foods she or he should eat from each group.

The Three Principles of the Food Guide Pyramid

• *Proportionality (balance).* Eat the recommended number of servings from each group. (See student resource 1.)

• *Variety.* Select a variety of foods within each of the five food groups. For example, while selecting from the grains food group, select bread, rice, tortillas, pasta, and other grains, and choose some whole grain varieties. No single food supplies all the nutrients you need, and foods within the same food group have different amounts of nutrients. Eating many different foods will ensure that you meet the nutritional recommendations.

• *Moderation.* Eat the appropriate number of servings from each food group in the appropriate quantities. Eat fats, oils, and sweets sparingly. These foods in the tip of the pyramid are low in essential vitamins and minerals and high in calories from fat or sugar. Eat fats, oils, and sweets in moderation only to lower the risk of developing

The Food Guide Pyramid
A Guide to Daily Food Choices

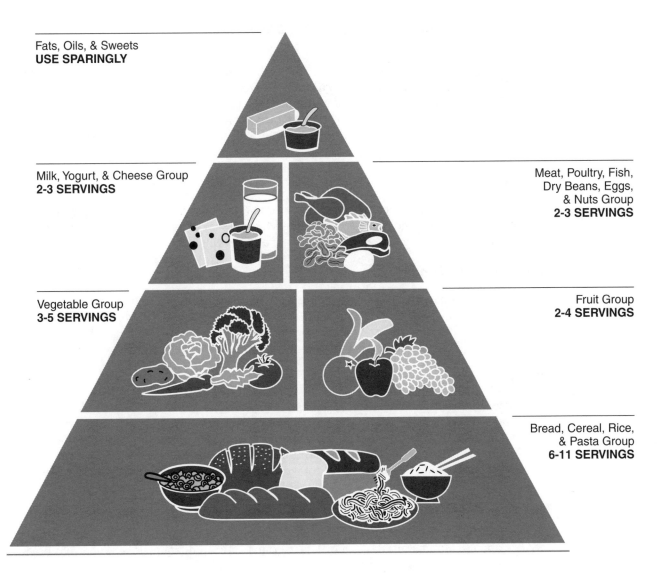

Fats, Oils, & Sweets
USE SPARINGLY

Milk, Yogurt, & Cheese Group
2-3 SERVINGS

Meat, Poultry, Fish,
Dry Beans, Eggs,
& Nuts Group
2-3 SERVINGS

Vegetable Group
3-5 SERVINGS

Fruit Group
2-4 SERVINGS

Bread, Cereal, Rice,
& Pasta Group
6-11 SERVINGS

Looking at the Pieces of the Pyramid

The Food Guide Pyramid emphasizes foods from the five major food groups shown in the three lower sections of the Pyramid. Each of these food groups provides some, but not all, of the nutrients you need. Foods in one group can't replace those in another. No one of these major food groups is more important than another—for good health, you need them all.

many health problems in adulthood. Animal fats, such as those found in meat, butter, and whole milk, are the major source of saturated fat listed on food labels. Solid margarines and shortenings, also called partially hydrogenated vegetable oils in ingredient lists, are the primary sources of trans fat.

The FGP applies to diets around the world. For example, 1/2 cup of mango juice from Brazil is a serving of juice.

Number of Servings From Each Food Group

The FGP suggests a range of servings for each group. It provides a chart that explains how many servings you will need from each group based on your age and sex. The FGP can be used by anyone—girls, boys, men, or women—regardless of age. The amount of food people eat differs by age, sex, and activity level. At a given level of activity, most boys and men need more food than most girls and women. Also, growing, active teenagers need more food than many sedentary adults. Review student resource 1 *Daily Servings*.

Serving Size

To understand that recommendations for number of servings are realistic, review the foods included in each food group and serving sizes for different foods and food groups (student resource 1). Review what counts as 1 serving for each food.

Combination Foods

Combination foods are made from ingredients that fit into more than one food group. One example is pizza, which provides refined grains, dairy, and vegetable servings. Learning the constituents of combination foods can help with comparing intake to the FGP.

Keeping Fat to a Suitable Level

The U.S. Dietary Guidelines recommend consuming no more than 30% of calories from total fat (unsaturated, saturated, and trans fat) and no more than 10% of calories from saturated fat. Although the guidelines don't mention an upper limit for trans fat, new scientific evidence points to the harmful effects of trans fat. Therefore, it is particularly important to limit trans fat intake as well as saturated fat intake. The recommended upper limits for daily fat intake for adolescents are

- about 73 grams per day (24 or fewer grams saturated fat) for 11–14-year-old girls (based on a 2,200 calorie diet), and
- about 83 grams per day (28 or fewer grams saturated fat) for 11–14-year-old boys (based on a 2,500 calorie diet).

Not All Fat is Created Equal

The fat in foods contains a mixture of saturated and unsaturated (monounsaturated and polyunsaturated) fatty acids, commonly called fats. Many animal products, such as fatty meat, whole milk, butter, and lard, are high in saturated fat. This kind of fat is typically solid at room temperature. Eating too much saturated fat increases the risk of developing heart disease. Therefore, the *Dietary Guidelines for Americans* recommends eating a diet low in saturated fat. Most of the fat you eat should be unsaturated since substituting unsaturated fat for saturated decreases the risk of developing heart disease. Most plant fats or oils are high in unsaturated fat and generally are liquid at room temperature. Vegetable oils (olive, canola, corn, peanut), most nuts, olives, and avocados are good sources of unsaturated fat. However, eating lots of any type of fat may not be healthy, so try to get no more than 30% of your calories from total fat (saturated, unsaturated, and trans fat).

There are exceptions to the rule. Not all plant fats are healthy. Through a commercial process called hydrogenation, plant oils can be converted into solids called trans fats (also called partially hydrogenated vegetable oil). This is how some margarines are made. Not surprisingly, foods high in trans fats have been found to increase the risk of heart disease also. To avoid these fats, check the ingredient lists on packaged foods such as cookies and crackers for partially hydrogenated vegetable oil. Also watch out for coconut oil and palm oil since these oils naturally are high in saturated fat.

Also, not all animal foods are high in saturated fats. Some ocean fish, such as salmon, mackerel, and tuna, are high in a polyunsaturated fat—called omega-3 fatty acid—that may protect you against heart disease. So choose to eat fish when you get the chance.

Why Is Eating a Balanced Diet Important?

1. Balanced diets provide the vitamins, minerals, fat, fiber, protein, and carbohydrates you need for good health today.
2. Diets based on the FGP help you maintain a healthy body weight.
3. A balanced diet can reduce the risk of developing certain conditions and diseases like obesity, diabetes, certain cancers, hypertension, cardiovascular disease, and osteoporosis.

References

National Dairy Council. 1994. *Leader guide to the guide to good eating and daily food guide pyramid.* Rosemont, IL: National Dairy Council.

U.S. Department of Agriculture and U.S. Department of Health and Human Services. 2000. *Nutrition and your health: Dietary guidelines for Americans* 2000, 5th edition. **www.usda.gov/cnpp**

U.S. Department of Agriculture and U.S. Department of Health and Human Services. Food Guide Pyramid.

U.S. Department of Health and Human Services. 2000. Healthy People 2010, conference edition, vols. I and II. **www.health.gov/healthypeople**

Willett, W. 2000. Got fat? Exploding nutrition myths. World Health News. **www.worldhealthnews.harvard.edu**

▶▶ Answer Key

Selected Answers to Activity 1

Step 2

1. *How many servings of each group have you eaten?* Total the servings listed in the table for each food group. Solution: Number of servings eaten.

- Grain: 6
- Fruits: 3.5
- Veggies: 1
- Meat: 1
- Dairy: 2
- Other: 1
- Fat: 47 grams

2. *What do you need to eat for dinner to achieve the Food Guide Pyramid daily recommendations? How many grams of fat should you try to limit your dinner to?* Plan: Daily FGP recommendation – number of servings eaten = what needs to be eaten. Solution:

	Girls	Boys
Grain	9 – 6 = 3	11 – 6 = 5
Fruits	3 – 3.5 = –0.5	4 – 3.5 = 0.5
Veggies	4 – 1 = 3	5 – 1 = 4
Meat	3 (upper limit) – 1 = 2	3 (upper limit) – 1 = 2
Dairy	2.5 – 2 = 0.5	2.5 – 2 = 0.5
Fat	73 – 47 = 26g	83 – 47 = 36g

3. *Which menu selections should you make? Hint: Tables can help you keep track of information. You might want to make a table that resembles the fast-food menus to keep track of the nutritional information for each of your choices.* Answers will vary. Students will find that there are not many fruit options.

Selected Answers to Activity 2

Step 2

1. *Based on the information in the problem, how many servings of each food group have you already eaten today? How much fat have you eaten? (Round your answers to the nearest 1/2 serving. A table might help you organize these numbers.)* Plan: 2/3 × daily FGP recommended number of servings for girls OR boys (student resource sheet). Solution:

	Girls	Boys
Grain	2/3 × 9 = 6	2/3 × 11 = 7.3 ~ 7
Veggies	2/3 × 4 = 2.7 ~ 3	2/3 × 5 = 3.3 ~ 3
Fruit	2/3 × 3 = 2	2/3 × 4 = 2.7 ~ 3
Dairy	2/3 × 2.5 = 1.7 ~ 2	2/3 × 2.5 = 1.7 ~ 2
Meat	2/3 × 3 (upper limit) = 2	2/3 × 3 (upper limit) = 2
Fat	2/3 × 73 = 48.7 ~ 49	2/3 × 83 = 55.3 ~ 55

Recommended Number of Servings for Girls and Boys Aged 11–14

Food group	Girls (2,200 calories/day)	Boys (2,500 calories/day)
Bread, cereal, rice, and pasta	9	11
Vegetable	4	5
Fruit	3	4
Milk, yogurt, and cheese	2.5	2.5
Meat, poultry, fish, dry beans, eggs, and nuts	2.5	2.5

What Counts as One Serving?

Food group	One serving
Bread, cereal, rice, and pasta	1 slice of bread 1 tortilla, roll, muffin 1/2 bagel, English muffin, hamburger bun 1/2 cup cooked cereal, grits, rice, pasta 1 oz (about 1 cup) ready-to-eat breakfast cereal
Vegetable	1 cup raw leafy vegetables 1/2 cup other chopped vegetables 1/2 cup other cooked vegetables 3/4 cup vegetable juice
Fruit	1 medium apple, banana, orange, pear 1/2 grapefruit 1/4 cantaloupe 1/2 cup of raw, canned, cooked, frozen fruit 1/4 cup raisins, dried fruit 3/4 cup of fruit juice
Milk, yogurt, and cheese	1 cup milk or yogurt 1.5 oz natural cheese (e.g., cheddar) 2 oz processed cheese (e.g., American) 1/2 cup pudding 1/2 cup ice cream, ice milk, frozen yogurt

Food group	One serving
Meat, poultry, fish, dry beans, eggs, and nuts	2.5 oz. of cooked, lean meat, poultry, or fish
	1/2 cup cooked dry beans, peas
	1 egg
	2 tablespoons peanut butter
	1/3 cup nuts, seeds

How Much Fat is Okay?

The U.S. Dietary Guidelines recommend consuming no more than 30% of calories from total fat (unsaturated, saturated, and trans fat) with no more than 10% from unsaturated fat. Individual foods may have more or less fat than this. Don't worry about occasional indulgences but try to keep your average at 30%. On average, adolescents should consume

- about 73 grams/day (24 or fewer grams saturated fat) for 11–14-year-old girls (based on a 2,200 calorie diet), and
- about 83 grams/day (28 or fewer grams saturated fat) for 11–14-year-old boys (based on a 2,500 calorie diet).

McDonald's

| Product | Fat (grams) | Number of servings | | | | | | Price $ * |
		Grain	Veggie	Fruit	Meat	Dairy	Other **	
Apple pie	13			1			1	.89
Big Mac	31	3			1.5	1	1	2.22
Cheeseburger	13	2			0.75	1		.85
Chicken McNuggets (6 pieces)	17				1			2.06
Quarter Pounder	21	2			1			2.22
Fish Filet Deluxe	28	2			1	1		2.27
French fries, small	10		1				1	.91
Hamburger	9	2			1			.70
Small milkshake, vanilla	1					1		1.26
Milk, 1% low-fat 8 oz	2.5					1		.42
Orange juice 6 oz	0			1				1.05
Coca-Cola 12 oz	0						1	1.05
Apple juice	0			1				.83
Side salad	0		1					2.30
Ranch dressing	21						1	Free
Reduced calorie French dressing	8						1	Free

*   Prices are estimates because they vary with location.

**   Products high in fat and/or sugar get categorized as "other" and would fit in the tip of the pyramid.

Domino's Pizza

Product	Fat (grams)	Number of servings						Price $ *
		Grain	Veggie	Fruit	Meat	Dairy	Other **	
Cheese pizza[1]	9	1				1		2.00
Green pepper and mushroom pizza[1]	10	1	1			1		2.50
Pepperoni pizza[1]	15	1			1	1		2.50
Small garden salad	0.25		1 or 2					2.50
Italian dressing	24						1	Free
Thousand Island dressing	20						1	Free
Light Italian dressing	1						1	Free

[1] Information is based on 2 slices of a large pizza.

Pizzas quoted above are on hand-tossed crust. Many locations do not sell pizza by the slice.

*   Prices are estimates because they vary with location.

**   Products high in fat and/or sugar get categorized as "other" and would fit in the tip of the pyramid.

Subway

| Product | Fat (grams) | Number of servings | | | | | | Price $ * |
		Grain	Veggie	Fruit	Meat	Dairy	Other **	
Garden salad	1		2					1.99
Ham sandwich	5	2.5	1		1			2.49
Turkey sandwich	4	2.5	1		1			2.49
Subway club	5	2.5	1		1.5			2.69
Meatball sandwich	16	3	1		1			1.99
Steak and cheese sandwich	13	2.5	1		2.5	1		2.49
Vegetarian sandwich	3	2.5	1					1.59
Fruit juice, 16 oz	0			2.5				.95
Creamy Italian dressing (1 Tbsp)	6						1	Free
Fat-free Italian (1Tbsp)	0						1	Free
Mustard	0						1	Free
Mayonnaise (1 tsp)	4						1	Free
Cheese	3					1		Free
Soda, small	0						1	.99

All sandwiches are 6". Values do not include cheese or condiments.

All standard sandwiches include lettuce, tomato, onions, green peppers, pickles, and olives.

*   Prices are estimates because they vary with location.

**   Products high in fat and/or sugar get categorized as "other" and would fit in the tip of the pyramid.

Use the five-step problem-solving process to help you reach a decision.

Situation

You are at the mall with a group of friends. You promised your Mom you would buy a nutritious meal with the $6 she gave you to spend on dinner. McDonald's, Domino's Pizza, and Subway are your favorite restaurants. Is it possible to buy a meal at one of these fast-food restaurants that is well-balanced and contains only a moderate amount of fat? Look at the guidelines outlined by the Food Guide Pyramid and the fast-food menus on the student resource sheets. Plan a meal that allows you to fulfill the Food Guide Pyramid daily recommendations. Assume you've eaten breakfast, lunch, and snack foods that contained 47 grams of fat and have provided you with the food servings listed in the table below. Defend your fast-food menu choices by explaining how the meal helps you fulfill the recommended number of food servings in each of the food groups and meet the fat recommendations.

Number of servings you've eaten today

Meal	Grains	Fruits	Veggies	Meat	Dairy	Other
Breakfast	2	1-1/2			1	
Lunch	2	2	1	1	1	
Snack	2					1
Total servings	6	3-1/2	1	1	2	1

Step 1: Explore

1. What is the question?

2. What data are presented that will help you answer the question?

Step 2: Plan

Making the best meal choice requires you to solve three smaller problems. Design a strategy to answer each question.

1. How many servings of each group have you eaten? How many grams of fat?

2. What do you need to eat for dinner to achieve the Food Guide Pyramid daily recommendations? How many grams of fat should you try to limit your dinner to?

3. Which menu selections should you make? Hint: Tables can help you keep track of information. You might want to make a table that resembles the fast-food menus to keep track of the nutritional information for each of your choices.

Step 3: Solve

Try your strategy. Make your meal choice.

1. Show your work on a separate sheet of paper.
2. Report your decisions and complete the analysis on the next page.

Step 4: Examine/Defend Your Decision

Defend your menu selections by comparing the Food Guide Pyramid daily recommended number of servings in each food group with the total number you would eat for this day. Would you eat more or less than the recommended number of servings for the day? Also, compare your total fat intake to the amount recommended for people your age. Include a discussion of the differences between the recommendations and your actual consumption. Use separate paper if necessary.

For example: My meal selection provided me with enough servings to fulfill the recommended number of servings in each food group except fruits. I ate only two servings of fruit, one less than the recommended number. I also ate one more than the recommended number of meat servings and two "sometimes" foods. My fat consumption was 10 grams more than recommended.

Step 5: Extend

What have you learned? How can you apply it?

1. What was the most difficult part of making this decision for your group? How could you have improved your approach to solving this problem?

2. Is it possible to eat at fast-food restaurants and still have a healthy diet overall? Explain your opinion.

3. Why is it important to eat a balanced diet?

Menu Analysis

This healthy menu is served at _____.

Menu selections: _____.

Total cost: _____.

Total grams of fat: _____.

How many servings of each food group are provided by your fast-food meal? Record your answer in the pyramid below.

A = Other
B = Milk group
C = Meat group
D = Vegetable group
E = Fruit group
F = Grain group

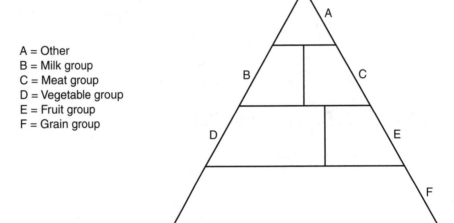

On the pyramid below, sum the servings provided by the menu you designed and the servings provided by the food you ate the rest of the day. Repeat this for each food group.

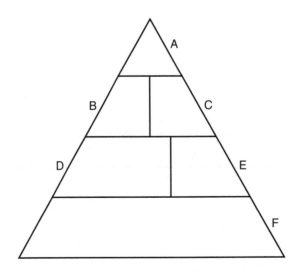

Use the five-step problem-solving process to help you reach a decision.

Situation

You are at the mall with a group of friends. You promised your Mom you would buy a nutritious meal with the $6 she gave you to spend on dinner. McDonald's, Domino's Pizza, and Subway are your favorite restaurants. Is it possible to buy a meal at one of these fast-food restaurants that is well-balanced and contains only a moderate amount of fat? Look at the guidelines outlined by the Food Guide Pyramid and the fast-food menus on the student resource sheets. Plan a meal that provides you with 1/3 the recommended servings in each food group and 1/3 the recommended daily grams of fat. Assume you've eaten two meals and one snack that provided you with approximately 2/3 of the recommended servings and grams of fat. Defend your choices by explaining how the meal helps you fulfill the recommended number of food servings in each of the food groups and meet the fat recommendations.

Step 1: Explore

1. What is the question?

2. What data are presented that will help you answer the question?

Step 2: Plan

Making the best meal choice requires you to solve three smaller problems. Design a strategy to answer each question.

1. Based on the information in the problem, how many servings of each food group have you already eaten today? How much fat have you eaten? (Round your answers to the nearest 1/2 serving. A table might help you organize these numbers.)

2. What do you need to eat for dinner to achieve the Food Guide Pyramid daily recommendations? How many grams of fat should you try to limit your dinner to?

3. Which menu selections should you make? Hint: Tables can help you keep track of information. You might want to make a table that resembles the fast-food menus to keep track of the nutritional information for each of your choices.

Step 3: Solve

Try your strategy. Make your meal choice.

1. Show your work below or on a separate sheet of paper.

2. Report your decisions and complete the analysis on the next page.

Step 4: Examine/Defend Your Decision

Defend your menu selections by comparing the Food Guide Pyramid daily recommended number of servings in each food group with the total number you would eat for this day. Also, compare your total fat intake to the amount recommended for people your age. Express these comparisons in words and fractions. Use separate paper if necessary.

For example: My meal selection provided me with enough servings to fulfill the recommended number of servings in each food group except fruits. I ate 8 servings of grain and 8 were recommended (expressed as 8/8 servings of grain.) I also ate 4/4 servings of milk, 3/2-3 servings of meat, and 4/4 servings of vegetables. I ate only 2/3 of the recommended number of fruit servings, but that's okay because the 5-A-Day rules say I should try to eat 5 servings of fruits and vegetables combined. I ate 80 grams of fat, 7 grams more than recommended (80/73).

Step 5: Extend

What have you learned? How can you apply it?

1. What was the most difficult part of making this decision for your group? How could you have improved your approach to solving this problem?

2. Is it possible to eat at fast-food restaurants and still have a healthy diet overall? Explain your opinion.

3. Why is it important to eat a balanced diet?

Menu Analysis

This healthy menu is served at _____.

Menu selections: _____.

Total cost: _____.

Total grams of fat: _____.

What fraction of the total number of recommended servings is provided by your fast-food meal? Record your answer for each food group in the pyramid below.

A = Other
B = Milk group
C = Meat group
D = Vegetable group
E = Fruit group
F = Grain group

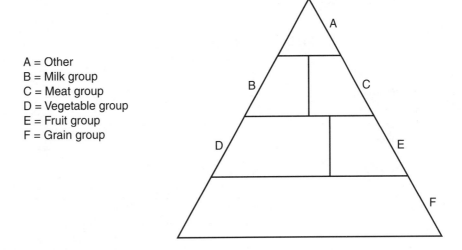

For example: If your menu selections provided 1 dairy serving and 4 were recommended, write 1/4 in the dairy food group.

On the pyramid below, sum the fraction of servings provided by the menu you designed and the fraction of servings provided by the food you ate the rest of the day. Repeat this for each food group. Remember, we assumed you ate 2/3 of the recommended number of servings during breakfast, lunch, and a snack. For example: Dairy 1/4 + 2.5/4 = 3.5/4.

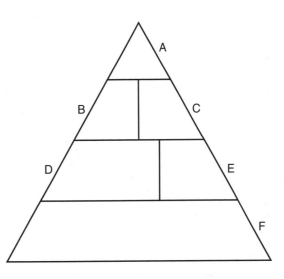

Name_____

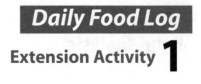

Keep a log of your food consumption for one day. Record the number of servings of each food you eat. Use the student resource sheet to help you figure out serving size.

Food	Food group (number of servings)					
	Grains	**Fruits**	**Veggies**	**Meat**	**Dairy**	**Sometimes foods**
Example: 1 large slice of pizza with green peppers (1/8 of 14" large pizza)	1		1		1	
Breakfast						
Lunch						
Dinner						
Snacks						
Total number of servings						

Analyzing the Data

Analyze the completeness of your diet by comparing it to the recommendations made by the Food Guide Pyramid.

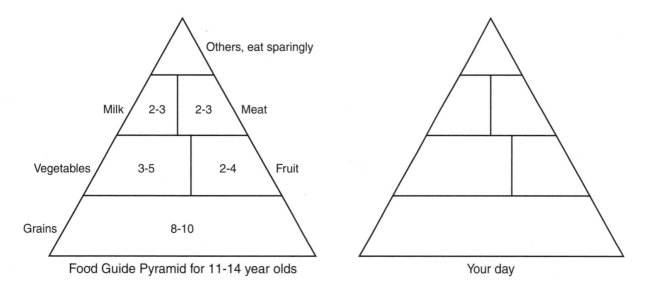

Food Guide Pyramid for 11-14 year olds   Your day

Write an inequality to express any differences between your diet and the servings recommended by the Food Guide Pyramid. Indicate which number in the inequality represents your number of servings and which represents the number of recommended servings.

	Student	<, >, =	Food Guide Pyramid
Example: Grains	5	<	10
Grains			
Vegetables			
Fruits			
Milk			
Meat			
Other			

Discussion

1. Describe the differences between your diet and the one recommended by the Food Guide Pyramid.

2. Was this a typical day's diet for you? Explain.

3. What were the highest-fat foods you ate today? Suggest some possible substitutions.

Figuring Out Fat

This lesson contains paired group activities. Calculators are recommended. Students will use percentages to examine the fat content of two imaginary diets. This lesson is designed to infuse information about eating fat in moderation into a unit on percentages.

▶▶ Behavioral Objective

To choose a diet low in saturated and trans fat and moderate in total fat.

▶▶ Learning Objectives

Students will be able to

1. calculate percent of calories from fat and saturated fat (activity 1),
2. interpret tables and graphs, and
3. make inferences about fat intake.

▶▶ Materials

- Activity 1 *Fat: It All Adds Up,* part I and part II
- Calculators recommended
- *Optional:* student resource 1 *What's the Rap on Fat?* from lesson 49 (page 334)

▶▶ Procedure

1. (3 minutes) Point out the goals of this lesson:
   - to practice calculating percentages by figuring out how much fat is in foods,
   - to learn the upper limits for total fat and saturated fat intake, and
   - to choose a diet low in saturated and trans fat and moderate in total fat.
2. Review the fat recommendations with students. Ask them:
   - What percentage of your total calories should come from fat? (*Answer: No more than 30% of total calories, with no more than 10% of calories from saturated fat.*)
   - Why should we eat less saturated and trans fat than unsaturated fat? (*Answer: Eating too much saturated and trans fat increases the risk of developing heart disease.*)

Make sure students understand that total fat refers to the sum of unsaturated, saturated, and trans fat consumed. You may choose to have students read *What's the Rap on Fat?* (Lesson 49, page 335). This student resource describes the different types of fat.

3. (5 minutes) Using examples 1 and 2, review math techniques needed to calculate percent of calories from fat.

Ask students how many of them have had a bagel in the past week, and if they think bagels are high-fat foods. Read the following two examples aloud and demonstrate how to calculate the percentage of the total fat in foods. Note: 1 gram (g) of fat = 9 calories (cal).

Example 1. A cinnamon and raisin bagel has 250 calories and 2 grams of fat. If 1 gram of fat provides 9 calories, what percentage of the calories in the bagel come from fat?

$2 \text{ g} \times 9 \text{ cal/g} = 18 \text{ cal}$

$18 \text{ cal} / 250 \text{ cal} = 0.072$

$0.072 \times 100 = 7.2\%$

7.2% of the bagel's calories come from fat (total fat). This is a low-fat food.

Example 2. A fried chicken breast has 412 calories and 24 grams of fat. What percentage of the calories in the chicken breast come from fat?

$24 \text{ g} \times 9 \text{ cal/g} = 216 \text{ cal}$

$216 \text{ cal} / 412 \text{ cal} = 0.524$

$0.524 \times 100 = 52.4\%$

52.4% of the chicken breast's calories come from fat. Fried chicken is a high-fat food.

4. (5 minutes) Have the class work in pairs. Copy examples A-D on the board. Have students calculate the percentage of calories from fat in each of the foods. Go over the answers to the examples with students.

Example A. 2% milk (8 oz): 110 calories and 4 grams of fat.

$4 \text{ g} \times 9 \text{ cal} = 36 \text{ cal}$

$36 \text{ cal} / 110 \text{ cal} = 0.327$

$0.327 \times 100 = 32.7\%$

Example B. Whole milk (8 oz): 157 calories and 9 grams of fat.

$9 \text{ g} \times 9 \text{ cal} = 81 \text{ cal}$

$81 \text{ cal} / 157 \text{ cal} = 0.516$

$0.516 \times 100 = 51.6\%$

Example C. Plain baked potato with skin: 212 calories and 1 gram of fat.

$1 \text{ g} \times 9 \text{ cal} = 9 \text{ cal}$

$9 \text{ cal} / 212 \text{ cal} = 0.042$

$0.042 \times 100 = 4.2\%$

Example D. French fries (4 oz): 360 calories and 17 grams of fat.

$17 \text{ g} \times 9 \text{ cal} = 153 \text{ cal}$

$153 \text{ cal} / 360 \text{ cal} = 0.425$

$0.425 \times 100 = 42.5\%$

Review calculations and answers with class to ensure correct data.

5. (5 minutes) The bar chart shows the percent of calories from fat for the items in examples A-D. Draw the chart on the board or enlarge the one shown below and make a transparency. Discuss the differences in percent calories from fat.

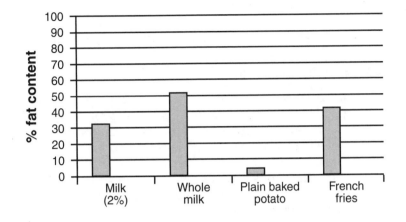

6. (15 minutes) Hand out parts I and II of the student activity. Read the directions as a class. In the previous examples, students calculated the percentage of calories from fat in one serving of food. Make sure students understand that in this activity, they will calculate the percentage of calories from fat in food eaten in one day and compare it to fat intake on a second day. They will also calculate the percentage of calories from saturated fat in food eaten on days 1 and 2. In part II, make sure students understand that they are multiplying by 9 because each gram of fat provides 9 calories. Have students work together in pairs to complete the activity. Calculators are strongly recommended.

7. (10 minutes) Discuss the imaginary diets. Look at the actual fat intake compared to the recommended amounts. Ask students what they learned from this exercise. On day 1, imaginary total fat intake was slightly below 30% and total saturated fat intake was just below 10%. On day 2, both total fat and saturated fat intake were way above recommended levels. Advise students to reduce fat intake by cutting back on foods high in saturated and trans fat. Discuss substitutions that could have been made to keep total fat intake at about 30% and saturated fat intake at about 10%. Examples of substitutions are a bagel instead of a cinnamon nut Danish, low-fat or skim milk instead of whole milk, grilled chicken instead of fried chicken, brown rice instead of French fries, and low-fat frozen yogurt with fresh fruit instead of a banana split. Suggest that when students choose a high-fat food (like a hamburger), they pair it with a lower-fat food (like a salad with dressing) instead of another high-fat food (like French fries). These substitutions would reduce saturated fat and total fat intake.

8. Discuss question 6 from activity 1: Is one day of high-fat eating a bad thing? (Answer: No, don't worry about occasional indulgences, and don't starve yourself to make up for them. Keep your average total fat intake at 30% of calories and average saturated fat intake at 10% of calories. Average refers to a period of a few days.)

▶▶ Teacher Resources

General Background Material

In preparing for this lesson, you may want to refer to the following resources:

• *Nutrition and Your Health: Dietary Guidelines for Americans.* See appendix A for information on how to obtain these resources.

• *Fat: Where It's At* (page 252)

Specific Background Material

Refer to student resource 1 *What's the Rap on Fat?* in lesson 49 (page 335).

Fat Recommendations

The U.S. Dietary Guidelines recommend consuming no more than 30% of calories from total fat with no more than 10% of calories from saturated fat. Although the guidelines do not mention an upper limit for trans fat, new scientific evidence points to the harmful effects of this type of fat. Therefore, it is important to limit trans fat intake as well as saturated fat intake, since both increase risk of heart disease.

Individual foods may have more or less fat than the recommended levels. To eat a total diet that stays within the recommendations, balance higher-fat food selections with lower-fat choices.

The recommended maximum number of total fat and saturated fat grams per day depends on the amount of calories eaten daily. An individual who eats 2,000 calories should try to get no more than 600 calories (30% of 2,000) from total fat and 200 calories (10% of 2,000) from saturated fat. Since fat provides 9 calories per gram, a person eating 2,000 calories a day should eat no more than 67 grams of total fat (600 calories / 9 calories per gram) and no more than 22 grams of saturated fat (200 calories / 9 calories per gram) each day. (Note: Nutrition labels round numbers to the nearest 5 grams.)

The recommended fat intakes for adolescents are

• about 73 grams per day total fat with 24 or fewer grams saturated fat for 11–14-year-old girls (based on a 2,200 calorie diet), and

• about 83 grams per day total fat with 28 or fewer grams saturated fat for 11–14-year-old boys (based on a 2,500 calorie diet).

Remind students that some fat in the diet is beneficial. Students should aim for fat to be 30% of their total calories, not at removing fat entirely from their diets. Thirty percent is okay. If they need to reduce fat intake to meet this level, encourage them to cut back on saturated and trans fat.

Tips for Lowering Saturated Fat Intake

The *Dietary Guidelines for Americans* offers these tips for lowering saturated fat intake:

• Eat plenty of grains, fruits, and vegetables.
• Cook with vegetable oils instead of butter.
• Add little or no butter to foods.
• Check food labels. Choose foods lower in saturated fat.
• Trim fat from meat and remove skin from poultry.
• Choose fat-free or low-fat milk, yogurt, and cheese.
• Choose fruit desserts most often.
• Choose 2 to 3 servings of fish or other lean meats daily.
• Choose dried beans, peas, or lentils often

- Limit intake of processed meats such as sausage, salami, and hot dogs.
- Limit intake of candy, cookies, cake, and chips.
- Limit intake of foods with creamy sauces.
- Limit intake of liver and other organ meats.
- Use egg yolks and whole eggs in moderation. Use egg whites and egg substitutes freely when cooking since they contain no cholesterol and little or no fat.

Comparing Saturated Fat in Foods

According to the *Dietary Guidelines for Americans 2000*, the following food categories are among the major food sources of saturated fat for U.S. adults and children (the bottom food in each category is the lower saturated fat alternative):

Cheese
- Regular cheddar cheese (1 oz.): 6.0 grams saturated fat
- Low-fat cheddar cheese (1 oz.): 1.2 grams saturated fat

Ground beef
- Regular ground beef (3 oz. cooked): 7.2 grams saturated fat
- Extra-lean ground beef (3 oz. cooked): 5.3 grams saturated fat

Milk
- Whole milk (1 cup): 5.1 grams saturated fat
- Low-fat (1%) milk (1 cup): 1.6 grams saturated fat

Bread
- Croissant (1 medium): 6.6 grams saturated fat
- Bagel (1 medium): 0.1 grams saturated fat

Frozen desserts
- Regular ice cream (1/2 cup): 4.5 grams saturated fat
- Frozen yogurt (1/2 cup): 2.5 grams saturated fat

Table spreads
- butter (1 tsp.): 2.4 grams saturated fat
- soft margarine (1 tsp.): 0.7 grams saturated fat

Calculating % Daily Value for Fat

Food labels list the % Daily Value (%DV) for nutrients next to the amount (grams) of each nutrient. This percentage lets you know what portion (how much) of the recommended daily amount is present in a serving of the food. The %DV listed on food labels is always based on a 2,000-calorie diet, the recommended diet for adult females. The average 11–14-year-old girl requires a 2,200-calorie diet; the average 11–14-year-old boy requires 2,500 calories. Therefore, the %DV for adolescents for a given food will be lower than the one listed on the food label. In other words, a serving of food with provide them with a smaller portion of the recommended daily amount than is indicated on the label. Even so, the %DV listed on food labels is a safe, approximate guideline for adolescents to use to compare nutrient content of similar foods.

To calculate %DV for total fat, divide the number of grams of total fat per serving by the daily allowance for total fat and multiply by 100.

(grams of total fat / daily recommended grams of total fat) × 100 = %DV

For example, a person eating a 2,000-calorie diet needs no more than 65 grams of total fat. This person chooses to eat chicken nuggets that have 15 grams of total fat.

What percentage of total fat will this food provide?

$15 \text{ g} / 65 \text{ g} = 0.23$

$0.23 \times 100 = 23\%$

The chicken nuggets will provide this person 23% of his or her total fat %DV.
To calculate the %DV of saturated fat, divide the grams of saturated fat by the daily recommended total grams of saturated fat and multiply by 100.

(grams of saturated fat / daily recommended grams of saturated fat) $\times$ 100 = %DV

The chicken nuggets have 3.5 grams of saturated fat. The daily recommended total of saturated fat for a person eating a 2,000-calorie diet is 20 grams. What percentage of the daily value of saturated fat will this person get from the nuggets?

$3.5 \text{ g} / 20 \text{ g} = 0.175$

$0.175 \times 100 = 17.5\%$ (round up to 18%)

The nuggets will provide 18% of the daily value of saturated fat for this person. As mentioned previously, the recommended fat intakes for adolescents are slightly higher since their calorie needs are higher.

References

Bierer, L.A., Warner, L., Lawson, S., and Cohen, T. 1991. *Life science: The challenge of discovery.* Lexington, MA: Heath.

U.S. Department of Agriculture and U.S. Department of Health and Human Services. 2000. *Nutrition and your health: Dietary guidelines for Americans 2000,* 5th edition. **www.usda.gov/cnpp**

U.S. Department of Health and Human Services. 2000. Healthy people 2010, conference edition, vols. I and II. **www.health.gov/healthypeople**

Willett, W. 2000. Got fat? Exploding nutrition myths. *World Health News* **www.worldhealthnews. harvard.edu**

▶▶ Answer Key

Activity 1 Fat: It All Adds Up

Day 1 totals

- 2,266 total calories
- 73 grams total fat
- 23.7 grams saturated fat

Day 2 totals

- 2,415 total calories
- 105 grams total fat
- 42 grams saturated fat

5. Day 1: both % of calories from fat and % of calories from saturated fat were below recommended levels. Day 2: both % of calories from fat and % of calories from saturated fat were above recommended levels.

6. No, don't worry about occasional indulgences, and don't starve yourself to make up for them. Keep your average total fat intake at 30% of calories and average saturated fat intake at 10% of calories. Average refers to a period of a few days.

1	2	3	4	5
Diet	Calories	Total Fat (grams)	Total Fat (grams) $\times$ 9 = calories from fat	Calories from fat / total calories $\times$ 100 = % calories from fat
Day 1	2,266	73	73 $\times$ 9 = 657	657 / 2,266 = 0.2899382 (round to 0.29) 0.29 $\times$ 100 = 29%
Day 2	2,415	105	105 $\times$ 9 = 945	945 / 2,415 = 0.3913043 (round to 0.39) 0.39 $\times$ 100 = 39%

1	2	3	4	5
Diet	Calories	Sat. Fat (grams)	Sat. Fat (grams) $\times$ 9 = calories from sat. fat	Calories from sat. fat / total calories $\times$ 100 = % calories from sat. fat
Day 1	2,266	23.7	23.7 $\times$ 9 = 213.3	213.3 / 2,266 = 0.0941306 (round to 0.09) 0.09 $\times$ 100 = 9%
Day 2	2,415	42	42 $\times$ 9 = 378	378 / 2,415 = 0.1565217 (round to 0.16) 0.16 $\times$ 100 = 16%

Name _____

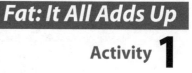

Activity **1**

Part I

Look at the two imaginary daily menus below. The total calories, grams of total fat, and grams of saturated fat are listed for each food item.

Calculate totals for calories, grams of fat, and grams of saturated fat for the imaginary day 1 and day 2 diets. Transfer totals to tables A and B in part II.

Day 1

Food	How much	Calories	Total fat (grams)	Sat. fat (grams)
Breakfast				
Shake: 1/2 cup skim milk, 1/2 cup strawberries, 6 oz. lowfat yogurt, ice cubes	12 oz.	275	5	3
Cinnamon raisin bagel	1	194	1	0.2
Cream cheese	2 Tbsp.	100	10	6
Lunch				
Chicken fajita	1	260	4	1
Milk (2% lowfat)	8 oz.	121	5	3
Small garden salad	1	80	4	1
Lite vinaigrette salad dressing	2 oz.	48	2	0
Split pea with ham soup	6 oz.	131	3	1
Snacks				
Apple	1	81	1	0
Milk (2% lowfat)	8 oz.	121	5	3
Dinner				
Baked potato with skin	1	220	0	0
Coleslaw	3 oz.	83	7	0
Carrot sticks	1/2 cup	24	0	0
Tuna sandwich with regular mayonaise	1	339	23	4
Strawberry frozen yogurt (lowfat)	5 oz.	189	3	1.5
Day 1 totals	**N/A**			

		Day 2		
Food	**How much**	**Calories**	**Total fat (grams)**	**Sat. fat (grams)**
Cinnamon nut danish	1	280	16	4
Whole milk	8 oz.	150	8	5
Fried chicken breast	1	436	17	5
French fries	4 oz.	350	17	3
Orange juice	8 oz.	112	0	0
Chocolate chip cookie	2	92	6	2
Hot dog with cheese	1	335	22	10
Whole milk	8 oz.	150	8	5
Banana split	13 oz.	510	11	8
Day 2 totals	**N/A**			

Part II

1. Transfer the total calories and total grams of fat for day 1 and day 2 to columns 2 and 3 in table A.
2. Using the formulas in columns 4 and 5, calculate total calories from fat and % calories from fat for day 1 and day 2.

Table A

1	2	3	4	5
Diet	Calories	Total fat (grams)	Total fat (grams) × 9 = calories from fat	Calories from fat / total calories × 100 = % calories from fat
Day 1				
Day 2				

3. Transfer the total calories and total grams of saturated fat for day 1 and day 2 to columns 2 and 3 in table B.
4. Using the formulas in columns 4 and 5, calculate total calories from saturated fat and % calories from saturated fat for day 1 and day 2. Round to the nearest whole percent (less than 0.5 round down; 0.5 or greater, round up).

Table B

1	2	3	4	5
Diet	Calories	Sat. fat (grams)	Sat. fat (grams) × 9 = calories from sat. fat	Calories from sat. fat / total calories × 100 = % calories from sat. fat
Day 1				
Day 2				

5. Compare the total fat and saturated fat intakes with the recommended amounts (30% of calories from total fat with 10% from saturated fat). Were the recommendations met on day 1? How about day 2?

6. Is one day of high-fat eating a bad thing?

Workspace

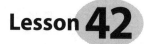
Looking for Patterns: What's for Lunch?

In this lesson, students will use statistics and graphs to look for evidence of healthy patterns in the foods being offered for lunch at the school cafeteria. In an attempt to provide activities that are accessible and challenging to a wide range of math students, we have included two case studies to choose from. The analysis of case study 1 can be completed at two levels of difficulty, depending on your students' abilities. The goal of this lesson is to promote the idea that healthy eating does not require following a strict, inflexible diet. It means establishing a balanced "total diet" that takes into account food consumed over several days or a week. Students will be encouraged to eat a variety of foods and will learn to eat "sometimes foods" occasionally without feeling guilty.

▶▶ Behavioral Objective

For students to establish healthy eating patterns.

▶▶ Learning Objectives

Students will be able to

1. solve problems that involve collecting and analyzing data from real-world situations,
2. use inequalities to compare recommendations with actual number of servings provided (activity 1 case study 1),
3. construct and interpret tables and histograms (activity 2 case study 2),
4. calculate the range, average, difference, and percentage of a data set (case study 1),
5. make inferences and convincing arguments that are based on data analysis,
6. explain why statistical methods are powerful aids for decision making,
7. think critically about what eating patterns are necessary to maintain a balanced "total diet," and
8. work cooperatively to solve problems.

▶▶ Materials

Calculators are recommended for both case studies.

For **case study 1**, you need

- one copy of student resource 1 per group of three,
- one copy of activity 1 case study 1 per group, and

- the section from activity 1 for inequality analysis *OR* statistical analysis.
  For **case study 2**, you need
- one student resource 2 *Fat: Where It's At* per group, and
- one activity 2 case study 2 sheet per group.

▶▶ Procedure

1. Overview

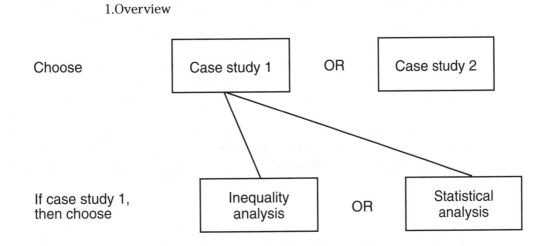

Choose | Case study 1 | OR | Case study 2

If case study 1,
then choose | Inequality analysis | OR | Statistical analysis

2. Choose whether you are going to use case study 1 or case study 2. If you decide to use case study 1, then please proceed here. If you decide to use case study 2, proceed to that section.

Case Study 1

All students should begin the activity by completing the first page of activity 1. Use either the inequalities analysis section of case study 1 *OR* the statistical analysis section of case study 1 to analyze the results of this case. Choose the one that best fits your students' skills.

1. (5 minutes) Ask students to complete the following statement in writing: *"A balanced diet is . . . ."* Have students share their answers. This will give you an idea of what information students remember from previous lessons and will set the stage for you to correct their misconceptions and clarify the idea of a balanced "total diet."

2. (5 minutes) Explain the American Heart Association's idea of a balanced "total diet." To make sure students understand what is meant by "balanced," briefly review the three principles of the Food Guide Pyramid dietary guidelines (see Teacher Resources). You may wish to display an overhead transparency of the Food Guide Pyramid (FGP) while you do this. You do not need to spend a great deal of time reviewing the FGP because students have been exposed to it in previous lessons and a student resource sheet will be available to them during the activity.

3. (3 minutes) Introduce the case study. Point out the goals of the activity:

- To work cooperatively as a class to examine one week's school lunch menu
- To analyze the patterns of foods offered in a week
- To determine in what ways school lunches help or hinder you from eating a balanced "total diet"

4. Divide the class into five groups. Assign one day's school lunch menu to each group.

5. Hand out student resource 1 and case study 1 to each group. Give each group inequalities *or* statistical analysis, but not both.

6. (5 minutes) Have each group complete the analysis of the lunch menu assigned to them and record their results on the board. Remind students that in order to complete this problem in the time allowed, they must work together as a team. You might suggest that each student be responsible for determining the food group and serving size of an equal number of foods in their menu. If students have difficulty determining serving size, they can talk to the food services staff or you can refer them to the resource *Seven Ways to Size Up Your Servings* (see appendix A).

7. (20 minutes) Have students complete the analysis of the class data using inequalities or statistics. (*Note on inequalities analysis*: Students may need you to clarify what they should do for the food groups that contain ranges for the recommended servings. Example #1: Monday's lunch had 3 servings of vegetables. Three is greater than the 1-2 servings recommended, so they should put a > in the column for Monday. Example #2: Tuesday's lunch had 0 servings of meat. Zero is less than 0.5-1, so students would put a < in the column for Tuesday.)

8. (5-10 minutes) Discuss the students' conclusions (questions 1-3 on case study 1).

Case Study 2

1. (5 minutes) Ask students to complete the following statement in writing: *"Eating a moderate amount of fat means . . . ."* Have students share their answers. This will give you an idea of what information students remember from previous lessons and will set the stage for you to correct their misconceptions and clarify the idea of moderating fat consumption in the context of a balanced "total diet."

2. (5 minutes) Review the fat recommendations and explain the American Heart Association's idea of a balanced "total diet." Try to get students to understand that generally they should get no more than 30% of their calories from total fat and no more than 10% of their calories from saturated fat, but that there will be some fluctuation with the variety of foods they eat. Encourage students to replace saturated fat and trans fat primarily with unsaturated fat. Eating too many saturated fats (found mainly in animal products such as meat, butter, and whole milk) and/or trans fats (found in fried and packaged foods that contain partially hydrogenated vegetable oil) increases the risk of developing heart disease. Substituting unsaturated fat (found in vegetable oil, nuts, olives, and avocados) decreases the risk of developing heart disease. The type of fat eaten is more important than the total number of calories from fat. (See lesson 49, student resource 1 *What's the Rap on Fat?* (page 335) for more information on the different kinds of fat.)

3. (3 minutes) Introduce the case study. Point out the goals of the activity:

• To work cooperatively as a class to examine one week's school lunch menu

• To use statistics to analyze the patterns of foods offered in a week

• To determine whether school lunches are helping you moderate fat consumption in your "total diet"

This lesson looks at total fat in the diet, though saturated and trans fats are discussed at the end of the lesson.

4. Divide the class into at least five groups. (To keep the groups small, you may need to have more groups, with several groups working on a particular menu.) Hand out

Fat: Where It's At (student resource 2) and case study 2. Tell students that this resource lists the total amount of fat (saturated, unsaturated, and trans fats) present in foods. You may want to read the case study instructions out loud to the class. (Suggestion: Collect the *Fat: Where It's At* sheet at the end of the period and keep one class set to be used the next time you do the activity.)

5. (5 minutes) Have each group complete the analysis of the lunch menu assigned to them and record their results on the board. Remind students that in order to complete this problem in the time allowed, they must work together as a team. You might suggest that each student be responsible for determining the fat content of an equal number of foods in their menu. (*Note:* You may wish to make an overhead transparency of the histogram below to show students.)

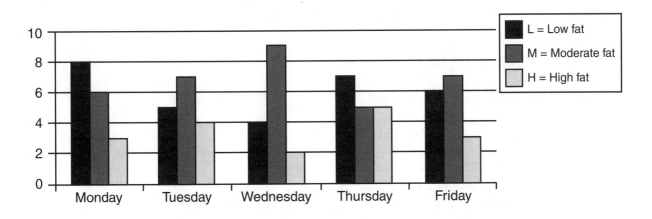

6. (20 minutes) Have students complete the analysis of the class data.

7. (5-10 minutes) Discuss the students' conclusions (questions 1-3). Ask students to go back to the menu and circle all the foods that are likely to contain high amounts of saturated fat (for example, meat, whole milk, butter) and trans fats (fried foods and bakery goods). Remind them that these are the fats they want to try to limit. Ask them to make suggestions for ways they can change the menu to decrease saturated and trans fats. (See Teacher Resources in this lesson and in lesson 41 for ideas.)

▶▶ Extension Activities

Case Study 1 or 2

1. Have students make predictions about the patterns of food selections they would expect to see in next week's cafeteria menus.
2. Have them test the accuracy of their predictions. Is there a lot of variability in the patterns observed from one week to the next?
3. Make a poster of their results and ask if you can post it in the cafeteria. Compliment the cafeteria staff on their effort to provide healthy menus.

Case Study 1

In question 3 of case study 1, students calculated the number of servings of fruits and vegetables they would need to eat on average outside of school to reach the 5-A-Day recommendations. Based on their findings, have students plan two days of breakfast, dinner, and snack menus that would provide them with the balance of the number of fruits and vegetables they need. They should provide the names and serving sizes of foods they enjoy eating.

Case Study 2

Have students analyze the fat content of the food they eat outside of school by doing the following:

1. Record what they eat for breakfast, dinner, and snacks on two days.
2. Make a frequency table to tally the number of servings that fall into each of the following categories: low (0-5 g), moderate (5-15 g), and high (>15 g) fat.

►►Teacher Resources

General Background Material

In preparing for this lesson, you may want to refer to the following resources:
• *Nutrition and Your Health: Dietary Guidelines for Americans.* See appendix A for information on how to obtain this resource.
• *Fat: Where It's At,* page 252
• *Guide to Good Eating* (appendix A)
• *Seven Ways to Size Up Your Servings* (appendix A)

Specific Background Material

Balancing Our "Total Diet"

The American Heart Association's *Dietary Guidelines for Healthy American Adults* (published in 1996) recommends that people rethink the meaning of a balanced *total diet.* "Until now, *total diet* has referred to the balance of foods eaten at a single meal or on a single day. Now the American Heart Association suggests that people take into account the food consumed over the course of several days or a week. This strategy allows some flexibility in choosing foods and fits the theme of consuming a variety of foods and reducing the guilt from eating something 'bad' now and then" (Harvard Medical School 1997).

School Lunch Program

The National School Lunch Program was established in 1946 "to safeguard the health and well-being of the nation's children and to encourage domestic consumption of nutritious agricultural commodities and other food" (Knutson et al. 1983, 309). In June 1995, the U.S. Department of Agriculture finalized a new policy ensuring that by the fall of 1996 school meals would meet the *Dietary Guidelines for Americans,* lowering the amount of fat and sodium and increasing the variety of foods. Some schools may have received waivers to postpone implementation until no later than school year 1998–1999.

President Bill Clinton had the following to say about the policy:

For the last five decades, the School Lunch Program has prepared children for a healthier tomorrow. . . . Building on this history, USDA has renewed the National School Lunch Program's original health and nutrition mission (USDA 1996).

Case Study 1: Specific Background

Bear in mind that *Planet Health* lessons in other subjects teach students about using the FGP to eat balanced diets. Hence, assuming that students have already been exposed to at least one of those lessons, this lesson can serve as a practical application, and math teachers need to spend only a few minutes reminding students about the key principles of the FGP and the new concept presented here: balancing the "total diet."

The Food Guide Pyramid
A Guide to Daily Food Choices

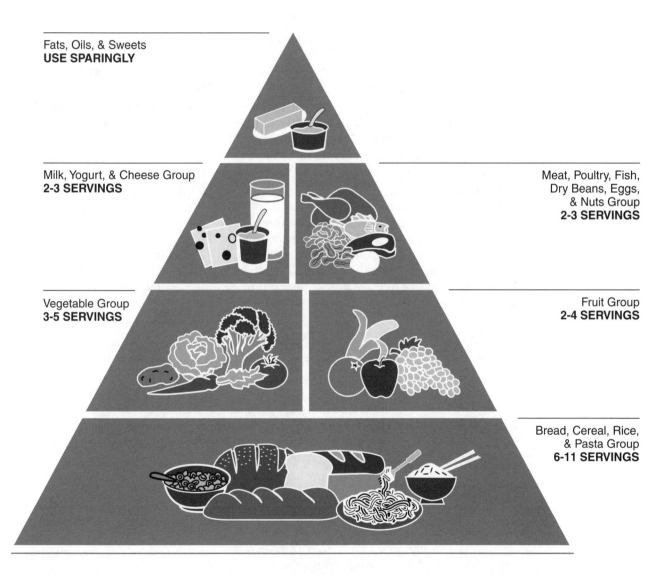

Fats, Oils, & Sweets
USE SPARINGLY

Milk, Yogurt, & Cheese Group
2-3 SERVINGS

Meat, Poultry, Fish,
Dry Beans, Eggs,
& Nuts Group
2-3 SERVINGS

Vegetable Group
3-5 SERVINGS

Fruit Group
2-4 SERVINGS

Bread, Cereal, Rice,
& Pasta Group
6-11 SERVINGS

Looking at the Pieces of the Pyramid

The Food Guide Pyramid emphasizes foods from the five major food groups shown in the three lower sections of the Pyramid. Each of these food groups provides some, but not all, of the nutrients you need. Foods in one group can't replace those in another. No one of these major food groups is more important than another—for good health, you need them all.

Highlights of the Food Guide Pyramid

• The FGP was designed by the U.S. Department of Agriculture (USDA) and released in 1992. The FGP is an eating guide that helps people understand the five food groups as well as the importance of variety, proportionality, and moderation in the diet. Following the FGP recommendations ensures consuming essential nutrients sufficient to meet the dietary needs of most people.

• The position of the food groups in the FGP reflects the number of servings people should eat from each food group *every day*. The pyramid has a wide base and a small tip, showing that the food group requiring the most daily servings is at the bottom, and the group requiring the least is at the top. Specifically, the grain group is the largest size food group and forms the pyramid's base, indicating we should eat more servings of grain products, especially whole grains, than of any other food groups. The tip includes foods such as fats, oils, and sweets. These foods should be consumed only in small amounts.

The Three Principles of the Food Guide Pyramid

• *Proportionality (balance).* Eat the recommended number of servings from each group daily. (See student resource 1.)

• *Variety.* Select a variety of foods within each of the five food groups. For example, when selecting from the grains food group, select bread, rice, and pasta, and select some whole grain varieties. No single food supplies all the nutrients you need, and foods within the same food group have different amounts of nutrients. Eating many different foods will ensure that you meet the nutritional recommendations.

• *Moderation.* Use the FGP serving sizes as a guide for determining how much you should eat. Eat fats, oils, and sweets sparingly. The foods in the tip of the pyramid are low in essential vitamins and minerals and high in calories from fat or sugar. Eating fats, oils, and sweets in moderation only can lower the risk of developing many health problems in adulthood. Animal fats found in foods such as meat, butter, and whole milk are the major source of saturated fats listed on food labels. Partially hydrogenated vegetable oils or trans fats are found in margarine, vegetable shortening, baked goods, and fast foods.

Number of Servings From Each Food Group

The FGP suggests a range of servings for each group. It provides a chart that explains how many servings you will need from each group based on your age and sex. The FGP can be used by anyone—girls, boys, men, or women—regardless of age. The amount of food people eat differs by age, sex, and activity level. At a given level of activity, most boys and men need more food than most girls and women. Also, growing, active teenagers need more food than many sedentary adults. Review the recommendations for adolescents on student resource 1.

5-A-Day Recommendations

Getting five or more servings per day of fruits and vegetables (combined, not of each) is important to help you maintain your health. Eat at least two servings of fruit and at least three servings of vegetables (with at least one serving of a dark green or orange vegetable) for a total of five servings each day.

Combination Foods

Combination foods are made from ingredients that fit into more than one food group. One example is pizza, which provides refined grains, dairy, and vegetable servings.

Learning the constituents of combination foods can help with comparing intake to the FGP.

Why Is Eating a Balanced Diet Important?

1. Balanced diets provide the vitamins, minerals, fat, fiber, protein, and carbohydrates you need for good health today.
2. Diets based on the FGP help you maintain a healthy body weight.
3. A balanced diet can reduce the risk of developing certain conditions and diseases like obesity, diabetes, certain cancers, hypertension, cardiovascular disease, and osteoporosis.

Case Study 2: Specific Background

Bear in mind that other *Planet Health* lessons teach students about the importance of choosing a diet low in saturated fat and moderate in total fat. Hence, assuming that students have already been exposed to at least one of those lessons, this lesson can serve as a practical application, and math teachers need to spend only a few minutes reminding students about fat recommendations and moderating their "total diet."

Keeping Fat to a Suitable Level

The U.S. Dietary Guidelines recommend consuming no more than 30% of calories from total fat (unsaturated, saturated, and trans fat) and no more than 10% of calories from saturated fat. The recommended upper limits for daily fat intake are

- about 73 grams total fat (24 or fewer grams of saturated fat) per day for 11–14-year-old girls (based on a 2,200 calorie diet), and
- about 83 grams total fat (28 or fewer grams of saturated fat) per day for 11–14-year-old boys (based on a 2,500 calorie diet).

Not All Fat Is Created Equal

The fat in foods contains a mixture of saturated and unsaturated (monounsaturated and polyunsaturated) fatty acids commonly called fats. Many animal products, such as fatty meat, whole milk, butter, and lard, are high in saturated fat. This kind of fat typically is solid at room temperature. Eating too much saturated fat increases the risk of developing heart disease. Therefore, the *Dietary Guidelines for Americans* recommends a diet low in saturated fat (less than 10% of calories). Most of the fat you eat should be unsaturated since substituting this type of fat for saturated fat decreases the risk of developing heart disease. Most plant fats or oils are high in unsaturated fats and generally are liquid at room temperature. Vegetable oils (such as olive, canola, corn, and peanut), most nuts, olives, and avocados are good sources of unsaturated fat. However, eating a lot of any kind of fat may not be healthy, so try to get no more than 30% of your calories from total fat (unsaturated, saturated fat, and trans fat).

There is an exception to the rule that plant fats are more healthy than animal fats. Through a commercial process called hydrogenation, the more healthy plant oils can be saturated and converted into solids called trans fats (also called partially hydrogenated vegetable oil). This is how some margarines are made. Not surprisingly, foods high in trans fats also have been found to increase the risk of heart disease. To avoid trans fats, check the ingredients lists on packaged foods such as cookies and crackers for partially hydrogenated vegetable oil. Also watch out for coconut oil and palm oil since these oils are naturally high in saturated fat.

Also, not all animal foods are high in saturated fat. Some ocean fish, such as salmon, mackerel, and tuna, are high in a polyunsaturated fat—called omega-3 fatty acid—that may protect you against heart disease. So choose to eat fish when you get the chance.

Why Should We Moderate Fat Intake?

Excess saturated fat increases the risk of certain diseases and health problems, particularly cardiovascular disease. Eating too many calories from any source can lead to weight gain.

Be Cautious About Consuming a Very Low-Fat Diet

Very low-fat diets might result in nutritional deficiencies, especially in children, growing teens, pregnant women, and the elderly. Students should aim for a total fat intake of no more than 30% of their total calories, and a saturated fat intake of no more than 10% of their total calories. Fat provides essential fatty acids and transports vitamins A, D, E, and K. It is also an important energy source, providing 9 calories per gram. Fat makes food more palatable and flavorful and provides a feeling of fullness.

"Sometimes Foods" Are Okay Now and Then

The American Heart Association's *Dietary Guidelines for Americans* recommends balancing your "total diet," but allows for occasional indulgences in high-fat or sugar foods.

"Sometimes foods" is a simple way to describe foods that should be eaten in moderation because they are high in fat or sugar, are low in nutrients, or are not nutrient dense (i.e., the ratio of nutrients to calories is low). Examples include corn chips or potato chips (high in fat, low in nutrients), grilled cheese sandwiches (lots of nutrients but high in saturated fat), bacon (high in saturated fat), and most candy bars (high in fat and sugar, low in nutrients). A healthier substitute for chips, baked goods, and other high-fat foods would be to choose varieties that have been prepared with healthier oils. Then an occasional indulgence would be less important.

How Do You Moderate Fat in Your Diet?

Here are some ways to reduce total fat and saturated fat consumption:

- Eat smaller amounts of high-fat sauces or toppings with pasta and salad.
- Select snack foods wisely.
- Reduce trips to fast-food restaurants.
- Bake or roast food instead of frying.
- Remove poultry skin and trim visible fat from red meats.
- Use less or no butter or margarine on breads or potatoes.
- Choose low-fat menu selections to complement higher-fat foods (e.g., choose a salad instead of French fries to go with hamburger).

To reduce your risk of heart disease, replace saturated fats like butter with unsaturated fats like vegetable oils or margarine made with no trans fats.

References

Bierer, L.A., Warner, L., Lawson, S., and Cohen, T. 1991. *Life science: The challenge of discovery*. Lexington, MA: Heath.

Harvard Medical School. 1997. Heart Association dietary guidelines. *Harvard Heart Letter* 7(6):4-6.

Knutson, R.D., Penn, J.B., and Boehm, W.T. 1983. *Agricultural and food policy.* Englewood Cliffs, NJ: Prentice-Hall.

Krauss, R.M., Deckelbaum, R.J., Ernst, N., Fisher, E., Howard, B.V., Knopp, R.H., Kotchen, T., Lichtenstein, A.H., McGill, H.C., Pearson, T.A., Prewit, T.E., Stone, N.J., Van Horn, L., and Weinberg, R. 1996. Dietary guidelines for healthy American adults: A statement for health professionals from the Nutrition Committee, American Heart Association. *Circulation* 94:1795-1800.

National Dairy Council. 1994. *Leader guide to the guide to good eating and daily food guide pyramid.* Rosemont, IL: Author.

U.S. Department of Agriculture. 1996. *Team Nutrition Connections* 3(2).

U.S. Department of Agriculture and U.S. Department of Health and Human Services. Food Guide Pyramid.

U.S. Department of Agriculture and U.S. Department of Health and Human Services. 2000. *Nutrition and your health: Dietary guidelines for Americans 2000*, 5th edition. **www.usda.gov/cnpp**

U.S. Department of Health and Human Services. 2000. Healthy People 2010, conference edition, vols. I and II. **www.health.gov/healthypeople**

Name _____

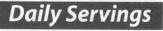

Recommended Number of Servings for Girls and Boys Aged 11-14

Food group	Girls (2,200 calories/day)	Boys (2,500 calories/day)
Bread, cereal, rice, and pasta	9 servings	11 servings
Vegetable	4	5
Fruit	3	4
Milk, yogurt, and cheese	2.5	2.5
Meat, poultry, fish, dry beans, eggs, and nuts	2-5	2.5

What Counts as One Serving?

Food group	1 serving
Bread, cereal, rice, and pasta	1 slice of bread 1 tortilla, roll, muffin 1/2 bagel, English muffin, hamburger bun 1/2 cup cooked cereal, grits, rice, pasta 1 oz (about 1 cup) ready-to-eat breakfast cereal
Vegetable	1 cup raw leafy vegetables 1/2 cup other chopped vegetables 1/2 cup other cooked vegetables 3/4 cup vegetable juice
Fruit	1 medium apple, banana, orange, pear 1/2 grapefruit 1/4 cantaloupe 1/2 cup of raw, canned, cooked, frozen fruit 1/4 cup raisins, dried fruit 3/4 cup of fruit juice
Milk, yogurt, and cheese	1 cup milk or yogurt 1.5 oz natural cheese (e.g., cheddar) 2 oz. processed cheese (e.g., American)

Planet Health: Looking for Patterns

Food group	One serving
Meat, poultry, fish, dry beans, eggs, and nuts	2.5 oz. of cooked, lean meat, poultry, or fish
	1/2 cup cooked dry beans, peas
	1 egg
	2 tablespoons peanut butter
	1/3 cup nuts, seeds

How Much Fat is Okay?

The U.S. Dietary Guidelines recommend consuming no more than 30% of calories from total fat and no more than 10% of calories from saturated fat. For adolescents this translates to

- about 73 grams per day total fat (24 or fewer grams saturated fat) for 11–14-year-old girls (based on a 2,200 calorie diet), and
- about 83 grams per day total fat (28 or fewer grams saturated fat) for 11–14-year-old boys (based on a 2,500 calorie diet).

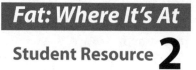

Table 1 Fat in the Five Food Groups

Fat (grams)	Food group				
	Grain	**Fruit**	**Vegetable**	**Milk**	**Meat**
0 g	Cold cereal (1 oz) Hot cereal (1/2 cup) Macaroni, plain (1/2 cup) Rice, white (1/2 cup)	Apple (1 medium) Applesauce (1/2 cup) Banana (1 medium) Cantaloupe (1/4 melon) Fruit cocktail (1/2 cup) Grapefruit (1/2 medium) Grapes (1/2 cup) Orange (1 medium) Orange juice (1/2 cup) Peaches (1/2 cup) Pear (1 medium or 1/2 cup) Pineapple (1/2 cup) Raisins (1/4 cup) Strawberries (1/2 cup) Watermelon (1/2 cup)	Broccoli (1/2 cup) Cabbage (1/2 cup) Carrot (1) Cauliflower (1/2 cup) Celery (1) Corn, frozen, cooked (1/2 cup) Greens (1/2 cup) Green beans (1/2 cup) Green peas (1/2 cup) Green pepper (1/2 pepper) Lettuce (1/2 cup) Baked potato (1 large) Sweet potato, baked (1/2 medium) Fresh tomato (1) Tomato juice (1/2 cup) Tossed salad, no dressing (1/2 cup) Zucchini (1/2 cup)	Chocolate milk, nonfat (1 cup) Skim milk (1 cup)	Black-eyed peas (1/2 cup) Pinto beans, dried, cooked (1/2 cup)
1 g	Plain bagel (1/2 bagel) Bran flakes (1 oz) Pita bread (1/2 pita) White, whole wheat bread (1 slice) Graham crackers (2) Saltine crackers (4) French bread (1 slice) Hamburger, hot dog bun (1/2 bun) Hard roll (1/2 roll) English muffin (1/2 muffin)		Corn, canned, cream style (1/2 cup) Corn on the cob, fresh, cooked (1 ear) Winter squash, fresh, baked (1/2 cup)	Cottage cheese, 1% lowfat (1/2 cup)	Flounder/sole, baked (3 oz) Refried beans, canned (1/2 cup)

			Food group		
Fat (grams)	**Grain**	**Fruit**	**Vegetable**	**Milk**	**Meat**
	Oatmeal, instant (1/2 cup) Raisin bran (1 oz) Brown rice (1/2 cup) Corn tortilla (6")				
3 g	Biscuit (1) Whole wheat crackers (2) Dinner roll (1) Pancake, plain (4") Flour tortilla (8")		Coleslaw (1/2 cup) Sweet potato, candied (1/2 medium)	Cottage cheese 2% lowfat (1/2 cup) Parmesan cheese, grated (1 Tbsp) Ice milk (1/2 cup) Milk 1% lowfat (1 cup) Yogurt, frozen (1/2 cup) Yogurt, fruit flavored, lowfat (1 cup)	Chicken, roasted, no skin (3 oz) Halibut, baked (3 oz) Tuna, canned in water (3 oz)
5 g	Snack crackers (4) Croissant, plain (1/2 roll) Granola (1 oz) Blueberry muffin (1 small) Bran muffin (1 small)		French-fried potatoes, oven-heated (10) Mashed potatoes (1/2 cup)	Cottage cheese, creamed (1/2 cup) Mozzarella cheese, part skim (1 oz) Ice cream, store brand (1/2 cup) Milk, 2% lowfat (1 cup) Chocolate milk, 2% lowfat (1 cup) Pudding (1/2 cup)	Bologna, turkey (1 oz) Canadian bacon (2 slices) Chicken, roasted, with skin (3 oz) Egg, hard-cooked (1) Egg, scrambled (1) Roast beef, lean (3 oz) Tofu (1/2 cup) Tuna, canned in oil (3 oz) Turkey (3 oz)
10 g	Waffle, homemade (7")		French-fried potatoes, fried (10) Hash brown potatoes (1/2 cup)	American cheese (1 oz) Cheddar cheese (1 oz) Monterey cheese (1 oz) Swiss cheese (1 oz) Ice cream, premium (1/2 cup) Ice cream soft serve (1/2 cup)	Bacon (3 slices) Bologna (1 oz) Chicken, fried, batter dipped (3 oz) Egg, fried (1) Fish sticks, oven-heated (3 oz) Ham (3 oz) Hot dog, chicken (2 oz) Salmon, baked (3 oz)

(continued)

Table 1 Fat in the Five Food Groups *(continued)*

Fat (grams)	Grain	Fruit	Vegetable	Milk	Meat
10 g *(cont.)*				Whole milk (1 cup) Milkshake (10 fl. oz)	Sausage, link (2) Sausage, patty (1) Shrimp, breaded and fried (3 oz) Steak, rib eye, broiled (3 oz) Steak, sirloin, broiled (3 oz) Steak, T-bone, broiled (3 oz)
15 g			Avocado, sliced (1/2 medium)		Ground beef, extra lean, broiled (3 oz) Hot dog, beef (2 oz) KFC's original recipe chicken (3 oz) McDonald's chicken McNuggets (6) Peanut butter (2 Tbsp) Pork chop, broiled (3 oz) Roast beef, lean and fat (3 oz) Sunflower seeds, no shell (1/4 cup)
25 g					Polish sausage (3 oz) Spareribs (3 oz)

Note: 1 oz of cheese = 1 1/2" square; vegetables are prepared without added fat.

Adapted from *Fat: A Balancing Act*, Washington State Dairy Council.

Table 2 Fat in Combination Foods and Extras

Fat (grams)	Combination foods	Extras
0 g		Angel food cake (1/12 cake) Barbeque sauce (1 Tbsp) Catsup (1 Tbsp) Coffee (1 cup) Gelatin, flavored (1/2 cup) Honey (1 tsp) Iced tea (12 fl. oz) Jelly (1 tsp) Maple syrup (1 Tbsp) Pickle (1) Popcorn, air-popped, no butter (1 cup) Soft drink, cola (12 fl. oz) Sugar (1 tsp) Tea (1 cup)
1 g	Baked beans (1 cup)	French dressing, low calorie (1 Tbsp) Beef gravy, canned (1/4 cup) Mustard (1 Tbsp) Pretzels (1 oz)
3 g	Chicken noodle soup, canned (1 cup) Clam chowder soup, with water or skim milk (1 cup) Cream of tomato soup, with water or skim milk (1 cup)	Coffee creamer, nondairy, liquid (1 Tbsp) Cream half-and-half (1 Tbsp) Popcorn, oil-popped, no butter (1 cup) Sour cream (1 Tbsp)
5 g	Cheese pizza (1/4 of 12") Clam chowder soup, with whole milk (1 cup) Cream of tomato soup, with whole milk (1 cup)	Brownie, with nuts (1 small) Butter (1 tsp) Chocolate chip cookies (2 small) French dressing, regular (1 Tbsp) Granola bar, plain (1 oz) Italian dressing (1 Tbsp) Margarine (1 tsp) Popcorn, oil-popped, buttered (1 cup) Popcorn, microwave, light (3 cups)
10 g	Beef and vegetable stew (1 cup) Beef burrito (1) Chili (1 cup) Chicken chow mein (1 cup) Macaroni and cheese, frozen, cooked (1 cup) McDonald's Egg McMuffin (1) Cheese and Pepperoni pizza (1/4 of 12") Spaghetti with meatballs (1 cup) Sub sandwich, with meat (2 oz) and cheese (1 oz) Taco Bell's bean burrito (1)	Chocolate cake (1/16 cake) Chocolate candy bar, plain (1 oz) Corn chips (1 oz) Cream cheese (1 oz) Doughnut, cake-type, plain (1) Mayonnaise (1 Tbsp) Oil and vinegar dressing, homemade (1 Tbsp) Pie, chocolate cream (1/8 of 9" pie) Potato chips (1 oz) Tortilla chips (1 oz) Popcorn, microwave (3 cups)

(continued)

Table 2 Fat in Combination Foods and Extras *(continued)*

Fat (grams)	Combination foods	Extras
	Taco Bell's taco (1) Tuna salad (1/2 cup) Turkey sandwich (3 oz meat) Wendy's chili (9oz)	
15 g	Arby's roast beef sandwich (1) Chef salad, no dressing (1 1/2 cups) Beef chop suey Dairy Queen's hot dog (1) Lasagna, no meat (2.5″ × 2.5″) Peanut butter (2 Tbsp) and jelly sandwich (1) Roast beef sandwich (3 oz meat) Wendy's single hamburger, plain (1)	Doughnut, yeast, glazed (1) Pie, apple (1/8 of 9″ pie) Sweet roll, cinnamon (1)
20 g	Burger King's Croissan'wich (1) Cheeseburger, regular (1) Chicken stir fry, with rice (1 1/2 cups) Dairy Queens chili dog (1) Cheese enchilada (1) Cheese and beef enchilada (1) Lasagna, with meat (2.5″ × 2.5″) Macaroni and cheese, homemade (1 cup) Quiche, without bacon (1/8 pie) Taco (1 small)	Cheesecake (1/12 cake)
25 g	Burger King's Whaler (1) Chicken pot pie, frozen, baked (1) Chicken salad (1/2 cup) McDonald's Filet-O-Fish (1) Quiche, with bacon (1/8 pie) Wendy's broccoli and cheese potato (1)	Pie, pecan (1/8 of 9″ pie)
30 g	Fish sandwich, with cheese (1) McDonald's Big Mac (1) McDonald's biscuit with sausage (1) Pizza Hut's supreme personal pan pizza (1)	
35 g	Arby's roast chicken club (1) Burger King's Whopper (1) Cheeseburger, large (1) Wendy's Big Classic (1)	

Adapted from *Fat: A Balancing Act*, Washington State Diary Council

School lunch programs work hard to provide healthy, good tasting meals for students. Of course, it's hard to please everybody! This is your opportunity to analyze the nutritional content of your school's lunches and appreciate the people who prepare them. What's for lunch this week? Can you choose from a variety of foods with selections from each of the food groups in the Food Guide Pyramid? To answer these questions, you will analyze this week's lunch menus (5 days) and report your findings on the attached form. You will work in groups to complete this assignment. Each group will evaluate one day's menu; then the class will pool all the findings.

Group Assignments

1. In the table, list all the foods from the meal assigned to your group. If your school offers multiple entrees for a given day, choose one meal.

2. Use student resource 1 to determine which food groups are represented and the number of servings of each food group provided by this meal.

Food	Quantity	Food group					
		Grain	Fruit	Veggie	Meat	Dairy	Other
Example: cheese pizza, with peppers	1 large slice	1		1		1	
Total							

3. Figure out the total number of servings for each food group. Record your findings in the food pyramid below.

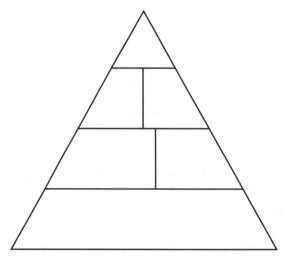

4. Report your findings to the rest of the class, and record their findings in the food pyramids below.

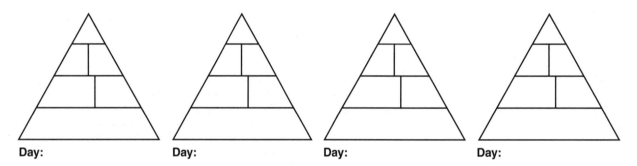

Day: Day: Day: Day:

5. Analyze your findings below using either inequalities OR statistics.

Inequalities Analysis

Because lunch is one of our three daily meals, it should provide approximately 1/3 of the recommended daily servings for each food group. Use the following table to compare the number of servings provided in each lunch menu with the number of recommended servings.

- If the number of servings provided in the lunch is **less than** 1/3 the Food Guide Pyramid recommendations, put a (<) sign in the appropriate column.
- If the number of servings provided in the lunch is **greater than** 1/3 the Food Guide Pyramid recommendations, put a (>) sign in the appropriate column.
- If the number of servings provided in the lunch is **equal to** 1/3 the Food Guide Pyramid recommendations, put an (=) sign in the appropriate column.
- Total the number of (>), (<), and (=) signs for each food group.

For example: If 3 servings of meat were served on Monday, you should put a (>) sign in the row for meat because 3 > 0.5-1 servings recommended.

Food groups	1/3 FGP daily recommended servings	Days of the week					Total		
		Mon.	Tues.	Wed.	Thurs.	Fri.	>	<	=
Grains	3								
Vegetables	1–2								
Fruits	1								
Dairy	1–2								
Meat	0.5–1								
Sometimes foods	Eat sparingly								

Analyzing Your Results

What patterns do you notice for each food group? *For example: Is the number of vegetables offered usually greater than, less than or equal to the Food Guide Pyramid recommendations for lunch? Are a variety of vegetables served (look at the menus)?*

Grain:

Vegetables:

Dairy:

Meat:

Other:

Statistical Analysis

Complete the analysis of your school lunch menus by doing the following calculations:

1. Record the **range** of servings offered for each food group in the following table.
2. Calculate the **average** number of servings offered for each food group. Record your results in the table below.
3. Calculate the **difference** between the number of daily servings recommended by the Food Guide Pyramid (choose male or female recommendations) and the average number of servings offered for each food group.
4. Calculate the **percentage** of the daily recommended servings (choose male or female recommendations) offered in the average lunch menu.

Food group	1/3 FGP daily recommendation	Range	Average	Difference (average − recommendation)	Percent (average \ recommendation × 100)
Grain	3				
Vegetables	1–2				
Fruits	1				
Dairy	1–2				
Meat	0.5–1				
Sometimes foods	Eat sparingly				

Looking for Patterns: Interpreting Your Findings

1. Is a large range of servings offered in any food groups? Which ones?

2. Are there any food groups that are offered an **average** of less than 1/3 of the recommended number of servings? Which groups?

3. Which column of numbers tells you **how many more servings** of each food group you need to eat to reach the recommended number of servings for a given day?

Conclusions

1. What comments would you make to the United States Department of Agriculture about your school's lunch program? Cite specific information that demonstrates your school lunches are designed with the Food Guide Pyramid in mind. Explain how they are adhering to the three guiding principles of :

- **Proportionality:** offering foods from all of the food groups.
- **Variety:** offering a variety of foods from each food group.
- **Moderation:** offering appropiate serving sizes and offering high-fat foods and sweets sparingly.

2. Based on your analyses, what recommendations for improvements would you make?

3. How many more servings of fruits and vegetables do children who eat lunch at your school need to consume on average at breakfast, dinner, and snacks to reach the 5-A-Day fruit and vegetable recommendation?

School lunch programs work hard to provide healthy, good tasting meals for students. Of course, it's hard to please everybody! Your class has been hired by the United States Department of Agriculture (USDA) to examine the fat content of your school cafeteria lunch menus. Are the meal selections generally low, moderate, or high in fat? To answer this question you will look at the fat content of this week's lunch menus (5 days) and report your findings on the attached form. You will work in groups to complete this assignment. Each group will evaluate one day's menu, then the class will pool all the findings.

Group Assignments

1. List the foods from the meal assigned to your group in the table below.
2. Use student resource 2 *Fat: Where It's At* to determine how many grams (g) of fat are in each of the foods. Put a check in the column that corresponds to the fat content of each food item. If you eat two servings of a food item, put two checks in the corresponding column (two slices of pizza = ✔✔ in the 5 g column). You may have to estimate the fat content of combination foods by comparing them to similar foods listed in the charts.
3. Determine the total number of servings in each category by counting the number of checks in each column. Report your findings to the class.

Day of Week

Foods	Low (0–3 grams of fat)	Moderate (5–15 grams of fat)	High (20–35 grams of fat)
Example: 1 slice cheese pizza		✔	
Total number of servings			

4. Use the information from the other groups in the class to complete the following frequency table. Record the total number of servings in each category.

Day of the week	Low (0–3 grams of fat)	Moderate (5–15 grams of fat)	High (20–35 grams of fat)
Monday			
Tuesday			
Wednesday			
Thursday			
Friday			
Weekly total			

5. Make a histogram to display the data from the frequency table above.
   • Label the *y*-axis **Number of servings** and the *x*-axis **Day of the week.**
   • Use a different color bar to represent each of the categories of fat content.
   • Plot the frequency for each category in Monday's menu.
   • Leave a space between Monday's and Tuesday's bars. Repeat for each day of the week.

Complete the analysis of your school lunch menus as directed below.

1. Look at the histogram. What patterns do you notice? Is there variability in the number of servings offered in each category?

2. Which day of the week were the following offered:
   • The largest number of high-fat food servings?

   • The lowest number of high-fat food servings?

   • The largest number of low-fat food servings?

   • The lowest number of low-fat food servings?

3. What percentage of the weekly total of servings were in the high-fat category? (Number of high-fat servings/total number of servings × 100 = % in high-fat category.)

4. What percentage of the weekly total servings were in the low-fat category? (Number of low-fat servings/total number of servings × 100 = % in low-fat category.)

5. Based on your analysis, write a paragraph that defends or refutes the following statement: *"Although our school lunches contain some foods high in fat, most of the food selections contain low to moderate quantities of fat."*

Apples, Oranges, and Zucchini: An Algebra Party

This lesson uses individual and group math activities. Calculators are desirable. Students will use algebra to plan a real-life activity (budgeting and buying food for a party) that incorporates the 5-A-Day theme of eating at least five fruits and vegetables every day. This lesson is designed to infuse information about choosing healthy foods into a classroom pre-algebra or algebra unit.

▶▶ Behavioral Objective

To gain skills and practice in selecting at least five fruits and vegetables a day.

▶▶ Learning Objectives

Students will be able to

1. write and solve one- and two-variable equations combining addition with multiplication,
2. apply math skills to using a budget, and
3. use unit pricing for fruits and vegetables.

▶▶ Materials

- Activity 1 *Plan Your Party!*
- Calculators (optional)

▶▶ Procedure

1. (3-5 minutes) Review the 5-A-Day recommendation with students, making sure they understand that eating at least five a day refers to fruits and vegetables *combined,* not to eating five fruits and five vegetables. Encourage students to eat at least two servings of fruit and at least three servings of vegetables (with at least one serving of a dark green or orange vegetable) for a total of five servings per day. Make sure students are familiar with the terms "sometimes foods" and "everyday foods" (see Teacher Resources).

2. (5-10 minutes) As needed, review algebra used in this lesson: two-step equations combining addition with multiplication.

3. (10 minutes) Scenario: Read aloud and use the board: *Your class deserves to have a party! You can have the party at your house, as long as you pay for the food. Searching*

for ways to raise money, you ask around and find out that your neighbors will pay you 75¢ for every bag of leaves that you rake.

Example 1: Using algebra, write an expression that shows how much money you can earn for the party by raking leaves. Let x be the number of bags of leaves that students rake. Then,

$0.75x$ = party budget in dollars

You are allowed to serve a few "sometimes foods" at the party (foods you should try not to eat every day, like potato chips). If you also serve five different fruits and vegetables, everyone will get an extra 10¢ for every bag of leaves they rake and be allowed to stay an hour longer at the party! Hooray! Eating five a day will help keep you healthy. In fact, nutrition experts say everybody should try to eat at least five fruits and vegetables every day.

Example 2: With the extra 10¢ per bag, the math formula for your party budget has changed. What is it now?

$0.75x + $0.10x$ = new party budget in dollars

SIMPLIFY: $0.85x$ = new party budget in dollars

Example 3: Your goal as a class is to raise $50 for the party. How many bags of leaves does your class need to rake? Use math to figure it out. Let x = the number of bags of leaves.

$0.85x = $50

x = $50 / $0.85

x = 58.8 bags of leaves.

Round off 58.8 to the nearest whole number. As a group, you need to rake 59 bags of leaves. *Bonus:* How many bags does each person need to rake? Make up and solve the math expression for this question.

$59 / x$, where x = the number of students in the class

   4. (15-20 minutes) Carry out the group activity below:

   A. Divide class into groups of up to four.

   B. Pass out activity 1 *Plan Your Party!* to each group. Review the worksheet.

   C. On the board, work out the following example with the class:

Example 1: How many pounds of apples can you buy with $4, if apples cost $1 per pound ($1/lb)? Write this as an equation, using x to stand for the number of pounds you can buy:

$1/lb $\times$ x lb = $4

$1/lb / $1/lb $\times$ x lb = $4 / $1/lb

x = 4 lb

Example 2: If you substitute y for the unit price of apples, you have a two-variable expression you could use to figure out how many pounds of any item (for example, oranges or zucchini) you can buy with $4. Remember that x still stands for the solution in pounds:

$y / lb $\times$ x lb = $4

D. Complete activity 1 *Plan Your Party!* in groups.

E. Discuss answers to the activity with entire class.

▶▶ Extension Activity

Have a class party and serve the food from one of the groups' menus.

▶▶ Teacher Resources

General Background Material

In preparing for this lesson, you may want to refer to *Time to Take Five.* See appendix A for information on how to obtain this resource.

Specific Background Material

Definitions:

• "Sometimes foods" is a simple phrase describing foods that should be eaten in moderation because they are high in fat or sugar, are low in vitamins or minerals, or are not nutrient dense (i.e., the ratio of vitamins or minerals to calories is low). Examples include corn chips or potato chips (high in fat, low in vitamins and minerals), grilled cheese sandwiches (high in protein and calcium but also high in fat), bacon (high in fat), and most candy bars (high in fat and sugar, low in vitamins and minerals).

• "Everyday foods" is a simple way to describe foods like fruits, vegetables, whole grain foods, fish or chicken, and so on that can be eaten daily because they provide plenty of nutrition and adequate amounts of fat and calories for health.

Bear in mind that *Planet Health* lessons in other subjects teach students about the 5 A Day recommendation in more depth. Hence, assuming that students have already been exposed to at least one of those lessons, this lesson can serve as a practical application, and math teachers need to spend only a few minutes reminding students about the 5 A Day theme.

Name _____

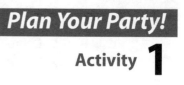
Apples, Oranges, and Zucchini: An Algebra Party

You've finished raking and you have $50! Congratulations! So now it's party time! You've spent $30 on chips, dips, drinks, cups, napkins, balloons, and streamers, and now you have $20 left for your five fruits and vegetables. That's $4 for each type of fruit or vegetable you pick. Each group will spend the $20 using algebra and following the directions below. Here is a list of fruits and vegetables and their unit prices. (Remember, lb = pound.)

Item	Unit price	Item	Unit price
Apples	$1.50 / pound	Green beans	$1.00 / pound
Bananas	$0.75 / pound	Oranges	$1.25 / pound
Broccoli	$1.00 / pound	Mangoes	$1.50 / pound
Carrots	$1.00 / pound	Red peppers	$3.00 / pound
Cauliflower	$1.50 / pound	Strawberries	$2.50 / pound
Celery	$1.10 / pound	Watermelon	$0.75 / pound
Cherry tomatoes	$1.50 / pound	Zucchini	$0.75 / pound
Grapes	$1.50 / pound		

1. Pick any combination of five fruits and vegetables (four fruits and one vegetable, two fruits and three vegetables, etc.).
2. Write your five picks in the table below and fill in the rest of the table.
3. Using the unit prices (y), figure out how many pounds of each of your choices you can buy (x).
4. Remember, $x = \$4 / y$.

Item name	$4 ÷ Y		= X pound(s)
Example: green beans	*$4 ÷*	*$1.00*	*= 4 pounds*
1.	$4 ÷		= pound(s)
2.	$4 ÷		= pound(s)
3.	$4 ÷		= pound(s)
4.	$4 ÷		= pound(s)
5.	$4 ÷		= pound(s)

Bonus

1. Which two items can you buy the most of with $4?
2. Which two items can you buy the least of with $4?

Plotting Coordinate Graphs: What Does Your Day Look Like?

In this lesson, students learn that a healthy body weight can be maintained by balancing the amount of energy they consume with the amount of energy they expend. Students will examine their own activity patterns and energy expenditure by making coordinate graphs of a given day's activity intensity. This lesson is designed to complement a graphing unit.

▶▶ Behavioral Objective

For students to be more aware of their own activity levels and to be more physically active.

▶▶ Learning Objectives

Students will be able to

1. construct a coordinate system with a labeled *x*-axis and *y*-axis,
2. graph ordered pairs on a coordinate system,
3. draw inferences and reason with tables and graphs that summarize personal activity data,
4. discuss the role physical activity plays in maintaining a healthy body weight, and
5. describe the physical activity recommendations for adolescents.

▶▶ Materials

- Overhead transparency masters 1, 2, and 3 (or handout or use chalkboard)
- Activity 1 *What Does Your Day Look Like?*
- Graph paper
- Ruler

▶▶ Procedure

1. (2-3 minutes) Get students thinking about why physical activity is important by displaying overhead transparency 1. *(The words that complete each of the blanks are "physical activity.")*
2. (2 minutes) Point out the goals of this activity:
    - To discuss the role physical activity plays in maintaining a healthy body weight

• To discuss the physical activity recommendations

• To graph physical activity intensity for yesterday

3. (5-7 minutes) Use overhead transparency 2 to explain the concept of energy balance and the role physical activity plays in maintaining a healthy body weight. Elicit student responses to fill in the blanks on the transparency. Test their understanding of your explanation by asking selected students to complete the sentences on overhead transparency 3. *(Answers: decreases, increases, increases, decreases.)*

4. (3 minutes) Display the activity recommendations for adolescents listed at the bottom of overhead transparency 3. Discuss some examples of activities that require moderate to vigorous levels of exertion.

5. (3 minutes) Hand out activity sheets. Review the definition of MET units described at the top of activity 1.

6. (25-45 minutes) Have students complete the activity sheets and the corresponding coordinate graphs of their activity data. *(Note:* In part II, do not try to have students estimate the average METs expended over half-hour intervals. Have students record what they were doing at each time point only.)

7. (5 minutes) Discuss student responses to the discussion questions at the end of activity 1.

▶▶ Extension Activity

Have students design and implement a plan for increasing their daily activity. Require them to keep a diary of their activity for one, two, or three days during this time and graph their data. How has their energy expenditure changed as a result of their increase in activity?

▶▶ Teacher Resources

General Background Material

In preparing for this lesson, you may want to refer to the following resources:

• *Centers for Disease Control and Prevention Fact Sheets on Physical Activity*

• *Healthy People 2010*

• *Compendium of Physical Activities: Classification of Energy Costs of Human Physical Activities*

See appendix B for information on how to obtain these resources.

Specific Background Material

Maintaining an Energy Balance

The human body requires energy for physical activity, growth, digestion, respiration, and many other body functions. Food provides us with our energy supply as well as other essential minerals and vitamins. Energy is stored in the carbohydrates, fats, and proteins contained in food. The amount of energy stored in foods is measured in calories. Fat provides 9 calories per gram, while carbohydrates and proteins each provide 4 calories per gram. To maintain an energy balance, the amount of calories consumed *(energy input)* in food must equal the amount of calories expended *(energy output)*. If more calories are taken in than are expended, they are stored by the body primarily as fat and a person gains weight.

In children or youth, excess fat stores would be evident from weight gain greater than that expected for healthy growth. The amount of energy required to contract muscles during physical activity accounts for the second largest component (20-50%) of total energy expenditure (the largest component being metabolic processes) and the largest component that we have control over. Growth adds only 1% to daily energy requirements. We can use or "burn" more of the calories that we consume by increasing our physical activity. More vigorous activities require more energy expenditure and therefore "burn" more calories than less vigorous activities over the same time period.

Calorie Requirements and Dietary Sources of Energy

People have different energy requirements depending on age and sex. The *Recommended Dietary Allowances,* 10th edition, notes that 11–14-year-old girls need 2,200 calories per day, while boys this age need 2,500. These are averages that can vary a bit from day to day. They also vary according to an individual's activity level and size. Compared to her peers who don't exercise, an athletic adolescent girl may need an additional 300-1,000 calories, and an athletic adolescent male may need an additional 600-1,500 calories per day! These active teens are using their energy stores at a faster rate than less inactive teens.

The Food Guide Pyramid reminds us to eat a certain number of servings from each of the five major food groups each day. People with higher energy needs require more servings than less active people do in order to get all the calories they need. Notice that the extra calories come from a healthy balance of foods, maintaining the balance of fat, carbohydrate, and protein. Active adolescents need more calories than their less active peers; they should choose to get them by increasing overall consumption, not by filling up on high-fat snacks. Athletes who consistently need lots and lots of extra calories look to complex carbohydrates (starchy foods like bread and pasta), not fats or proteins, to take up the slack.

Some daily dietary variation in energy and food intake is normal. Exercise helps regulate appetite. Your body will need more energy and will tell you by feeling hungrier!

Planet Health's Activity Message

Physical activity promotes health and well-being, and offers opportunities to socialize and have fun. Adolescents should be moderately active for at least 30 minutes every day or nearly every day as part of play, games, sports, chores, transportation, or planned exercise, AND they should participate in at least three sessions per week of vigorous physical activity lasting 20 minutes or more. Adolescents should aim for a total of 60 minutes or more of activity on five to seven days a week.

What is a MET value?

(*Note:* Students do not need to understand how METs relate to calories to complete this activity. They need only to understand that it is a unit used to compare the exercise intensities or energy expenditures of various activities.) A *MET* is an intensity unit assigned to all activities and is based on the rate of energy expenditure required for a given activity. Vigorous activities require more energy or METs than less intense activities. Sitting quietly requires 1 MET of energy expenditure and is defined as your resting metabolic rate, or RMR (Ainsworth et al. 1993). For the average adult, the RMR is approximately 1 kilocalorie (kcal) per kilogram (kg) body weight per hour. Activities "are classified as multiples of one MET or the ratio of the . . . metabolic rate for a specific activity divided by the resting metabolic rate" (Ainsworth et al. 1993). Dancing requires five times as much energy as sitting, or 5 METs of energy expenditure.

Pate and associates (1995) define moderate activity as 3.0-6.0 METs and vigorous activity as more than 6 METs.

By multiplying the body weight in kilograms by the MET value and duration of activity, it is possible to estimate the energy expenditure (kcal) for a specific person. For example, bicycling at a 4 MET value expends 4 kcal/kg body weight/hour. A 60-kilogram person (approximately 132 pounds) bicycling for 40 minutes expends the following:

$$4 \text{ METs} \times 60 \text{ kg body weight}) \times (40 \text{ min} / 60 \text{ min}) = 160 \text{ kcal}$$

What are the risks of a sedentary lifestyle?

Activity is required for health. Studies suggest that physically active individuals enjoy lower risks of developing cardiovascular disease, diabetes, colon cancer, osteoporosis, and anxiety and depression relative to sedentary individuals. TV viewing, a major component of inactivity, is one of the major causes of overweight among youth. TV watching also has been associated with elevated cholesterol levels and poor cardiovascular fitness.

What are the benefits of a more active lifestyle?

Activity helps children develop and retain cardiovascular fitness, muscle strength, and confidence in their physical ability. Regular activity helps individuals maintain a healthy weight, build lean muscle, and reduce fat. It can reduce stress and brighten a person's mood. Regular exercise helps develop and maintain dense bones, and thereby helps prevent osteoporosis. Likewise, active adults have a lower risk of developing diabetes, high blood pressure, and colon cancer, and are at lower risk of dying prematurely.

What are some examples of things you can do to increase your activity and decrease your inactivity?

Take the stairs; don't park next to the building; walk or ride your bike to school if there is a safe route; walk around the mall or the neighborhood with friends; watch only your favorite TV shows; remove or unplug the TV in your bedroom; play catch with a sibling, a friend, or a parent.

References

Ainsworth, B.E., et al. 1993. Compendium of physical activities: Classification of energy costs of human physical activities. *Medicine and Science in Sports and Exercise* 25(1): 71-80.

Bierer, L.A., Warner, L., Lawson, S., and Cohen, T. 1991. *Life science: The challenge of discovery*. Lexington, MA: Heath.

National Dairy Council. 1994. *Leader guide to the guide to good eating and daily food guide pyramid*. Rosemont, IL: Author.

National Research Council. 1989. *Recommended dietary allowances*. 10th ed. Washington, D.C.: National Academy Press.

Pate, R., et al. 1995. Physical activity and public health: A recommendation from the Centers for Disease Control and Prevention and the American College of Sports Medicine. *Journal of the American Medical Association* 273(5): 402-407.

U.S. Department of Health and Human Servcies. 2000. Healthy People 2010, conference edition, vols. I and II. **www.health.gov/healthypeople**

▶▶ Answer Key

Answers to Blanks on Overhead Transparencies

Overhead 1: Physical activity
Overhead 2: Increases, decreases
Overhead 3: Decreases, increases, increases, decreases

Answers to Activity 1, Part I

1. B, 1.5 METs
2. C, 10
3. D, 4
4. A, 2.5
5. E, 1.0

What two words can be used to start each of these sentences?

_____ _____ is fun!!!

_____ _____ puts you in a better mood.

_____ _____ helps your heart get stronger.

_____ _____ builds strong muscles and bones.

_____ _____ uses energy which helps you maintain a healthy body weight.

Maintaining an Energy Balance

Energy input = Food

Energy output = Physical activity + Growing + Other body functions

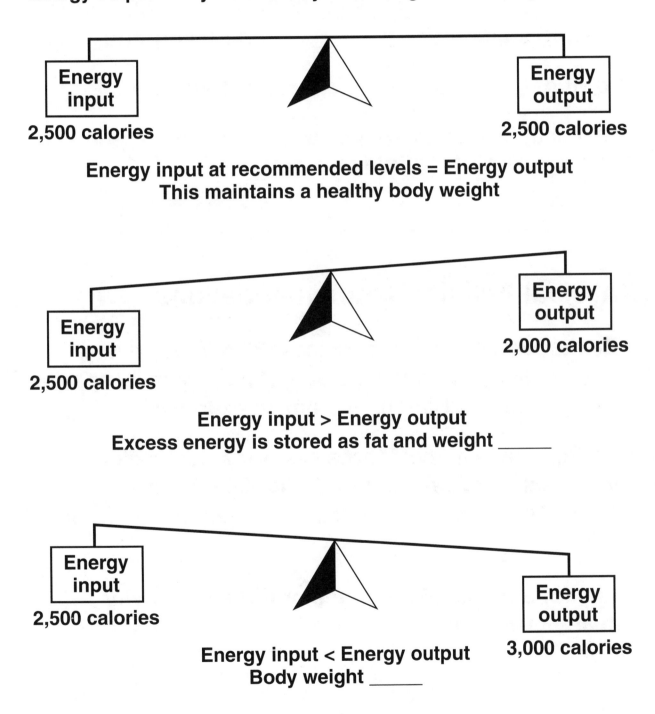

Energy input — 2,500 calories

Energy output — 2,500 calories

Energy input at recommended levels = Energy output
This maintains a healthy body weight

Energy input — 2,500 calories

Energy output — 2,000 calories

Energy input > Energy output
Excess energy is stored as fat and weight _____

Energy input — 2,500 calories

Energy output — 3,000 calories

Energy input < Energy output
Body weight _____

Choose the word <u>INCREASES</u> or <u>DECREASES</u> to complete each of the sentences below.

Watching TV _____ energy output.

Climbing stairs _____ energy output.

Growing _____ energy output.

If physical activity increases and food consumption stays the same, then body weight _____.

Physical Activity Recommendations

- **Be moderately active for at least 30 minutes every day or nearly every day as part of play, games, sports, chores, transportation, or planned exercise.**

- **Participate in at least three sessions per week of vigorous physical activity lasting 20 minutes or more. These activities make you sweat and breathe hard.**

- **Aim for a total of 60 minutes or more of activity nearly every day.**

Definition

A MET is a unit used to compare the amount of energy required by different activities to the amount required to sit quietly. Vigorous activities require more energy or METs than less intense activities. Sitting quietly requires 1 MET of energy expenditure. Dancing requires five times as much energy as sitting or 5 METs of energy expenditure.

Part I: Interpreting Line Graphs

Sometimes a graph is used to describe a series of events. A seventh-grade girl wore an electronic monitor which recorded her activity during a typical school day. Below is a graph illustrating her activity intensity (METs) for the day. When did the events below occur? Record the letter that corresponds to each event and the MET value for the activity.

    1. The girl listened intently to her teachers.

    2. She participated in a soccer game during gym class.

    3. She quickly walked to the store for her mother.

    4. She got dressed.

    5. She watched TV.

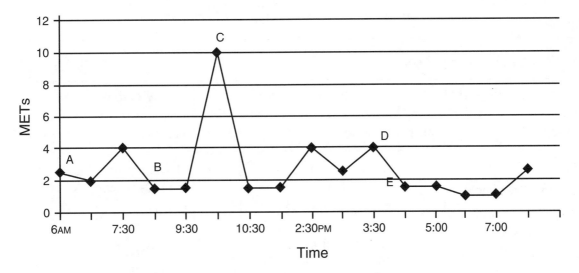

Part II: Constructing Coordinate Graphs

What did you do yesterday? In this activity you will make a coordinate graph to illustrate your activity intensity (METs) yesterday. Be as accurate as possible. Complete table 1 as follows:

    1. List the event/activity you were engaged in at each of the times listed. If you were involved in more than one activity for a given time interval, list the one activity that took **most** of the interval.

    2. Use table 2 to estimate the number of METs you were expending at each time point.

Table 1 What Did You Do Yesterday?

Time	Event	METs	Time	Event	METs
6:00 AM			2:00 PM		
6:30			2:30		
7:00			3:00		
7:30			3:30		
8:00			4:00		
8:30			4:30		
9:00			5:00		
9:30			5:30		
10:00			6:00		
10:30			6:30		
11:00			7:00		
11:30			7:30		
12:00 PM			8:00		
12:30			8:30		
1:00			9:00		
1:30			9:30		

Table 2 Examples of MET Scores

Inactivity/light activities*		Moderate activities*		Vigorous activities*	
Activity	METs	Activity	METs	Activity	METs
Sleep	0.9	Walking at a moderate pace (3.0 mph)	3.5	Shoveling snow, bicycling (10–12 mph)	6.0
Watching TV, reading	1.0	Raking, walking at a brisk pace (3.5 mph), bicycling for pleasure, horseback riding, volleyball (competitive)	4.0	Skating, rowing (moderate effort)	7.0
Sitting in class, eating, doing homework	1.5	Dancing, carrying heavy objects, skateboarding, heavy chores, baseball/softball	5.0	Basketball, football, hockey, swimming laps, calisthenics (push-ups, sit-ups), jogging, walking upstairs, tennis, bicycling (12–14 mph)	8.0
Dressing, grooming, self care, cooking, washing dishes, straightening-up, sweeping, walking at a slow pace (2 mph)	2.5			Soccer	10
				Running (8 minute mile)	12.5
				Running (6 minute mile)	16

* MET levels may be higher or lower depending on your effort.

Planet Health: Plotting Coordinate Graphs

Use graph paper to make a coordinate graph of your activity.

1. Label the *x*-axis **Time (hours)** and the *y*-axis **MET score.**
2. Number both axes as follows: *x*-axis (6 AM–10 PM); *y*-axis (0–10 or higher).
3. Graph each ordered pair from table 1 above.
4. Use your ruler to draw a line connecting adjacent data points.
5. Divide the graph into three parts by plotting the lines y = 3 and y = 6. Label the space above the *y*-axis **Inactive to light activity.** Label the space between the lines **Moderate activity.** Label the top section **Vigorous activity.** See the figure below.

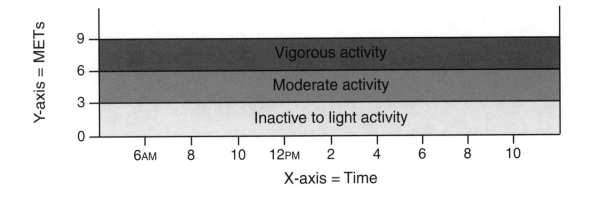

Interpreting Your Activity Patterns

1. During what part of the day were you most active?

2. During what part of the day were you least active?

3. Use the graph to estimate how much time you spent doing
   Moderate activity _____
   Vigorous activity _____

Discussion Questions

1. What fun things could you do to break up the periods of inactivity?

2. What lifestyle changes could you make to increase the amount of energy you expend doing moderate physical activity? *For example: Take the stairs instead of the elevator.*

3. What are the benefits of a very active lifestyle?

4. What are the health risks of a sedentary lifestyle?

Survey the Class

In this lesson, students assess the amount of time they spend being physically active and use this information to practice calculating means, medians, and ranges. They then pool their results to develop statistics for groups of students. This lesson is designed to infuse information about the health benefits of physical activity into a classroom unit on basic statistics.

►► Behavioral Objective

To be physically active on a regular basis.

►► Learning Objectives

Students will be able to

1. review and characterize the types and frequency of physical activity for individuals and small groups, and
2. calculate statistics and apply basic concepts of statistical analysis to survey data.

►► Materials

- Activity 1 *Personal Data Record*
- Activity 2 *Group Data*
- Activity 3 *Analyzing Class Data*

►► Procedure

1. (3-5 minutes) Discuss the importance of physical activity and its benefits. Give examples of physical activity (e.g., walking, basketball, cleaning).

2. (3-5 minutes) Discuss population surveys and how they are used to describe the opinions or behaviors of a total population (e.g., political polls, diet and activity surveys). Review specific math terms, such as mean, mode, and range.

3. (8-10 minutes) Distribute and review activity 1 *Personal Data Record*. This activity asks students to record (a) physical activities that they have done over the past seven days, and (b) the amount of time (in hours) that they have spent doing these activities over the past seven days. Have students complete activity 1. While students are working on activity 1, pass out activity 3 *Analyzing Class Data*. Have students complete the questions under Personal Data.

4. (10-15 minutes) Distribute and review activity 2 *Group Data*, which summarizes data for the group. Divide the class into several groups with approximately six

students per group. Using activity 2, tally data from the group and answer questions under Group Data on activity 3.

5. (5-8 minutes) Select a student representative from each group to describe the group findings. The teacher may assist by charting group findings (using chart from activity 2) to summarize entire class findings.

6. (5-8 minutes) Compare class findings with the recommended daily physical activity hours for the appropriate age group (see *Planet Health*'s Activity Message in Teacher Resources). Students may also be interested in comparing individual physical activity hours with recommendations. Are students moderately active every day for *at least* 30 minutes? Do they engage in vigorous activity at least three times per week for 20 minutes or more?

Note: Teachers who cannot photocopy worksheets can help students set up tables in their notebooks. Provide a sample on the board.

▶▶ Extension Activity

Have students review activity 1 *Personal Data Record* and write a data report. The report should consist of one paragraph that describes their personal activity choices and time spent being active over the past seven days. They should incorporate answers from questions 1–4 from activity 3 in their reports.

▶▶ Teacher Resources

General Background Material

In preparing for this lesson, you may want to refer to the following resources:

- *Healthy People 2010*
- *Centers for Disease Control and Prevention Fact Sheets on Physical Activity*
- *Planet Health* FitCheck sheets

See appendix B and part II (page 21) for information on these resources.

Specific Background Material

Planet Health's Activity Message

Physical activity promotes health and well-being, and offers opportunities to socialize and have fun. Adolescents should be moderately active for at least 30 minutes every day or nearly every day as part of play, games, sports, chores, transportation, or planned exercise, AND they should participate in at least three sessions per week of vigorous physical activity lasting 20 minutes or more. Adolescents should aim for a total of 60 minutes or more of activity on five to seven days a week.

To meet the minimum recommendation, students should be physically active 4-1/2 hours each week (30 minutes of moderate activity nearly every day plus 20 minutes of moderate to vigorous activity three times per week).

Planet Health's FitCheck

If PE teachers in your school are teaching *Planet Health,* they are using these sheets to help students track the amount of time they spend in moderately-intense physical activities, vigorously-intense physical activities, and inactivity. In addition, PE teachers are delivering five-minute *Planet Health* microunits on physical fitness themes, so your students should be familiar with our activity message. The FitCheck is the source of the activity list used in the survey in this lesson. It, too, should be familiar to students.

References

Sallis, J.F., and Patrick, K. 1994. Physical activity guidelines for adolescents: Consensus statement. *Pediatric Exercise Science* 6:302-314.

U.S. Department of Health and Human Services 2000. Healthy people 2010, conference edition, vols I and II. **www.health.gov/healthypeople**

In this table, record the physical activities that you have performed over the past seven days.

1. Under column 1, list the activities you have done over the past seven days. Use the FitScore Activities list to help you remember.
2. Under column 2, note how many hours you have spent doing each activity for each day that week.
3. When you are finished, sum the total time under column 3 and complete the row labeled "Total activity for the week."
4. Use this data to answer questions on activity 3 *Analyzing Class Data*.

Time spent doing each activity over the past week

Physical activity	Day 1	Day 2	Day 3	Day 4	Day 5	Day 6	Day 7	Total time
Example: swimming	*1/2 hour*			*1/2 hour*				*1 hour*
Total activity for the week								

FitScore Activities

shoveling snow	sledding
raking leaves	skateboarding
cleaning	playing soccer
vacuuming	swimming
running	playing hockey
doing sit-ups	playing basketball
jumping rope	walking
weightlifting	riding a bike
playing tag	in-line skating
skiing	climbing stairs

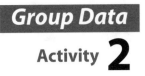

Use activity 1 to complete the chart below.

1. Under column 1, list the activities that each student has done over the past seven days. List each activity once.
2. Under column 2, write the number of hours that students in your group spent doing each physical activity over the past seven days.
3. Sum the "Total time spent by group on each activity."
4. Complete the row at the bottom of the chart labeled "Total time group spent active over the past 7 days" by summing the totals in the column "Total time spent by group on each activity."

Physical activity	Hours spent per week				Total time spent by group on each activity
	Student 1	Student 2	Student 3	Student 4	
Example: swimming	2	1	1/2	0	3.5 hours
Total time the group spent active over the past 7 days					

Personal Data (From Activity 1)

Use back of sheet for scratch paper.

1. Rank the three physical activities that you spent the most time doing:

   Highest time 1. _____

   Second highest time 2. _____

   Third highest time 3. _____

2. What percent of your total physical activity time was spent on each one? Time spent on activity / total activity time × 100 = % of total activity time.

   Example: 5 hrs walking / 10 hrs of total activity = 0.50 × 100 = 50% of activity time was spent walking.

3. What is the mean number of hours you spent doing physical activity per day? Does this answer surprise you? In what way? Mean = total activity time / 7 days per week.

   Example: 10 hrs of total activity / 7 = 1.43 hours per day spent on physical activity.

4. Review your physical activity list. Is there one activity that you did on more days than you did any other activity? (Example: if you walked every day for 1/2 hour and you swam four days a week for an hour, the answer would be walking.) The answer to that question is also called the *mode* (most commonly occurring response).

5. What was the range in hours spent in individual physical activities over the past 7 days?

Group Data (From Activity 2)

6. What is the total number of hours that the group participated in physical activity?

7. What is the mean number of hours the group spent doing physical activity per day? (See the formula from question 3.)

8. What is the mean number of hours each person spent being active in the last 7 days? Mean = total active time (for group) / total number in group.

9. Rank the three physical activities that the group spent the most time doing:

   Highest time 1. _____

   Second highest time 2. _____

   Third highest time 3. _____

10. What percent of their time did the group spend doing each physical activity? Compute this for the three activities listed in number 9. (See formula for percent from question 2.)

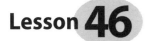

Circle Graphs: Where Did the Day Go?

Students will make circle graphs to illustrate the proportion of their day they spend doing vigorous, moderate, and inactive to light activities. This lesson is designed to help students become aware of the time they spend being inactive and to encourage them to make lifestyle changes that will increase their activity.

Constructing circle graphs will provide a review of the following math skills: expressing time as fractions of an hour, converting percentages to decimals, and calculating central angles and percentages. An alternative activity for less advanced math students is included. It provides students with a circle graph that has been divided into 24 sections. They must express their activities as fractions of a 24-hour day and shade the circle graph accordingly. This lesson may take one and a half periods, depending on the skill level of the students.

▶▶ Behavioral Objective

For students to be more aware of the amount of time they spend being inactive and to be more active.

▶▶ Learning Objectives

Students will be able to

1. construct a circle graph,
2. report time as fractions of an hour, calculate percentages, and convert fractions to decimals,
3. calculate central angles (advanced version of the activity only),
4. draw inferences and reason with tables and graphs that summarize personal activity data,
5. discuss the benefits of a more active lifestyle, and
6. describe the physical activity recommendations for adolescents.

▶▶ Materials

- Copies of worksheets for activity 1 OR activity 2 *Where Did the Day Go?*
- Five pieces of large paper or five overhead transparencies
- Calculator recommended
- Compass, protractor, plain paper (activity 1 only), colored pencils or crayons
- *Optional:* overhead transparencies 1, 2, and 3

►► Procedure

1. (10 minutes) To introduce the activity, have students complete a carousel brainstorming activity as described below. Write each of the questions below on the top of a different piece of large paper or overhead transparency. Spread the papers or transparencies out around the room.

- What changes in society have brought about a decrease in daily physical activity? Think about how your life is different from that of your grandparents.
- How much time do you think kids of your age spend watching TV? List some fun activities that you can do in place of watching TV.
- What are the risks of an inactive lifestyle?
- What are the benefits of an active lifestyle?
- How much activity do you think you should do to be healthy and fit?

Divide the class into five groups. Assign each group to one of the questions above. Give them a minute and a half to write their response to the question on the paper, then have the groups move to another question. Continue the process until each group has had the opportunity to respond to all five questions. It is important that you give the signal to move at precisely the allotted amount of time so that students do not waste time chatting. Incomplete answers are okay. The idea is to get them thinking. You also might consider giving each group a different color marker so you can track group responses. Requiring each person in the group to take a turn being the recorder is a good way to ensure that everyone participates.* (See Teacher Resources for answers to these questions.)

2. (5 minutes) Display and discuss student answers to each of the questions, filling in gaps in student knowledge where necessary.

3. (1-2 minutes) Point out the goals of the math lesson:

- To think about how much of their day they spend being inactive and how they might be more active.
- To make a circle graph to illustrate what portion of the day they spend being active and inactive.
- To apply and review math skills they have already learned (representing time as fractions of an hour, multiplying and adding fractions, converting fractions to decimals, calculating percentages and central angles). The skills needed for this activity vary depending on which version of the activity you have students do.

4. Hand out worksheets for activity 1 OR activity 2. Activity 1 is appropriate for students who have learned or are learning how to make circle graphs. Activity 2 is appropriate for less advanced math students. It does not require students to construct the circle graph. They will shade in an already prepared graph. The activities ask students to estimate the amount of time they spent doing different things "yesterday." If you are doing this lesson on a Monday, you may wish to replace "yesterday" with the words "last Friday" or "on a typical school day."

5. (3 minutes) *Optional:* Use overhead transparency 1 to work through one example of estimating time and the math calculations. You may need to remind students that $1/4 = .25$, $1/2 = .5$, and $3/4 = .75$.

6. (40 minutes for activity 1; 30 minutes for activity 2) Have students complete activity 1 or activity 2 and construct or shade in the circle graph, respectively. You may wish to display as an overhead transparency an example of a labeled and shaded

---

*Stern, A. *Instructional strategies and techniques to enhance motivation and achievement.* Workshop, 1996.

circle graph included in activity 2. (*Note:* The directions for labeling the circle graph are slightly different on the two versions of the worksheets.) Using calculators will decrease the amount of time needed for this activity.

7. (5 minutes) Have students get into groups of three or four to discuss their conclusions and share their circle graphs.

▶▶ Extension Activities

Have students interview an adult in their families to determine how he or she spends the day. Have students construct a circle graph to illustrate their findings. Have them write a report that compares and contrasts their individual activity and inactivity percentages with those of the adults they interviewed.

You may shorten the amount of class time spent on this activity by having students complete their circle graphs and conclusions for homework.

▶▶ Teacher Resources

General Background Materials

In preparing for this lesson, you may want to refer to the following resources:

- *Centers for Disease Control and Prevention Fact Sheets on Physical Activity*
- *Television Viewing as a Cause of Increasing Obesity Among Children in the United States, 1986-1990*
- *Healthy People 2010*

See appendix B for information on how to obtain these resources.

Specific Background Material

What changes in society have brought about a decrease in daily physical activity?

In the latter part of the 20th century, there was a dramatic reduction in the amount of physical activity performed in daily life. The growth of the economy resulted in a dramatic increase in the number of sedentary, white-collar jobs and a decrease in blue-collar and farming jobs that required physical work. Modern appliances, machinery, and motorized transportation have decreased the amount of activity required to complete household chores and work-related tasks. The growing contribution of technology to inactive leisure activities has also been enormous, with computers, video, and TV being the major factors. The Internet, CD-ROM, and continued expansion of the TV channel market will help these trends continue.

How much time do adolescents spend watching TV?

According to Dietz (1991), American children spend more time watching TV than they do engaging in any other activity except sleeping. In 1988, the average adolescent viewed approximately 22 hours per week. The percentage of youth watching TV and playing computer or video games for 5 or more hours per day has increased greatly, from 13% in the late 1960s to 43% in 1990. Essentially, TV watching for many children has become a full-time job! On average, adolescents spend more time watching TV than they spend in school. The American Academy of Pediatrics recommends limiting TV viewing to 2 hours or less per day.

What are the risks of a sedentary lifestyle? Activity is required for health. Studies suggest that physically active individuals enjoy lower risks of developing cardiovascular disease, diabetes, colon cancer, osteoporosis, anxiety, and depression relative to sedentary individuals. Sedentary habits increase the risk of death from these diseases. Television viewing is one of the major causes of overweight among youth. TV watching also has been associated with elevated cholesterol levels and lower cardiovascular fitness.

What are the benefits of a more active lifestyle? Activity helps children develop and retain cardiovascular fitness, muscle strength, and confidence in their physical ability. Regular activity helps individuals maintain a healthy weight, build lean muscle, and reduce fat. It can reduce stress and brighten a person's mood. Regular exercise helps build and maintain dense bones, which helps prevent osteoperosis. Active adults have a lower risk of dying prematurely and developing diabetes, high blood pressure, and colon cancer.

What are the alternatives to TV viewing? Anything that involves movement! Limiting TV time can ensure children do other activities that involve more physical activity. Also, you don't have to sit still while you watch TV—you can be dancing, cleaning, cooking, and so on. One easy way to cut down on TV time is to take the TV out of the room where you sleep. If you don't want to physically remove it, just unplug it. Watch TV only if your favorite show is on.

How much activity is needed to obtain health-related benefits? Moderate amounts of activity are recommended for people of all ages. However, physical activity need not be strenuous to be beneficial. Just a small increase in physical activity can generate genuine health benefits, such as reduction of body weight and the risk of heart attack, hypertension, and death. Thirty minutes or more of moderately intense activity, such as walking, is beneficial for your health. Regular vigorous activity, however, is the best way to improve cardiovascular fitness.

How much activity is needed for fitness? How long, how hard, and how often you are active will determine how fit you are! To be fit, you must work on your cardiovascular (aerobic) endurance, muscular strength (anaerobic fitness), and flexibility. Do strength training two to three times per week. Stretch and do cardiovascular training at least three times per week for at least 20 minutes. You can improve fitness by increasing the frequency (if you are not already exercising regularly), increasing the intensity (doing something faster, doing more repetitions or sets, or using heavier weights), or increasing the time you spend on each exercise. You might choose more types of exercise to do!

What are some examples of things you can do to increase your activity and decrease your inactivity? Take the stairs; don't park next to the building; walk or ride your bike to school if there is a safe route; walk around the mall or the neighborhood with friends; watch only your favorite TV shows; remove or unplug the TV in your bedroom; play catch with a sibling, a friend, or parent.

References

Blair, S. 1993. C.H. McCloy research lecture: Physical activity, physical fitness, and health. *Research Quarterly for Exercise and Sport* 64(4): 365-376.

Dietz, W. 1991. Physical activity and childhood obesity. *Nutrition* 7(4): 295-296.

Dietz, W.H., and Strasburger, V.C. 1991. Children, adolescents, and television. *Current Problems in Pediatrics* 21(1):8-31.

Gortmaker, S.L. 1990. National health examination survey, 1967-70. Unpublished data.

Gortmaker, S.L. 1990. National longitudinal survey of youth. Unpublished data.

Park, R. 1992. Human energy expenditure from *Australopithecus afarensis* to 4-minute mile: Exemplars and case studies. *Exercise and Sport Sciences Reviews* 20: 185-220.

Part I: Data Collection

The following activity will help you construct a circle graph to illustrate how much time you spent in a variety of activities over one day. A circle graph is used to compare parts of a whole. To begin, complete the table as follows:

1. Estimate the time you spend on a typical weekday doing each of the activities listed in column 1. Express your time estimates in hours or fractions of an hour rounded to the nearest quarter hour (example: eating = 1-1/4 hr). In the blank spaces at the bottom of column 1, write in other activities that you are involved in that are not included on the list.

2. Convert your time estimates to decimals and record your answers in column 3 (example: 1-1/4 = 1.25 hrs).

3. Sum column 3. If the sum is less than 24 hours, calculate the difference and put it in the row labeled "Other activities." If the sum is greater than 24 hours, reconsider the accuracy of your time estimates.

4. Express the time spent in each activity as a ratio of your total day and place this fraction (or decimal) in column 4 (example: sleep = 1.25 hrs / 24 hrs = .05).

5. Calculate the percentage of your day you spent doing each activity. Divide the time you spent doing the activity by 24 hours and multiply by 100 (example: 1.25 hours / 24 hours $\times$ 100 = 5%). Enter your answer in column 5.

6. To make a circle graph you must now figure out the central angle for each activity. Multiply the ratio (decimal) in column 5 by 360° and put the number in column 6 (example: $0.05 \times 360° = 18°$).

Table 1

1	2	3	4	5	6
Activity	**Time (hours) fraction**	**Time (hours) decimal**	**Ratio (x hours / 24 hours)**	**Percentage (%)**	**Central angle (°)**
Example: Eating	*1-1/4 hours*	*1.25 hours*	*1.25 / 24 = .05*	*.05 × 100 = 5%*	*.05 × 360° =18°*
Sleeping					
Working at a job					
Watching TV					
Eating					
Listening to your teachers					
Talking on the phone					
Playing computer games					

1	2	3	4	5	6
Activity	Time (hours) fraction	Time (hours) decimal	Ratio (x hours / 24 hours)	Percentage (%)	Central angle (°)
Hanging out with friends					
Homework					
Walking					
Playing a sport					
Household chores					
Showering, dressing					
Other activities:					
	Total				

Part II: Classification

Calculate what portion of your day is devoted to inactivity, light activity, moderate activity, and vigorous activity by doing the following:

1. Use table 2 to help you classify your activities as inactive, light, moderate, or vigorous.
2. Write the activities in the appropriate column in table 3. Don't include activities that you spend zero time doing on a typical day (example: If household chores = 0 hr, don't record in table 3). Also, record the % and central angle you calculated in table 1.
3. Total the percentages and the central angles for each activity category.

Table 2

Inactive	Lying down, sleeping, sitting, reading, watching TV, eating, listening to music
Light activity	Dressing, grooming, washing dishes, cooking, making beds
Moderate activity	Walking, carrying heavy objects, raking leaves, skating, bicycling, skateboarding, baseball/softball, dancing, climbing stairs
Vigorous activity	Running, swimming, basketball, football, tennis, fast bicycling, hockey, soccer, in-line skating, weight lifting

Table 3

Inactive/light activity			Moderate activity			Vigorous activity		
Activity	**%**	**Central angle**	**Activity**	**%**	**Central angle**	**Activity**	**%**	**Central angle**
Example: eating	5	18°						
Total						Total		

Part III: Construction

1. Use a compass to draw a circle large enough to write in. Mark the center with a dot.

2. Use a protractor to draw the central angle for each activity. Place all the events from a given activity category next to each other in the circle.

3. Put the name and % of each activity on or next to the corresponding section of the circle graph.

4. Choose a different color to represent each of the three activity categories. Make a legend next to the circle graph to indicate which color represents each category. Shade the circle to illustrate what portion of your day is spent doing inactive, moderate, and vigorous activities.

5. During what percentage of your day are you having fun? Draw diagonal lines through the sections of the circle which represent the activities you enjoy.

Part IV: Conclusion

Use the analysis from part III to write a paragraph describing your findings. Include 1–2 sentences that describe the amount of time you spent doing inactive/light, moderate, and vigorous activities. Include 1–3 sentences describing ways to decrease the amount of time you are inactive and increase the amount of fun moderate and vigorous activities you do.

Part I: Data Collection

How much of your day do you spend being active? Sitting around? Having fun? Watching TV? Talking on the phone? The following activity will help you answer these questions. You will complete a circle graph to illustrate your findings. A circle graph is used to compare parts of a whole. To begin, complete the table as follows:

1. Estimate the time you spend on a typical weekday doing each of the activities listed in column 1. Express your time estimates in hours or fractions of an hour rounded to the nearest quarter hour (example: eating = 1-1/4 hour). In the blank spaces at the bottom of column 1, write in other activities that you are involved in that are not included on the list.

2. Convert your time estimates to decimals and record your answers in column 3 (example: 1-1/4 = 1.25).

3. Sum column 3. If the sum is less than 24 hours, calculate the difference and put it in the row labeled "Other activities." If the sum is greater than 24 hours, reconsider the accuracy of your time estimates.

4. Express the time spent in each activity as a ratio of your total day and convert to a decimal. Place this decimal in column 4 (example: 1.25 hrs / 24 hrs = .05).

5. Calculate the percentage of your day you spent doing each activity. Divide the time you spent doing the activity by 24 hours and multiply by 100 (example: 1.25 hrs / 24 hrs × 100 = 5%). Enter your answer in column 5.

Table 1

1	2	3	4	5
Activity	**Time (hours) fraction**	**Time (hours) decimal**	**Ratio (x hours / 24 hours)**	**Percentage (%)**
Example: Eating	*1-1/4 hours*	*1.25 hours*	*1.25 / 24 = .05*	*.05 × 100 = 5%*
Sleeping				
Working at a job				
Watching TV				
Eating				
Listening to your teachers				
Talking on the phone				
Playing computer games				
Hanging out with friends				
Homework				
Walking				

1	2	3	4	5
Activity	Time (hours) fraction	Time (hours) decimal	Ratio (x hours / 24 hours)	Percentage (%)
Example: Eating	*1-1/4 hours*	*1.25 hours*	*1.25 / 24 = .05*	*.05 × 100 = 5%*
Playing a sport				
Household chores				
Showering, dressing				
Other activities:				
Totals				

Part II: Classification

Calculate what portion of your day is devoted to inactivity, light activity, moderate activity, and vigorous activity by doing the following:

1. Use table 2 to help you classify your activities as inactive, light, moderate, or vigorous.
2. Write the activities in the appropriate column in table 3. Don't include activities that you spend zero time doing on a typical day (example: if household chores = 0 hr, don't record in table 3). Also, record the % and time (fraction) you calculated in table 1.
3. Total the time and percentages for each activity category.

Table 2

Inactive	Lying down, sleeping, sitting, reading, watching TV, eating, listening to music
Light activity	Dressing, grooming, washing dishes, cooking, making beds
Moderate activity	Walking, carrying heavy objects, raking leaves, skating, bicycling, skateboarding, baseball/softball, dancing, climbing stairs
Vigorous activity	Running, swimming, basketball, football, tennis, fast bicycling, hockey, soccer, in-line skating, weight lifting

Table 3

Inactive/light activity			Moderate activity			Vigorous activity		
Activity	Time fraction	%	Activity	Time fraction	%	Activity	Time fraction	%
Totals								

Part III: Graphing

Shade in the circle graph as follows:

1. Each section of the circle represents 1 hour. Assign each activity a color. Shade in the portion of the circle which most accurately represents the amount of time you spent doing each activity. Place all the events from a given activity category (inactive, light, moderate, vigorous) next to each other in the circle.

2. Put each activity's name and % on or next to the corresponding section of the circle graph.

3. Assign each of the activity categories a color. Outline the portion of the circle which represents each category with the assigned color. Make a legend next to the circle graph to indicate which color represents each category. Write the total percentage of time spent doing each activity category in the legend.

4. During what percentage of your day are you having fun? Draw diagonal lines through the sections of the circle which represent the activities you enjoy.

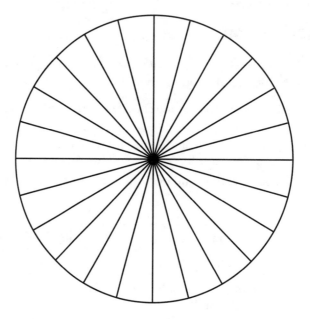

Part IV: Conclusion

Write a paragraph describing your findings. Include 1–2 sentences that describe the amount of time you spend doing inactive, light, moderate, and vigorous activities. Include 1–3 sentences that describe ways to decrease the amount of time you are inactive and increase the amount of fun moderate and vigorous activities you do.

Energy Equations

In this lesson, students learn that fat is one of our major sources of calories from food (protein and carbohydrate are the others). They learn that these macronutrients should be present in their diets in certain proportions on average. Students also learn that physical activity increases energy requirements, but the required proportions of fat, protein, and carbohydrate remain unchanged except at very high activity levels.

Through individual work and group discussion, students use addition, multiplication, and division to calculate averages, derive data for graphing, and figure out unknown variables or percentages of fat, protein, and carbohydrates.

This lesson is designed to infuse information about the relationship between physical activity and calorie intake into classroom work using pre-algebra level skills.

▶▶ Behavioral Objective

For students to be physically active and to balance their energy needs with their activity demands.

▶▶ Learning Objectives

Students will be able to

1. state that energy intake needs to increase with increasing activity,
2. state the dietary recommendations for protein, carbohydrates, and fat, and recognize that these percentages are the same at any calorie level, and
3. derive means and graph data.

▶▶ Materials

Activity 1 *Calculating Intake*

▶▶ Procedure

1. (5-15 minutes) Explain the following:

   • Fat, protein, and carbohydrates supply us with energy or calories, and all foods are made from them in varying amounts.
   • Fat should constitute 30% of daily calories.
   • About 10–15% of calories should come from protein, and the remaining 55–60% should come from carbohydrates.
   • An individual's energy needs increase with increasing amounts of activity. Example: If you play outside all afternoon, your body uses more energy than if you

watch TV for the same amount of time. (See Teacher Resources for additional review material on diet and activity.)

2. (5 minutes) Distribute activity 1 *Calculating Intake* and discuss bar graph A *Recommended Daily Nutrient Breakdown* at the top of the page. The activity requires students to review and evaluate their imaginary food intake over four days. They will

- calculate the number of calories consumed daily as carbohydrate, protein, and fat,
- calculate the average percent of total daily calories consumed as carbohydrate, protein, and fat and graph these results, and
- evaluate their imaginary food choices and make suggestions for improving their diet.

3. (30-40 minutes) Students complete the worksheet, with the teacher available for individual assistance. To save time, you may want to have students work in teams of two or three.

4. (5-10 minutes) Review the worksheet with the class (see Teacher Resources). As you review the answers to questions 2 and 3 in part I of the activity, discuss with students the importance of paying particular attention to the amount of saturated fat in the foods they eat, since eating too much saturated fat increases the risk of developing heart disease. Experts recommend getting no more than 10% of daily calories from saturated fat and replacing saturated fat and trans fat with unsaturated fat since this decreases the risk of developing heart disease. Because excessive intake of any kind of fat is not optimal for health, total fat intake should not exceed 30%. (See Teacher Resources for a discussion of the different types of fat and the foods that contain them.) Also, point out the importance of including plenty of whole grain foods, fruits, and vegetables in their daily meals, since these foods are generally high in fiber as well as other complex carbohydrates, vitamins, and minerals. Eating plenty of fiber decreases the risk of developing heart disease and diabetes.

▶▶ Extension Activities

Have students answer the following questions:

- If you run around for half an hour instead of watching a TV show, will your energy needs go up, go down, or stay the same?
- Will the percent of calories you need from carbohydrate, protein, or fat change? Why?

▶▶ Teacher Resources

General Background Material

In preparing for this lesson, you may want to refer to the following resources:

- *Centers for Disease Control and Prevention Fact Sheets on Physical Activity*
- *Healthy People 2010*
- *Guide to Good Eating*

See appendixes A and B for information on how to obtain these resources.

Specific Background Material

Planet Health's Activity Message

Physical activity promotes health and well-being and offers opportunities to socialize and have fun. Adolescents should be moderately active for at least 30 minutes every day or nearly every day as part of play, games, sports, chores, transportation, or planned exercise, AND they should participate in at least three sessions per week of vigorous physical activity lasting 20 minutes or more. Adolescents should aim for a total of 60 minutes or more of activity on five to seven days a week.

Calorie Requirements and Dietary Sources of Energy

People have different calorie requirements depending on age, sex, and activity level. The National Research Council's *Recommended Dietary Allowances,* 10th edition, notes that 11–14-year-old girls need 2,200 calories per day, while boys this age need 2,500. These are averages that can vary a bit from day to day. They also vary according to an individual's activity level and size. Compared to her peers who don't exercise, an athletic adolescent girl may need an additional 300-1,000 calories, and an athletic adolescent male may need an additional 600-1,500 calories per day! These active teens are using their energy stores at a faster rate than the inactive teens.

Serving Requirements

The Food Guide Pyramid reminds us to eat a certain number of servings from each of the five major food groups each day. People with higher energy needs require more servings than do less active people to get all the calories they need. For example, teenage boys on average need about 2,500 calories per day versus 2,200 for girls. To make up this difference, teenage boys are advised to eat a higher number of servings from the five major food groups compared to others with lower energy needs. Notice that the extra calories come from a healthy balance of foods, maintaining the balance of fat, carbohydrate, and protein. An active adolescent girl also needs more calories than her less active peers, so she also should get them by increasing overall consumption, not by filling up on high-fat snacks. Athletes who consistently need lots and lots of extra calories look to complex carbohydrates primarily from grains, fruits, and vegetables, not fats or proteins, to take up the slack.

Some daily dietary variation in energy and food intake is normal. Exercise helps regulate appetite. Your body will need more energy and will tell you by feeling hungrier!

Dietary Recommendations for Fat, Protein, and Carbohydrates

Fat provides 9 calories per gram. Fat is important for cell structure, transporting fat-soluble vitamins (A, D, E, and K), storing energy, and insulating our bodies. It's important to note that calories from any source—protein, carbohydrate, fat, or alcohol—are stored as fat when intake exceeds expenditure.

The fat in foods contains a mixture of saturated and unsaturated (monounsaturated and polyunsaturated) fatty acids, commonly called fats. Many animal products, such as fatty meat, whole milk, butter, and lard, are high in saturated fat. This kind of fat is typically solid at room temperature. Eating too much saturated fat increases your risk for developing heart disease. Therefore, the *Dietary Guidelines for Americans* recommends eating a diet low in saturated fat (less than 10% of calories). Most of the fat you eat should be unsaturated, since substituting this type of fat for saturated fat in your diet decreases your risk of developing heart disease. Most plant fats, or oils, are unsaturated fats and are generally liquid at room temperature. Vegetable oils, such as olive, canola, corn, and peanut oils, most nuts, olives, and avocados are good sources of unsaturated fat. However, eating lots of fat of any type may not be healthy, so the *Dietary Guidelines for Americans* recommends that you get no more than 30% of your calories from fat.

There are exceptions to the rule. Not all plant fats are healthy. Through a commercial process called hydrogenation, the more healthy plant oils can be converted into solids called *trans fats* (also called *partially hydrogenated vegetable oils).* This is how some margarines are made. Not surprisingly, foods high in trans fats have been found to also increase the risk of heart disease. To avoid these fats, check the ingredient list on packaged foods like cookies and crackers for partially hydrogenated vegetable oil. Also look out for coconut oil and palm oil since these oils are naturally high in saturated fat.

Not all animal foods are high in saturated fats. Some fish, such as salmon, mackerel, and tuna, are high in a polyunsaturated fat—omega-3 fatty acid—that may protect you against heart disease. So choose to eat fish when you get the chance.

Populations with higher saturated fat intakes have higher rates of chronic disease, particularly heart disease, relative to populations with lower intakes. Americans typically get about 33% of their total calories from fat and 11% from saturated fat, exceeding recommendations for no more than 30% total fat (saturated fat and unsaturated fat) and no more than 10% saturated fat.

It is easy to calculate the daily allowance of dietary fat for an adolescent girl who needs a total of 2,200 calories per day. Her total fat allowance is 30% of 2,200 total calories or

$$0.30 \times 2,200 = 660 \text{ calories per day.}$$

Fat contains 9 calories per gram, so to figure her fat allowance in grams

$$660 / 9 = 73 \text{ grams of fat per day.}$$

Her saturated fat allowance is 10% of 2,200 calories, or

$$0.10 \times 2,200 = 220 \text{ calories per day.}$$

Fat contains 9 calories per gram, so to figure her saturated fat allowance in grams

$$220 \text{ calories} / 9 \text{ calories per gram} = 24 \text{ grams.}$$

You can find out the amount of total fat and saturated fat in a product by looking at the food label.

Protein provides 4 calories per gram. Protein is essential to growth and to building and repairing cells, making enzymes and hormones, and so on. Protein is produced by cells. Dietary protein needs vary over the life span. Generally expressed in terms of grams needed per kilogram of body weight, protein needs are highest during infancy, at about 2.2 g/kg, and decline to 0.8 g/kg in adulthood. Adolescents need about 1 g/kg each day.

Experts recommend that 10–15% of daily calories should come from protein. During a growth spurt, adolescents may require more calories from protein. However, they should consult with their pediatricians before increasing their protein consumption. Americans usually exceed protein requirements and rarely have diets deficient in this nutrient.

Lean meats and low-fat dairy products are excellent sources of protein. Dried beans and peas (such as pinto beans, black-eyed peas, and canned baked beans) and nuts are also good sources. Eating the recommended servings of the meat group (2-3 servings) and the dairy group (2-3 servings) every day will provide you with adequate protein.

An adolescent boy who needs 2,500 total calories per day needs a minimum of 250 calories from protein each day, or 63 grams. Food labels list protein grams per serving.

Carbohydrates provide 4 calories per gram. Carbohydrates are our major source of energy and include simple carbohydrates (sugars) and complex carbohydrates (starches and fiber).

The rationale for the recommendation that 55–60% of daily calories come from carbohydrates is not based on a physiological requirement. Rather, it derives from the need to provide an upper limit on fat and protein intake. Thus, if fat and protein intake combined account for 40–45% of intake, the rest should be from carbohydrates.

Grains, especially whole grains, vegetables, and fruits are excellent sources of complex carbohydrates and naturally occurring sugars and are the foundation of a healthy diet. Eat six or more servings of grain products daily and include several whole grain varieties. Eat five or more servings of fruits and vegetables daily. Be sure to choose a variety of foods within these groups. This will help you get the nutrients and fiber you need. Go easy on sweet foods like soda, cookies, and candy. They provide carbohydrates but are usually low in vitamins and minerals and can be high in saturated and trans fats.

For an adolescent boy eating 2,500 calories per day, carbohydrate intake would be as much as 375 grams (60% of calories at 4 calories per gram). Grams of total carbohydrate per serving are listed on food labels.

Alcohol

Alcohol provides 7 calories per gram. There is no dietary requirement for alcohol. Evidence suggests that moderate consumption by healthy men and healthy, nonpregnant, nonlactating women (equivalent to one glass of wine per day for women, two for men) may lower the risk of heart disease in some individuals. Higher levels of alcohol consumption increase the risk for high blood pressure, stroke, heart disease, certain cancers, accidents, violence, suicide, birth defects, and death. Even moderate consumption may increase the risk of developing certain cancers. Alcohol should not be consumed by children and youth.

References

Bierer, L.A., Warner, L., Lawson, S., and Cohen, T. 1991. *Life science: The challenge of discovery.* Lexington, MA: Heath.

National Dairy Council. 1994. *The guide to good eating and daily food guide pyramid.* Rosemont, IL: National Dairy Council.

National Research Council. 1980. *Recommended dietary allowances.* 10th ed. Washington, D.C.: National Academy Press.

U.S. Department of Agriculture and U.S. Department of Health and Human Services. 2000. *Nutrition and your health: Dietary guidelines for Americans 2000*, 5th edition. **www.usda.gov/cnpp**

U.S Department of Health and Human Services. 2000. Healthy People 2010, conference edition, vols. I and II. **www.health.gov/healthypeople**

Willett, W. 2000. Got fat? Exploding nutrition myths. *World Health News.* **www.worldhealthnews.harvard.edu**

▸▸ Answer Key

Activity 1

Table A Average Daily Macronutrient Intake

	Carbohydrate %	Protein %	Fat %
Day 1	60	13	27
Day 2	40	12	48
Day 3	48	10	42
Day 4	60	15	25
Average daily intake (%)	**52**	**12.5**	**35.5**

Table B Total Daily Calorie Intake

	Carbohydrate		Protein		Fat		Total calories
	%	N	%	N	%	N	
Day 1	60	**1,170**	13	**253.5**	27	**526.5**	1,950
Day 2	40	**920**	12	**276**	48	**1,104**	2,300
Day 3	48	**1,056**	10	**220**	42	**924**	2,200
Day 4	60	**1,530**	15	**382.5**	25	**637.5**	2,550
Average daily intake		**1,169**		**283**		**978**	**2,250**

Selected Answers to Questions: Part I

2. My diet contains more fat than is recommended and not enough carbohydrates.

3. I could fix the imbalance by replacing some of the calories from **fat** with calories from **carbohydrates.**

Selected Answers to Questions: Part II

1. Day 1.

2. Day 2.

3. Physical activity requires energy (calories). The more active I am, the more energy I need. Since food gives me energy, I need to eat more when I'm physically active.

Part I

The bar graph below shows the percent of daily calories that experts recommend for protein, carbohydrates, and fat. These proportions help keep you healthy!

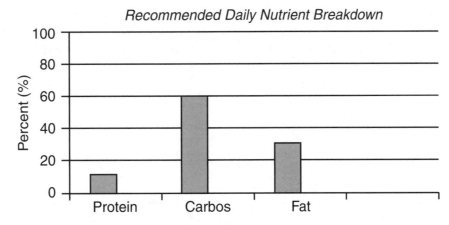

Recommended Daily Nutrient Breakdown

Table A breaks down the percent of calories from carbohydrates, protein, and fat you got from an imaginary diet over four days.

Table A Your Average Daily Macronutrient Intake

	Carbohydrate %	**Protein %**	**Fat %**
Day 1	60	13	27
Day 2	40	12	48
Day 3	48	10	42
Day 4	60	15	25
Average daily intake (%)			

1. What was your average daily intake for each of the macronutrients? Fill in the blanks in table A.

2. Make bars on the bar graph above for your average intake. How does your diet compare to the recommendations?

3. Which macronutrient do you need more of? Which do you need less of? How could you fix the imbalance in your diet? Hint: Replace some of the calories from _____ with calories from _____.

Part II

Table B is the same as table A, except that it also shows the total number of calories you ate each day of your imaginary diet. Read across each row. For example, on day 1 you ate 1,950 calories. Carbohydrates made up 60% of your total daily caloric intake, protein made up 13%, and fat made up 27%.

Calculate the number of calories from carbohydrate, protein, and fat that you consumed each day.

Table B Your Total Daily Calorie Intake From Your Imaginary Diet

	Carbohydrate		Protein		Fat		
	%	Calories	%	Calories	%	Calories	Total calories
Day 1	60		13		27		1,950
Day 2	40		12		48		2,300
Day 3	48		10		42		2,200
Day 4	60		15		25		2,550
Average daily intake							

1. One day you rested and weren't very hungry. Can you figure out which day? Justify your answer.

2. One day you played soccer for a long time. Can you figure out which day? Justify your answer.

3. What can you conclude about the effect of activity on your daily intake?

This unit contains eight lessons. Use the At A Glance chart below to help you select the lessons that best fit your curriculum objectives. Some of the lessons offer a choice of activities. Adapt the lesson procedures to fit your teaching style, students' skills, and time constraints.

Lessons in this unit meet many Massachusetts learning standards that may be similar to standards in your state. Refer to appendix E (page 508) to see which of the 1996-1999 Massachusetts Curriculum Frameworks (MCFW) each lesson incorporates.

Science At A Glance

Theme	Lesson	Level of difficulty (grade) *			Subject specific skills	Materials needed
		6th	7th	8th		
Balanced diet	48 Mighty Minerals: Calcium and Iron	M	M	L	Calcium function, bone development, skeleton	Scissors, paper, markers, chicken bone, 20% hydrochloric acid, beaker, and safety goggles (optional)
Balanced diet	49 Fat Functions	M	L-M	L	Testing for lipids, scientific process	Food items, paper towel
Balanced diet	50 Smart Snacks	M	L-M	L	Nutrition, reading food labels	Overhead transparencies
Fruits and vegetables	51 The Plants We Eat	M	M	L	Plant structure, classification, nutrition	Food items, magnifying glass, vitamin C tablet (optional)
Activity	52 Foods for Energy	H	M	M	Carbohydrate function	Tennis balls or textbooks (optional)
Activity	53 Muscle Mysteries	M-H	M	L-M	Muscle function	
Lifestyle	54 The Human Heart	H	M	M	Heart function, measuring heart rate, scientific process	Clock or watch with a second hand, tennis balls (optional)
Lifestyle	55 How Far Can You Jump?	M	M	M	Analyzing movement, scientific process	Tape measure, masking tape

* Level of difficulty: L = low, M = medium, H = high

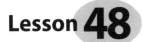

Lesson 48

Balanced Diet Theme

Mighty Minerals: Calcium and Iron

This lesson discusses the role of two minerals, calcium and iron, in the development, function, and maintenance of the bones and organs in the human body. Two activities are included; do one or both as time and interest permit. Both activities describe the health risks for adolescents who do not consume enough calcium and iron.

Activity 1 uses a game to teach students that the amount of calcium in bones is in constant flux (a great example of homeostasis), and that to ensure strong healthy bones, adequate supplies of calcium need to be ingested throughout life. Students learn what types of foods are high in calcium, how many servings they need to eat, and what enhances or inhibits calcium deposits in the bones. This lesson is designed to be incorporated into a unit on the human skeletal system and is appropriate for sixth-, seventh-, or eighth-grade students.

Activity 2 is designed to teach students about the function of iron in the human body. Students will learn what types of foods are high in iron and how much iron they need daily. They will create a comic strip that depicts the function of iron in the body. This lesson could be included in a unit on the cardiovascular system. It is appropriate for sixth or seventh grade.

▶▶ Behavioral Objective

For students to eat a variety of foods that give the body important minerals and nutrients for health.

▶▶ Learning Objectives

After activity 1, students will be able to

1. describe the functions of calcium in the body,
2. list some foods that are excellent sources of calcium,
3. discuss the negative effects of a diet low in calcium,
4. work together with other students to learn new information, and
5. recognize some of the bones in the human skeleton.

After activity 2, students will be able to

1. describe the functions of iron in the body,
2. list some foods that are excellent sources of iron,
3. discuss the possible negative effects of a lack of iron, and
4. create a comic strip that depicts the role of iron in the body.

▶▶ Materials

For activity 1:

- Student resource 1 *Filling Your Calcium Bank*
- Activity 1 *Building a Strong Skeleton: The Rules of the Game*
- Copies of bones (two sets per group)
- Scissors (one pair per person if possible)
- Answer key (one per group)
- Chicken bone (thigh or femur)
- Hydrochloric acid (20%)
- Beaker
- Safety goggles

For activity 2:

- Plain white paper
- Crayons or colored markers
- Activity 2 *Iron "Toons"*

▶▶ Procedure

Decide which activity best suits your curriculum.

Activity 1 Building a Strong Skeleton: The Rules of the Game

This activity will probably require one and a half to two periods. Please note: You will need about three to four days to allow the minerals to leach out of the bone.

Day 1

1. Point out the goals of this lesson:
   - To describe calcium's jobs in the body
   - To become familiar with some foods that are excellent sources of calcium
   - To discuss the negative effects of a diet low in calcium
   - To play a game that helps reinforce understanding of the importance of calcium

2. (2-3 minutes) Ask students the following:
   - Why do we need to eat foods with plenty of calcium? *(Most likely answer: To build strong bones and teeth.)*
   - What happens if we don't get enough calcium? *(Answer: Calcium leaves the bones and bones weaken.)*

3. (3-5 minutes) Pass around a fresh, clean, chicken leg bone. Have students touch the bone and observe its structure. Place the bone in a beaker of dilute hydrochloric acid. Ask students: *What do you think will happen to the bone as it sits in this weak acid?* Cover the beaker. Observe the change in the bone after three to four days. Use tongs to remove the bone from the beaker. Rinse the bone in water for 1 minute before allowing students to twist and bend the bone. *(The calcium will leave the bone, and it will become flexible; only the bone cells will be left behind. This shows students that calcium is essential for building strong bones.)*

4. (1 minute) Ask students whether they think the following statement is true or false: **Bones are alive and growing! They completely replace themselves every seven years.** *(True)*

Do not discuss students' opinions about the question until after they have read student resource 1, *Filling Your Calcium Bank.*

5. (5-10 minutes) Have students read student resource 1 *Filling Your Calcium Bank.* Have them put a check next to the foods they think are good sources of calcium. *(Answers: milk, yogurt, cheese, spinach, broccoli, tofu.)*

6. (5 minutes) Discuss their answers to the true/false question (please refer to step 4). Go over which foods are good sources of calcium. Make sure students understand what is meant by weight-bearing exercises. Mention some other lifestyles (habits) that increase or decrease calcium deposits in the bones. (See Teacher Resources.)

7. (5 minutes) Put students into groups of five. Tell them that they will play a game to help them learn more about calcium in a fun way. Pass out the necessary supplies to each group: scissors for cutting out the bone models, two copies of the bone models, copies of activity 1 *Building a Strong Skeleton: The Rules of the Game.*

8. (5-10 minutes) Go over the rules of the game. Make sure everybody understands the rules.

9. (5-10 minutes) Have students cut out the bone models.

Day 2

1. (5 minutes) Ask someone to summarize the game objective and the rules.

2. (1 minute) Display a human skeleton or an overhead transparency of the skeleton on page 318. Let students study the correct arrangement of bones for about 1 minute.

3. (5 minutes) Have students get into their groups and set up the game.

4. Pass out the answer key and skeleton to the master of ceremonies in each group.

5. (15 minutes) Students play the game.

6. (2-3 minutes) Students display their skeleton models for the rest of the class.

Activity 2 Iron "Toons"

1. Point out the goals of the lesson:
   - To describe the functions of iron in the body
   - To become familiar with some foods that are excellent sources of iron
   - To discuss the possible negative effects of a lack of iron
   - To create a comic strip that depicts the role of iron in the body

2. (5 minutes) Hand out activity 2 *Iron "Toons."* Have students read the top of the sheet.

3. (5 minutes) If possible, show students an object made out of iron. Discuss the reading. Ask them the following:
   - Why do we need to ingest this mineral? What is iron's job in our bodies?
   - What happens if you don't get enough iron?
   - Give some examples of foods that are high in iron?

4. (3-5 minutes) Go over the instructions for making the comic strips.

5. (Time will vary) Have students begin their comic strips. They may need to finish them as homework.

6. Display students' comic strips and give students an opportunity to walk around and read them.

▶▶ Extension Activities

1. Before the next class, check the calcium and iron content of some foods you see at home or in stores. Bring some labels to class. Make a collage of the labels from foods that provide good supplies of these minerals.

2. Write a rap song or poem describing the importance of iron or calcium. Share it with the class.

3. Your grandmother decides she wants to retire and build a house on the moon. However, her doctor will not sign the medical release form she needs for space travel. He says the trip will aggravate her osteoporosis. Explain to your grandmother why she should remain living on earth. Give her advice on how she can strengthen her bones.

▶▶ Teacher Resources

Specific Background Information: Calcium (Activity 1)

Functions of Calcium in the Body

Calcium plays an important role in

- bone and tooth growth, development, and structure,
- muscle contraction and relaxation,
- nerve functioning,
- the reduction of blood clotting,
- the reduction of blood pressure, and
- immunity to disease and infection.

Calcium Requirements for Adolescent Boys and Girls

The recommended daily intake of calcium for 9–18 year olds is 1300 mg. To meet this recommendation, consume 4 servings of milk or milk products each day or a combination of foods rich in calcium (see the table *Food Sources of Calcium*).

Vitamin D helps us absorb calcium from the foods we eat. Without enough vitamin D, our body will take calcium from our bones. The recommended daily intake of vitamin D is 5 micrograms. We can get vitamin D from two sources: (1) the sun, and (2) our diet. (Our skin makes vitamin D when we are exposed to direct sunlight.) Fortified dairy products, egg yolks, saltwater fish, and liver are good sources of vitamin D.

Other facts about calcium:

- Dairy foods contribute 75% of the calcium intake in the U.S.
- Dairy products and tofu are the best source of bio-available calcium in the diet. Plants considered high in calcium often contain oxalates and phylates that inhibit the absorption of calcium in the body. However, calcium is well absorbed from kale and broccoli.
- The amount of food needed to provide the same amount of calcium as 1 cup of milk is shown by these examples: 15.5 servings of spinach, 5.2 servings of broccoli, 3.5 servings of kale, 2.3 servings of soybeans, 1.2 servings of tofu.

Food Sources of Calcium

Food	Serving size	Calcium (mg)	Food	Serving size	Calcium (mg)
Dairy			**Meat**		
Yogurt, plain, low fat	1 cup	400	Tofu, raw firm	1/2 cup	258
Swiss cheese	1.5 oz	408	Sardines, canned with bones	3 oz	321
Cheddar cheese	1.5 oz	306	Almonds, dry roasted	1 oz	80
Skim milk	1 cup	302	**Green vegetables**		
Ice cream, hard, 10% fat	1/2 cup	85	Spinach, fresh, cooked	1/2 cup	122
Grains			Okra, frozen, cooked	1/2 cup	88
Waffle	7"	171	**Combination foods**		
Biscuit	1	58	Lasagna	2 1/4" × 2 1/4"	460
Cereal bar, calcium-fortified	1	200	Pizza, cheese	2 slices	277
Fruit					
Orange juice, calcium-fortified	8 oz	350			

- Calcium-fortified products, like orange juice and cereal bars, are also a good source of calcium, especially for individuals who don't like dairy products. An 8-ounce glass of calcium-fortified orange juice provides 35% of the daily recommended allowance (RDA) of calcium. An 8-ounce glass of milk provides 30% of RDA.

Lactose Intolerance

Some people have difficulty digesting dairy products. These people lack the enzyme lactase, which is needed to break down the milk sugar lactose. When these individuals consume milk, they experience cramping, bloating, gas, and diarrhea. This condition is called *lactose intolerance*. Most infants and children are capable of breaking down lactose, but as some people age they lose the ability to make lactase.

An estimated 30 to 50 million adults in the United States are lactose intolerant. As many as 75% of all African-Americans, Jews, Hispanics, and Native Americans and 90% of Asian-Americans are lactose intolerant. However, most Northern Europeans and some African tribes and Mediterraneans and their descendants produce sufficient quantities of lactase.

The severity of the condition varies from individual to individual. Most affected individuals can eat yogurt, hard cheeses, and milk that has been treated with commercially available lactase. Many can even drink small quantities of regular milk.

Calcium-fortified foods, tofu, soybeans, broccoli, and kale are also good sources of calcium for lactose-intolerant individuals

Are Calcium Supplements Necessary?

Calcium supplements may be necessary for people who are unable to consume milk and milk products. Likewise, they may be used as a part of therapy for osteoporosis. However, there are physiological risks (e.g., kidney stones and vomiting) associated with consuming excess calcium (beyond 2,500 mg per day). Supplements beyond the suggested daily levels are not recommended.

Calcium Deficiency Signs, Symptoms, and Risk Factors

In adults, osteoporosis or osteomalacia can result from calcium deficiency. Bone loss can occur without symptoms.

Bone Formation

• Calcium is continually being deposited in bones and reabsorbed from bones throughout life. In children and adolescents, a larger amount of calcium is deposited than is reabsorbed. However, after the age of 30, more calcium is reabsorbed than is deposited in bone and bones become progressively less dense.

• Almost 50% of bone mass is formed during teen years. Even when teenagers stop growing taller, calcium continues to be deposited in their bones, increasing bone density. If inadequate amounts of calcium are deposited, bones will be less dense, and the individual will be more likely to develop osteoporosis or to suffer bone fractures later in life.

• Peak bone mass is reached by age 30.

• An active lifestyle can save your bones! Regular exercise can help slow the rate your bones age. Active people have significantly greater bone mass than sedentary people. Researchers believe that bone behaves like a piezoelectric crystal, converting mechanical stress into electrical energy. When bone is mechanically stressed, the electrical charge created stimulates the activity of bone-forming cells, leading to a buildup of calcium (McArdle, Katch, and Katch 1991).

• Weight-bearing exercises (activities that force you to work against gravity) such as walking, dancing, or jogging and activities such as weightlifting in which muscular force is generated against the long bones of the body are especially good at enhancing calcium deposits in the bone.

• Prolonged bed rest, as well as the zero-gravity conditions of space travel, weakens bones. The longer an astronaut stays in orbit, the more calcium leaches out of bones. On long missions, astronauts must follow rigorous exercise programs and special diets to help counteract this problem.

• Smokers and alcoholics are at a higher risk of bone fractures than nonsmokers and those who don't drink or who drink in moderation.

• Underweight women and those with eating disorders are at a higher risk of fractures than individuals of average weight.

• At birth, humans have 300 bones. By the time adulthood is reached, the bones number 206, because some have fused.

• Half of your bones are in your hands and feet (Allison 1976).

Specific Background Information: Iron (Activity 2)

Iron Requirements for Adolescent Boys and Girls

Under the age of 10, schoolchildren need 10 milligrams of iron daily. Boys 10 and older require 12 milligrams per day; for girls 10 and older, 15 milligrams daily are recommended.

Functions of Iron in the Body

Iron is essential for transporting oxygen around the body. It is part of hemoglobin and myoglobin:

1. *Hemoglobin* (a protein) is the oxygen carrier in red blood cells. One red blood cell has almost 300 million molecules of hemoglobin.
2. In muscles, *myoglobin* (a protein) makes oxygen available for cellular respiration (ATP production) in muscle cells.

Food Sources of Iron

- Beef, pork, lamb, fish, poultry (especially dark meat), shellfish, eggs, liver, and other organ meats.
- Legumes such as lima beans and green peas; and dry beans and peas such as pinto beans, black-eyed peas, and canned baked beans.
- Dark green vegetables such as broccoli and kale.
- Yeast-leavened whole wheat bread.

Are Iron Supplements Necessary?

Iron supplements may be needed by pregnant women or by people not consuming meat. Supplements should be discussed with your doctor. Iron supplements often have a side effect—constipation.

Signs and Symptoms of Iron Deficiency

A lack of iron can affect us in many ways:

- The lack of oxygen transportation can reduce energy (ATP) production in cells, causing fatigue and reducing attention span.
- Iron deficiency reduces resistance to cold, lowers the ability to control body temperature, and can cause itchy skin.

Food Sources of Iron

Food	Serving size	Iron (mg)
Hamburger, lean, broiled	3.5 oz	2.45
Liver, beef, braised	3.5 oz	6.77
Chicken, thigh, roasted	1 thigh	0.83
Broccoli, boiled	1/2 cup	0.65
Baked beans	1 cup	3.60
Lima beans	1 cup	4.50

Other Important Information

- Consuming small amounts of meat and foods rich in vitamin C in a meal greatly increases iron absorption.
- There is a greater need for iron during rapid growth periods, such as the adolescent growth spurt. However, not all adolescents get enough iron. Studies including children have suggested that a lack of iron may be associated with poor school performance, short attention span, and decreased immune function.

References

Allison, L.1976. *Blood and guts.* Boston: Little, Brown.

American Dietetic Association. **www.eatright.org**

Bierer, L.A., Warner, L., Lawson, S., and Cohe, T. 1991. *Life science: The challenge of discovery.* Lexington, MA: Heath.

Chandler, D. 1991. Exploring life without gravity. *Boston Globe,* June 10.

Institute of Medicine Dietary Reference. 1997. I*ntakes for calcium, phosphorus, magnesium, vitamin D, and fluoride.* Washington, DC: National Academy Press.

McArdle, E., Katch, F., and Katch, V. 1991. *Exercise physiology: Energy, nutrition, and human performance.* 3d ed. Philadelphia: Lea & Febiger.

National Dairy Council. 1994. *The all-American guide: Thinking about calcium. Find it in food first.* 3d ed. Rosemont, IL: National Dairy Council.

National Digestive Diseases Information Clearinghouse. **www.niddk.nih.gov/health/digest/pubs/lactose.htm**

National Institute of Diabetes and Digestive and Kidney Diseases. **www.niddk.nih.gov**

New England Dairy and Food Council. 1996. *Healthy bones: Ideas for teaching children, teens, and adults about building healthy bones.* Boston: New England Dairy Council.

Calcium's Value

Most people know that calcium is a mineral that helps build strong bones and teeth. But did you know that calcium also

- helps your muscles contract and relax,
- helps your heart beat,
- helps your blood clot, and
- helps your nerves send messages.

So what happens if you don't supply your body with enough calcium to perform these important functions? Your body takes calcium it needs from your bones! Your bones act as a kind of savings account for calcium.

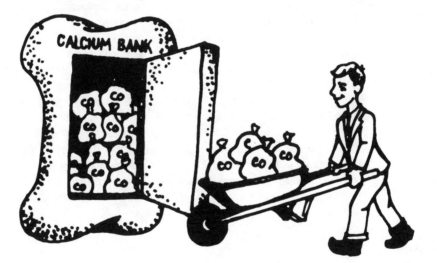

If your diet supplies enough calcium, your body deposits some in your bones.

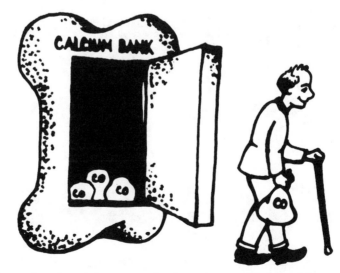

If your diet is low in calcium, your body makes a withdrawal from your bones.

Penalties for Not Keeping a Minimum Balance

A diet low in calcium has been linked to several health problems.

Osteoporosis—a crippling bone disease. Bones become so brittle that they break easily.

Bone loss in the jaw—this can lead to difficulty chewing, tooth loss, and poor-fitting dentures.

Hypertension—high blood pressure can lead to strokes and heart attacks in some people.

How to Make a Deposit

If you're like most Americans, you may not be getting all the calcium you need. To provide your body with enough calcium, you (9-18 year olds) need to make daily "deposits" of 1,300 mg. Milk and other dairy products (yogurt and cheeses) offer the largest amount of calcium per serving. Four glasses of milk daily will provide you with all the calcium your body needs. Tofu and small fish with bones, like sardines, are also excellent sources of calcium. Kale, broccoli, and other green leafy vegetables are good sources of calcium, but provide much fewer grams per serving than most milk products.

Calcium supplements may be necessary for people who are unable to consume milk and milk products. Talk to your physician before taking a calcium supplement. There are no benefits for taking more than the recommended daily allowance of calcium. In fact, excess doses of calcium can interfere with the absorption of nutrients like iron.[1]

Weight-bearing exercises such as walking, dancing, and jogging also enhance calcium deposits in the bone and are critical during adolescence to build peak bone mass. During the teen years, people go through a growth spurt—almost 50% of bone mass is formed then! Even if a teenager does not appear to grow, bones are still getting denser. If inadequate amounts of calcium are deposited, bones will be less dense, and the individual will be more likely to develop osteoporosis or to suffer bone fractures later in life.[2]

Problem

Put a check next to the foods below that are rich in calcium.

❏ red meat	❏ chicken
❏ cheese	❏ oranges
❏ milk	❏ tofu
❏ broccoli	❏ spinach
❏ yogurt	❏ apples

---

[1] *The All-American Guide to Calcium-Rich Foods,* 1990. Courtesy of National Dairy Council.

[2] *Healthy Bones: Ideas for Teaching Children, Teens, and Adults About Building Healthy Bones,* 1996. New England Dairy Association.

Objective

To collect ten human bones and assemble them correctly to form a skeleton.

Materials

2 sets of the bone models

1 answer key

5 (or more) people per group

scissors

tape

Setting Up the Game

1. Cut out the bone models.
2. Place them on a table so that the bone name is face up.
3. Decide who will be the master of ceremonies.
4. Form two teams.

Collecting the Human Bones

To collect a bone, a team must correctly answer the question on the back of the bone. The questions test your understanding of the role calcium and lifestyle play in building strong bones. Some questions ask students to name a food that is high in calcium. Others ask whether a particular lifestyle is likely to help deposit calcium in bones or remove calcium from bones. For example, "Does regular exercise help deposit calcium in bones or weaken bones by removing calcium from bones?" The master of ceremonies checks the answer key to see whether the team's answer is right or wrong. If they are right, they keep the bone. If they are wrong, the bone is left in play.

Note: For the femur, humerus, fibula and tibia, radius and ulna, hands, and feet, only one question is required to obtain both right and left bones.

Playing the Game

1. Flip a coin to see which team goes first.
2. Teams take turns choosing a bone to play for. A team is given 30 seconds to answer the question on the back of the bone. If their reply is correct, they keep the bone. If it is incorrect, the bone is turned back over, and the other team begins its turn.
3. The first team to collect all ten bones is given 30 seconds to assemble the bones correctly. After 30 seconds, they must stop manipulating the bones until their next turn. If they are unable to assemble the skeleton, or if they have made some mistakes, the master of ceremonies gives the competing team a chance to win another

bone. The first team receives a second chance to assemble the bones correctly on their next turn.

4. The first team to collect all ten bones AND correctly assemble them to form a human skeleton wins the game.

5. Have students tape their skeleton models together.

Master of Ceremonies

The master of ceremonies keeps time, allowing each team 30 seconds to answer the questions. He or she also checks the answer key to determine whether the response is accurate. If the response is incorrect, the master of ceremonies should NOT read the correct answer. The master of ceremonies also determines which team correctly assembles the skeleton first.

Building a Strong Skeleton: The Rules of the Game

Answer Key

Building a Strong Skeleton: The Rules of the Game

Bone	Question	Answer
Ribs and vertebrae	Name a food that is high in calcium. (It must be one that has not been mentioned yet in this game.)	Milk, yogurt, cheddar cheese, pizza, lasagna, macaroni and cheese, salmon, (canned with bones), dark green vegetables (like kale and broccoli), some tortillas, and some tofu.
Left and right femur	How many glasses of milk would you need to drink to get a full day's supply of calcium?	4 (9–18 year olds).
Left and right humerus	People who do not get an adequate supply of calcium when they are young are likely to develop _____	Osteoporosis or bone fractures.
Left and right fibula and tibia	Watching TV is a habit that _____ bones. Explain.	Weakens bones. Sedentary activity increases the amount of calcium that leaves the bones.
Left and right radius and ulna	Living in outer space would _____ your bones. Explain.	Weaken your bones. Putting weight on your bones helps deposit calcium in them. In outer space there is very little gravity; therefore, there is not much stress on your bones, so calcium leaves bones.
Skull and vertebrae	Does bed rest strengthen bones or weaken bones? Explain.	Weakens bones. Weight-bearing exercise is needed to help deposit calcium in bones.
Pelvis, sacrum, and vertebrae	Name a habit that would withdraw calcium from your bones, weakening them. (It must be one that has not been mentioned yet in this game.)	Skipping meals, drinking alcohol, smoking cigarettes, watching TV, starving yourself to lose weight.
Left and right hands	Name a habit that would help deposit calcium in your bones.	Eating a well-balanced diet, drinking 4 glasses of milk a day, regular exercise
Left and right feet	Which food group contains foods that have the most calcium per serving?	Dairy
Clavicle and scapula	Name one job that calcium does in your body besides build strong bones.	Helps muscles contract and relax, helps the heart beat, helps blood clot, and helps nerves send messages.

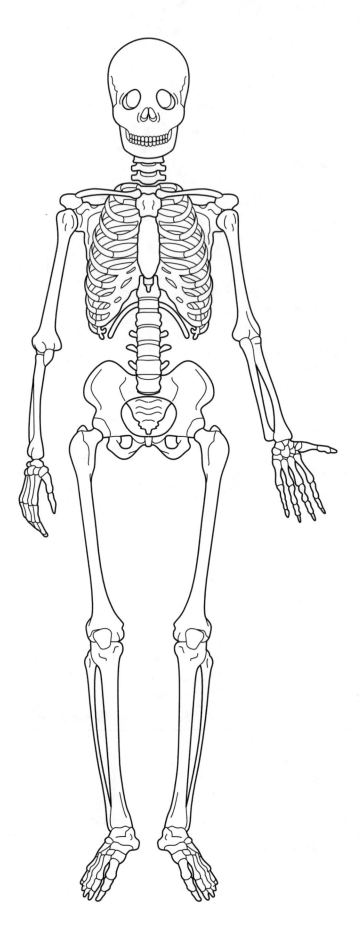

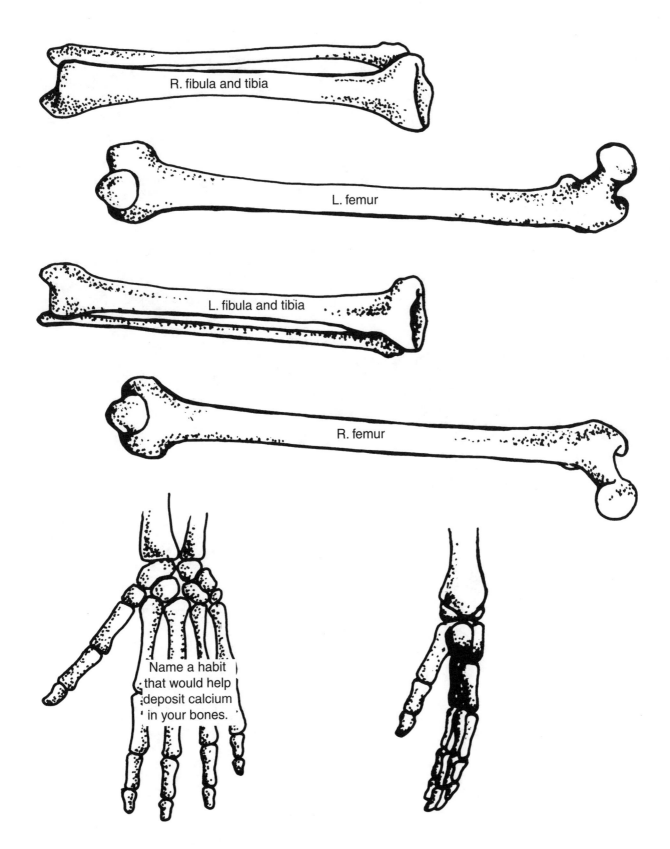

R. fibula and tibia

L. femur

L. fibula and tibia

R. femur

Name a habit that would help deposit calcium in your bones.

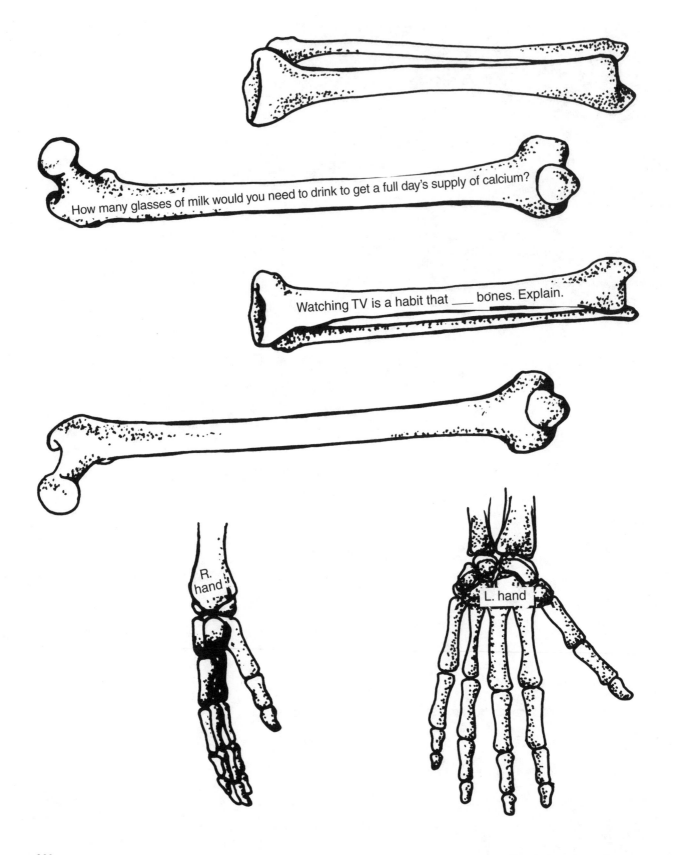

How many glasses of milk would you need to drink to get a full day's supply of calcium?

Watching TV is a habit that ___ bones. Explain.

R. hand

L. hand

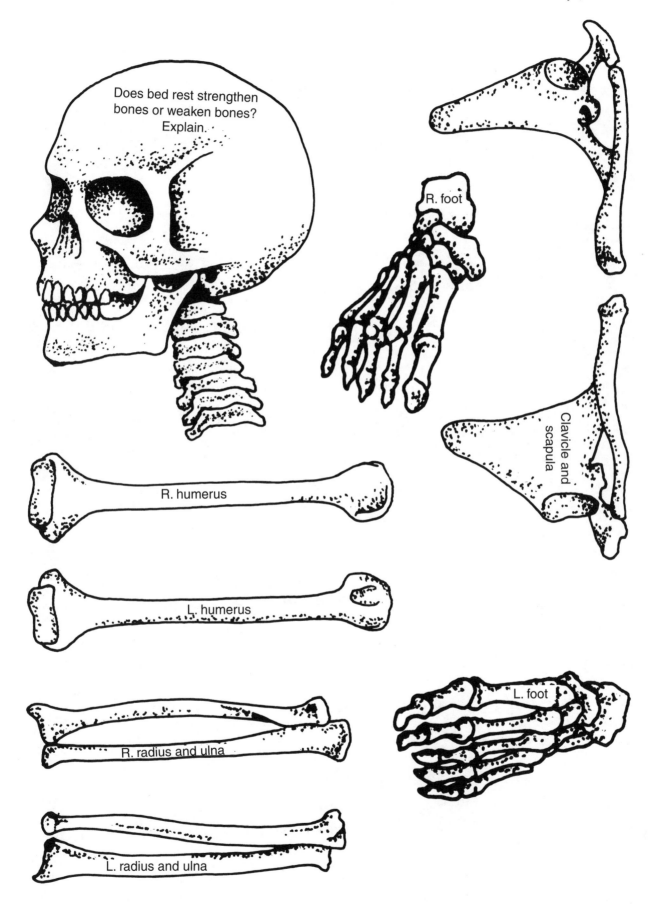

Does bed rest strengthen bones or weaken bones? Explain.

R. foot

Clavicle and scapula

R. humerus

L. humerus

R. radius and ulna

L. foot

L. radius and ulna

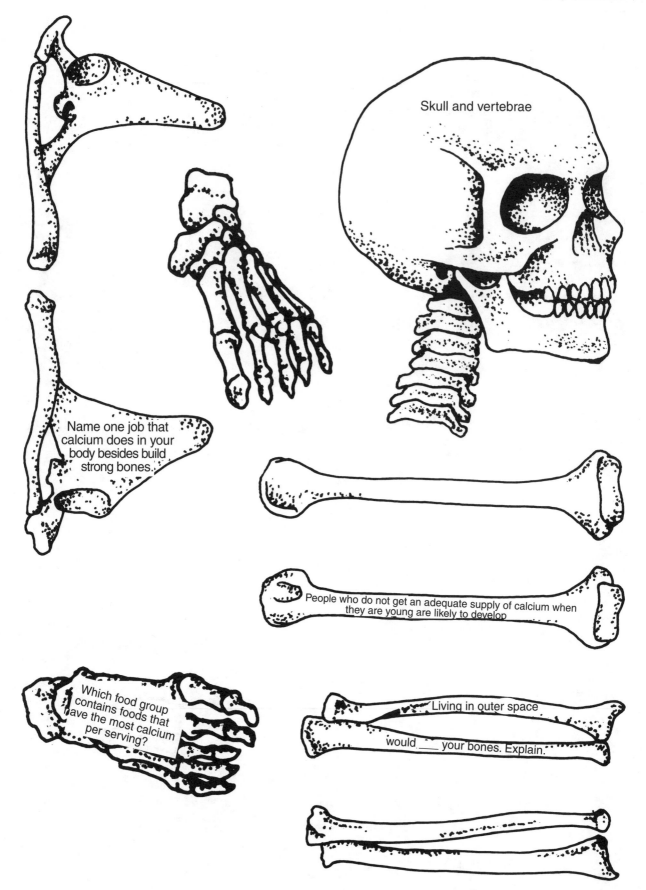

Skull and vertebrae

Name one job that calcium does in your body besides build strong bones.

People who do not get an adequate supply of calcium when they are young are likely to develop

Which food group contains foods that have the most calcium per serving?

Living in outer space

would ___ your bones. Explain.

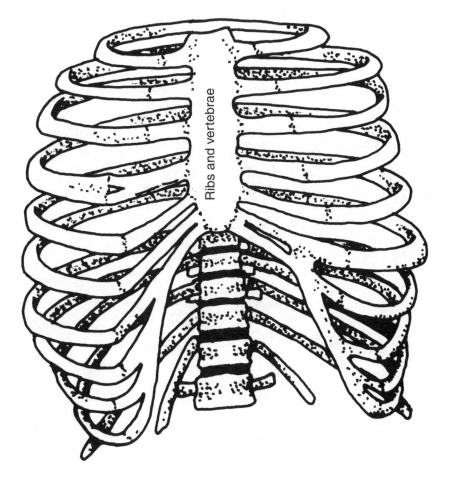

Ribs and vertebrae

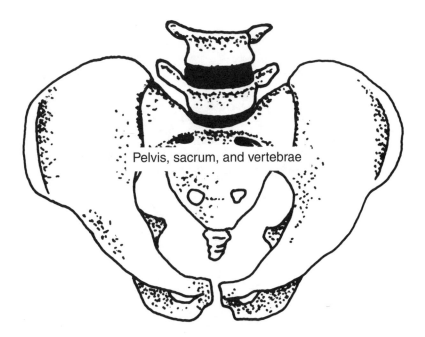

Pelvis, sacrum, and vertebrae

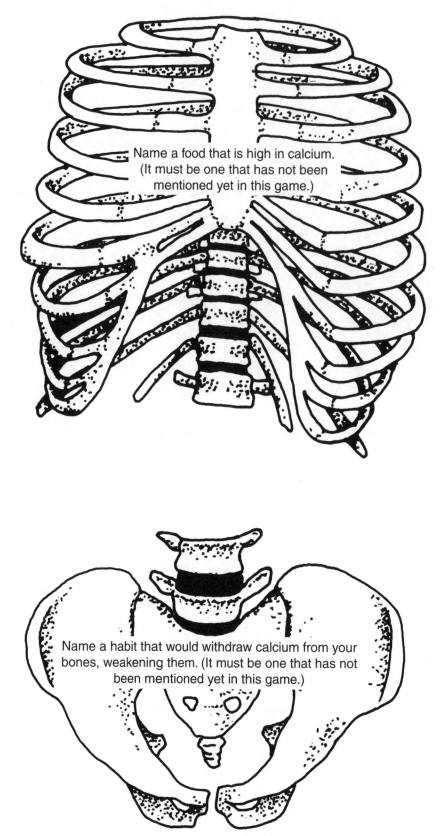

Name a food that is high in calcium. (It must be one that has not been mentioned yet in this game.)

Name a habit that would withdraw calcium from your bones, weakening them. (It must be one that has not been mentioned yet in this game.)

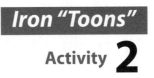

Do I really need to eat iron? It's a metal.

Yes! Iron is an important part of every red blood cell in your body. Red blood cells are filled with an iron-containing protein called hemoglobin. Oxygen binds to the iron and is carried around the body inside red blood cells. Iron also plays a role in the immune system.

How much iron do I need?

Under the age of eleven, school children need 10 milligrams of iron daily. Boys eleven and older require 12 milligrams per day; for girls eleven and older 15 milligrams daily are recommended. There is a greater need for iron during rapid growth periods, such as the adolescent growth spurt.

What foods are good sources of iron?

Lean meat and poultry, fish, leafy green vegetables from the cabbage family (broccoli, kale, and collards), dried beans and peas (pinto beans, black-eyed peas, and canned baked beans), and bread, pasta, rice, and cereals enriched with iron (iron is added during food preparation) are good sources of iron. Eating small amounts of vitamin C rich foods in a meal greatly increases the amount of iron absorbed from food into the blood.

Are iron supplements necessary?

Pregnant women or people who do not eat meat may need to ingest iron in tablet form. Many vitamin supplements include iron. Supplements should be discussed with your doctor.

What happens if I don't eat enough iron?

A lack of iron makes it difficult for your red blood cells to carry enough oxygen to your cells. The lack of oxygen reduces energy production in your cells, causing you to feel tired and weak. Eventually your body produces too few red blood cells, a condition called anemia. Very low iron intake also reduces your resistance to colds, your ability to control body temperature and can cause itchy skin. Studies with children have suggested that a lack of iron may be associated with short attention span, poor school performance, and short stature.

Directions

Use the information above to make a comic strip which illustrates iron's job in the body. Follow the guidelines listed below.

1. The comic strip must be at least 4 frames long.
2. Your story should include examples of food sources high in iron.
3. You must show what happens when not enough iron is eaten.
4. Helpful tips:
   - Red blood cells are disk shaped with dents in the middle. These cells flow through blood vessels.
   - The chemical symbol for iron is Fe.
   - The chemical symbol for oxygen is O_2.

Lesson 49

Fat Functions

In this lesson, students learn that fat is an essential nutrient needed by the human body, but that eating excess amounts of certain types of fats carries major health risks. Students will conduct a scientific investigation on invisible and visible fat to help them understand dietary sources of fat.

This lesson is designed to infuse information about consuming fat in moderation into a classroom unit on the role of fat in the body.

▶▶ Behavioral Objectives

- To understand the role of fat in the diet.
- To choose a diet low in saturated fat and moderate in total fat.

▶▶ Learning Objectives

Students will be able to

1. conduct a scientific investigation on invisible and visible fat, and
2. use results of an experiment to form conclusions about fat.

▶▶ Materials

- Butter; oil; a piece of cooked meat or poultry; hard-boiled egg; cooked beans; tofu; cheese; yogurt (not low fat); potato chips (regular, not low-fat); cereal; cake, donut, or croissant; and some fruits and vegetables for demonstration. *Be sure to include examples from each of the Food Guide Pyramid food groups so that you have foods with saturated fat, unsaturated fat, trans fat, and no fat.*
- Brown paper bags or brown paper towels
- Activity 1 *Understanding Visible and Invisible Fat*
- Student resource 1 *What's the Rap on Fat?*
- Overhead transparency 1 *Definitions* (or handout or chalkboard)
- Overhead transparency 2 *Role of Lipids* (or handout or chalkboard)
- *Optional:* Extension activity 1 *Moderation and Fat*

▶▶ Procedure

Pre-Lab Preparations

1. Assemble the following food items: butter; oil; cooked meat or poultry; hard-boiled egg (separate the yolk and white); cooked beans; tofu; cheese; potato chips

(regular, not low fat); cereal; cake, donut, or croissant; and some fruit and vegetables. Be sure to include examples from each of the Food Guide Pyramid food groups.

2. Cut or break up the food.

Lesson Procedure

1. (10 minutes) Have students read student resource 1 *What's the Rap on Fat?*

2. (10 minutes) Discuss the different types of fat (see the scientific terms in Teacher Resources) and discuss the importance of fat in the body. (Use overhead transparencies 1 and 2 or the chalkboard.)

3. (5 minutes) Discuss problems associated with consuming excess fat.

4. (5 minutes) Put students into groups of four or five. Distribute activity 1 *Understanding Visible and Invisible Fat.* Assign two or three foods to each group.

5. Have students make predictions. What will happen and why?

6. Ask students to place food on a brown paper towel or a brown grocery bag.

7. After 10 minutes, remove food and let the paper dry. (You may wish to have students work on extension activity 1 *Moderation and Fat* during this time.)

8. If the paper has dried and there is enough time before the end of the class period, record observations. Otherwise, save the papers and record observations the following day.

9. (10 minutes) In the next class, have students present the results of their experiment to the class. Record the class results on the chalkboard. Have students record the results and answer the conclusion questions.

10. (10 minutes) Observations and conclusions. Discuss the results of the experiment:

After the paper is dried up, those that contained the cereal, tofu, beans, egg white, and fruit or vegetable pieces should not have any fat stains on them. The papers that contained the butter or oil, meat, egg yolk, cheese, potato chips, cake, donuts, and croissant should have fat stains on the areas where the foods were kept. The stains may have even extended beyond the areas. These foods contain fat. Fat does not evaporate like the water found in the fruits and vegetables.

Most fruits and vegetables do not contain any fat and therefore do not leave a stain. (Olives and avocados are examples of fruits that do contain fat.) But cheese, meats, and bakery goods have invisible fat, and therefore leave a stain that is similar to the stain left by butter, which is visible fat.

Fat is an essential nutrient. If you compare the foods tested to the Food Guide Pyramid, it can be seen that a certain amount of fat is included in foods from all groups on the pyramid. Sometimes, the brown paper bag test does not show the fat contained within the food. That is why it is necessary to read labels to find fat sources.

Not all fats are created equal! Labels list not only the total fat grams, but the grams of saturated fats as well. Trans fats (partially hydrogenated vegetable oils) are hidden in the ingredients list. Unsaturated fats are healthier for our bodies than saturated fats or trans fats, which tend to raise blood cholesterol and increase the risk of developing heart disease. The paper bag test does not demonstrate the differences among trans fats, saturated fats, and unsaturated fats. They will appear the same. This is why it is necessary to read labels.

Cholesterol is found only in foods of animal origin. Cholesterol may also raise blood cholesterol, but not nearly as much as saturated fat. That is why the fat in coconut (mostly saturated fat) is less healthy than other oils, despite the fact that it has no cholesterol.

11. (5 minutes) Review key points from the lesson:

- Fat plays a major role in the body. However, too much, as well as too little, fat in the diet can result in health problems.

- We should make sure our diets contain a moderate amount of total fat with lower amounts of saturated and trans fats.

▶▶ Extension Activities

Choose one of the following:

1. Why does too much or too little fat in our diet result in health problems? (6-8 sentences)

2. Use extension activity 1 *Moderation and Fat* as a homework assignment or as needed during the lesson.

3. Have students choose three to five foods at home and repeat this experiment. Find out from labels or other resources how much fat is in a serving of each of the foods you tried.

▶▶ Teacher Resources

General Background Material

In preparing for this lesson, you may want to refer to the following resources:

- *Nutrition and your health: Dietary guidelines for Americans* (5th ed.).
  See appendix A for information on how to obtain this resource.

- *Fat: Where It's At,* page 252

Specific Background Material

Lipid: The scientific term for fats. Lipids include dietary fats and oils. While fats are solid at room temperature, most oils (excluding coconut) are liquid at room temperature. Fats provide 9 calories per gram.

Visible fat: Fat you can see. This includes fats we add to food: butter, margarine, oils, lard, drippings, and so on that we use for cooking, spreading on toast, or in salad dressings. This category also includes fat that you can trim from meat.

Invisible fat: Fats that are present in food that may be invisible to the eye. These include fats in meat, poultry, fish, eggs, dairy products, sweets and baked goods.

Saturated fats: Fats contained in animal products like high-fat dairy products (whole milk, butter, cream, ice cream, cheese), fatty fresh and processed meats, and lard, and in palm and coconut oil. This type of fat is generally solid at room temperature. Eating foods high in saturated fat raises blood cholesterol levels. Eating saturated fats in excess over time can increase the risk of developing heart disease. Experts recommend eating a diet low in saturated fats.

Unsaturated fats (polyunsaturated and monounsaturated): Fats or oils contained in plant products like vegetable oils (olive, canola, corn, peanut, soybean), most nuts, olives, and avocados, and in fatty fish like salmon. This type of fat is generally liquid at room temperature. Eating unsaturated fats does not raise blood cholesterol levels and, therefore, does not contribute to heart disease. In fact, some oils may lower LDL cholesterol (the "bad" cholesterol) and raise HDL cholesterol (the "good" cholesterol), thus decreasing the risk of developing heart disease. Some evidence indicates that omega-3 fatty acids, an unsaturated fat found in salmon, tuna, and mackerel, may protect against heart disease.

Trans fatty acids: Vegetable oils that have been converted from liquids into solids by a commercial process called hydrogenation. These fats are commonly called partially hydrogenated vegetable oils on ingredient lists. Solid margarines, shortenings, commerically fried foods, many crackers, and bakery goods are high in this type of fat. To identify these fats, check the ingredient lists on packaged foods like cookies and crackers. Avoid varieties made with partially hydrogenated vegetable oil. Choose margarines with liquid oil as the first ingredient. If eaten in excess over time, foods high in trans fats can increase the risk of developing heart disease.

Dietary cholesterol: Lipids (sterols) found only in animal products. Liver and other organ meats, eggs, and high-fat dairy products are high in cholesterol. Eating an excess of these foods increases blood cholesterol levels and can contribute to heart disease. Recent research indicates that individuals with normal blood cholesterol levels can eat an egg a day without increasing their risk of developing heart disease.

For a discussion of the different types of dietary fats, see student resource 1 *What's the Rap on Fat?*.

Role of Lipids in the Diet

- Fats and oils add flavor, aroma, and texture to food.

- Lipids provide a feeling of fullness because they remain in the stomach longer than carbohydrates and proteins and take longer to digest than other nutrients.

- Dietary fat is essential for the absorption of fat-soluble vitamins A, D, E, and K. Taking supplements of fat-soluble vitamins without eating any fat will not help prevent deficiencies of these vitamins.

- Fat is a major source of energy. While 1 gram of carbohydrate and 1 gram of protein provide 4 calories each, 1 gram of fat provides 9 calories.

Role of Lipids in Our Bodies

- Lipids include essential fatty acids (EFA). Humans can't synthesize these and therefore need to obtain them through the diet. Essential fatty acids are needed for normal tissue function throughout the body. Deficiency syndromes can develop if they are missing from the diet.

- Fat helps the body maintain its temperature. About one-half of the fat in the body is deposited just under the skin. This provides a layer of insulation to protect against changes in external temperature.

- Fat serves as a cushion for major organs such as the heart and kidney. These body organs are surrounded by fat, which holds them in place and also protects them from injury. For this reason, the fat stores next to the vital organs are the last to be used for energy in times of need.

- Increases in percent body fat are linked with development changes in females. Girls start menstruating and mature sexually after they have achieved a certain amount of body fat. If they do not have enough body fat, they may start menstruating late. Also, if a woman loses a lot of weight, she may stop menstruating.

- Some lipids are important hormone precursors.

- Phospholipids are the major component of all cell membranes in the body.

- Cholesterol is a lipid that helps transport fatty acids in the blood.

What's the chemical difference between saturated and unsaturated fat?

Food contains many types of lipids (triglycerides, cholesterol, phospholipids). Saturated and unsaturated fats are triglycerides. Triglycerides are composed of a glycerol molecule and three fatty acids. Fatty acids are classified as saturated (lacking double bonds between carbon atoms), monounsaturated (containing a single double bond), or polyunsaturated (containing more than one double bond). Hydrogenation is a commercial process that adds hydrogen to some of the double bonds in poly- and monounsaturated fatty acids, making them more like saturated fats. In addition, some of the remaining double bonds are converted from the *cis* to the *trans* form. Triglycerides are the most concentrated source of energy in the diet (9 calories per gram).

Facts Associated With Excess Fat Intake

- Habitual fat intake in excess of physiological needs increases risk for chronic disease in adulthood. This risk can begin in the teen years.
- Excess saturated fat consumption can cause blocked arteries and the development of heart disease as well as certain cancers in adult years.
- Atherosclerosis, the process of fatty substances building up in arteries, begins early in life.

What Are the Recommendations for Fat Intake?

The National Research Council's *Dietary Guidelines* and *Healthy People 2010* recommend consuming no more than 30% of calories from total fat and no more than 10% of calories from saturated fat. Individual foods can have more or less percent of calories from fat. It's the total percent of energy that counts.

Recommended fat intake:

- 11–14-year-old girls can have about 73 grams per day (30% of 2,200 calories) with 24 or fewer grams of saturated fat.
- 11–14-year-old boys can have about 83 grams per day (30% of 2,500 calories) with 28 or fewer grams of saturated fat.

References

Holt science. 1989. Austin, TX: Holt, Rinehart & Winston.

U.S. Department of Agriculture and U.S. Department of Health and Human Services. 2000. *Nutrition and your health: Dietary guidelines for Americans 2000,* 5th edition. **www.usda.gov/cnpp**

U.S. Department of Health and Human Services. 2000. Healthy People 2010, conference edition, vols. I and II. **www.health.gov/healthypeople**

Whitney, E.N., and Rolfes, S.R. 1993. *Understanding nutrition.* 6th ed. St. Paul: West.

▶▶ Answer Key

Extension Activity 1

1. FATS are SOLID and OILS are LIQUID at room temperature.
2. Oils, butter, and margarine are examples of VISIBLE fats.
3. Lipids are made up of FATTY ACIDS and GLYCEROL
4. One gram of fat provides NINE calories.
5. Lipids include ESSENTIAL fatty acids, which prevent FLAKING and DRYING of the SKIN.
6. When in food, fats add FLAVOR, TEXTURE, and AROMA to the food.
7. Body fat serves as a CUSHION for the major organs such as heart, kidney, etc.
8. Body fat provides a layer of INSULATION to protect the body from changes in the outside temperature.
9. Consuming EXCESS saturated fat can result in HEART problems as an adult.
10. Define visible and invisible fat. (See Teacher Resources.)

Lipid: The scientific name for fats, oils, hormones, cholesterol, fat-soluble vitamins, phospholipids, and other chemicals that do not dissolve in water.

Visible fat: Fat you can see. Includes fat we add to food: butter, margarine, oils, lard, and drippings. Also includes fat you can trim from meat.

Invisible fat: Fats that are present in food that may not be visible to the eye. These include fats we eat from meat, poultry, fish, eggs, dairy products, sweets and baked goods.

Saturated fats: Fats contained in animal products like high-fat dairy products (whole milk, butter, cream, ice cream, cheese), fatty fresh and processed meats, lard, and two plant oils: palm and coconut oil. This type of fat is generally solid at room temperature.

Unsaturated fats (polyunsaturated and monounsaturated):
Fats (or oils) contained in plant products like vegetable oils (such as olive, canola, corn, peanut, and soybean oils), most nuts, olives, avocados, and fatty fish like salmon. This type of fat is generally liquid at room temperature.

Trans fatty acids: Vegetable oils that have been converted into solids by a process called hydrogenation. These fats are commonly called partially hydrogenated vegetable oils on ingredient lists. Solid margarines, shortenings, commercially fried foods, and some bakery goods are high in this type of fat.

Role of lipids in the diet:

- Add flavor and texture to food.

- Provide a feeling of fullness.

- Essential for the absorption of fat-soluble vitamins, like A, D, E, and K.

- Provide major source of energy.

Role of lipids in the body:

- Fatty acids are essential for normal body function.

- Stored body fat helps the body maintain its temperature.

- Stored body fat serves as a cushion for major organs such as the heart, kidneys, etc.

- Every cell membrane is made up of phospholipids.

- Lipids give the body shape.

- Some lipids are necessary for hormone production.

- Cholesterol is a lipid that helps transport fatty acids in the blood.

Not All Fats Are Created Equal

Your body uses fat for energy, to transport vitamins, to protect your organs, and to make hormones. Every cell in your body is surrounded by a membrane made of fat, or lipid as scientists call it. Fat gives your body shape and insulates you from the cold. The bottom line is—you need to eat fat! But how much, and what kind?

Foods made from both animals and plants contain fat. These fats fall into two categories: saturated fat and unsaturated fat. Many animal products, like fatty meat, whole milk, butter, and lard, are high in saturated fat. This kind of fat is typically solid at room temperature. Eating too much saturated fat increases your risk of developing heart disease, so try to build your daily menu around foods that are low in saturated fat (grains, fruits, and vegetables). Eat low-fat dairy products and lean cuts of meat, and go easy on snacks made with butter and eggs (cookies and cakes). Think of high-saturated fat foods as "sometimes" foods.

To lower your intake of saturated fats:

- Cook with vegetable oils instead of butter.
- Trim fat from meat and take the skin off poultry.
- Choose fat-free or low-fat milk, yogurt, and cheese.
- Limit processed meats such as sausage, salami, and hot dogs.
- Limit creamy sauces.
- Check food labels. Choose foods lower in saturated fat.

Most of the fat you eat should be unsaturated, since this type of fat does not contribute to heart disease. Most plant fats, or oils, are unsaturated fats and are generally liquid at room temperature. Vegetable oils (like olive, canola, corn, and peanut oils), most nuts, olives, and avocados are good sources of unsaturated fat. However, eating lots of fat of any type may not be healthy, so try to get no more than 30% of your calories from fat.

Exceptions to the Rule!

Not all plant fats are healthy! Through a commercial process called *hydrogenation,* these more healthy liquid fats can be converted into solids called *trans fats* (also called partially hydrogenated vegetable oils). This is how some margarines are made. Not suprisingly, foods high in trans fat also have been found to increase the risk of heart disease. To avoid these fats, check the ingredient list on packaged foods like cookies and crackers. Avoid varieties made with partially hydrogenated vegetable oil. Also look out for coconut oil and palm oil since these oils are naturally high in saturated fat

Not all animal foods are high in saturated fat. Some ocean fish (like salmon and tuna) are high in a polyunsaturated fat called omega-3 fatty acid that may protect you against heart disease. So choose to eat fish when you get the chance.

Procedure

1. Place food items on a brown paper bag or paper towels. Write the name of food on the bag.
2. Let the food sit on the paper for 10 minutes.
3. Record your predictions (what you think will happen) on the table below.
4. Remove food and let the paper dry. (You may need to leave these to dry overnight.)
5. Record observations. Describe any stains left on the paper.
6. Exchange your results with other members of the class.

Results

Food item	Description of food item	Prediction of stain on the paper after 30 minutes	Description of stain on the paper after 30 minutes	Observations (quantitative)
Example: orange slice	Wet pulp, bumpy skins with soft white seeds	Small orange juice stain	No stain	14 cm × 6 cm × 10 cm, 4 seeds
1.				
2.				
3.				
4.				
5.				
6.				
7.				

Conclusions

Use the entire class's data to answer the following questions.

1. Which food items contained fat?

2. Of these foods, which are likely to be high in saturated fats? in trans fats?

3. If you compare the foods tested to the Food Guide Pyramid, which food groups contain fat?

Unscramble the letters to review some terms related to fats.

1. TAFS are DOSIL and LIOS are QLIIDU at room temperature.

2. Oils, butter, and margarine are examples of IIBVESL fats.

3. Lipids are made up of TTFAY DISAC and LLGRYECO.

4. One gram of fat provides NNEI calories.

5. Lipids include SSEETNLIA fatty acids, which prevent GNIKALF and GNIDRY of the NISK.

6. When in food, fats add OVRALF, EETTXUR, and MRAOA to the food.

7. Body fat serves as a CHNSIOU for the major organs such as heart, kidney, etc.

8. Body fat provides a layer of TINALIONSU to protect the body from changes in the outside temperature.

9. Consuming SESCXE saturated fats can result in TRHEA problems as an adult.

10. Define visible and invisible fat.

Lesson **50**

Smart Snacks

This lesson teaches students the importance of healthy snacks in the diet. The fast growth of adolescents makes snacks vital to maintaining a suitable energy balance. However, many snack foods are high in fat (especially saturated and trans fats), refined sugar, and salt, and low in other nutrients needed for health. The lesson makes students aware of food labels and how to read them and offers some options for healthy snack choices. By replacing some snacks with healthier choices, we are still able to eat favorite foods.

▶▶ Behavioral Objective

For students to eat healthy snack foods and learn to read food labels.

▶▶ Learning Objectives

Students will be able to

1. read food labels,
2. use food labels to compare and contrast the fat content of foods,
3. explain why it is important to choose healthy snacks, and
4. identify low-fat snacks.

▶▶ Materials

- Overhead transparency 1
- Overhead transparency of activity 1 answers and student resource 1, *Reading Food Labels* (or handout or use chalkboard)
- Activity 1 *Be Fat Wise*
- Activity 2 *Analyzing Food Labels*
- *Optional:* Food labels from home
- Optional: Student resource 1 *What's the Rap on Fat?* (lesson 49, page 335)

▶▶ Procedure

1. Point out the goals of this activity:
   - To discuss healthy snack options and the importance of eating healthy snacks
   - To learn to read and analyze food labels
2. (1-2 minutes) Have students make a list of their five favorite snack foods or beverages.
3. (2-3 minutes) Display overhead transparency 1. Have students identify the pyramid group to which each of their snack foods belong. Write selected student snack examples in the appropriate spaces on the pyramid.

4. (2-3 minutes) Ask and discuss the following questions:

• Into which group were most of your snacks placed?

• Were most of your snack choices low in saturated fat, salt, and/or sugar?

5. (2 minutes) Explain to students that foods in each food group may move to the top of the pyramid if they have large amounts of added fat and sugar. (For example, cakes are made from grains, but because of their high saturated fat and sugar content, they belong at the top of the pyramid.)

6. (2-3 minutes) Discuss the importance of selecting foods that are low in saturated fat and trans fat and moderate in total fat. (See Teacher Resources for a discussion of the different types of fat, or handout "What's the Rap on Fat," p. 335).

7. (2-3 minutes) To help students identify some healthy snack choices, have them complete activity 1 *Be Fat Wise.* This activity can be done as a class, individually, or in pairs. Review the answers by displaying a transparency of the answer key to activity 1. See Teacher Resources for more examples of healthy snacks.

8. (5-10 minutes) Hand out student resource 1 *Reading Food Labels* (or display it on the overhead projector) and explain the label information. Use the students' food labels from home for activity 2.

9. (15 minutes) Divide the class into groups of three or four. Give each group four to six food labels. These can include the ones they brought from home and/or the ones included with this lesson. Have students complete activity 2. They will locate and record the serving size, servings per container, amount of fat grams per serving, and percent of daily value recommended for fat contained per serving. Have groups exchange food labels so that they review at least 10 labels.

10. (5 minutes) Discuss students' findings. See the Teacher Resources to help you discuss the last question on saturated fat content.

11. (3 minutes) Ask students to write down three foods they might like to snack on that are low in saturated and trans fats and three high-fat foods they should try to limit to occasional indulgences.

▶▶ Extension Activities

1. Food Label Matching Game: Collect food labels. Separate the names of the products from the nutrient information on the labels. Divide the class into groups of four. Give each group five to eight labels. Have students try to match the nutrient information with the appropriate product name.

2. Bring in nutritious snacks from home to sample. Include snacks from each group of the Food Guide Pyramid.

▶▶ Teacher Resources

General Background Material

In preparing for this lesson, you may want to refer to the following resources:

• *Nutrition and Your Health: Dietary Guidelines for Americans*

• *Daily Food Guide Pyramid*

See appendixes A and B for information on how to obtain these resources.

• *Fat: Where It's At,* page 252

Specific Background Material

Do I need to stop eating any foods to be healthy?

"There are no 'bad' foods that should never be eaten, but most Americans tend to eat too many foods high in fat, salt, and refined sugars. These foods are at the top of the Food Guide Pyramid because it is ideal to eat only a limited amount of these foods and to eat more of the nutrient-rich foods located at the base of the pyramid. The purpose of this lesson is to help students make better snack choices by recognizing sources of fat. Reading food labels is an effective way to compare the fat and nutrient content of various snack foods" (*Eat Well and Keep Moving* 1996, 96).

Why do adolescents need snacks?

Adolescents are at a very important stage in their physical development, with each individual entering a rapid growth spurt according to his or her own internal time table. During growth, the body has higher nutrient needs. The prevalence of dietary inadequacies is higher during adolescence than at any other stage of the life cycle. Smaller, more frequent meals have been shown to have physiological and nutritional advantages for teenagers. Snacking is a way of life for adolescents, so we need to focus on improving the quality of those snacks. Snacks provide an energy boost and have a place in most people's daily diets.

What are some healthy foods adolescents can snack on?

Snacks can make an important contribution to the diet if they are monitored in terms of quality and amount. They can also provide up to 20-25% of an adolescent's energy intake and many nutrients. Each group on the Food Guide Pyramid offers healthy snack choices. Here are some healthy snacks:

- Whole grain breads, plain bread sticks, whole-grain crackers, rice cakes, cereal, bagels
- Fruits and fruit juices (except coconuts)
- Vegetables (plain or dipped in humus or low-fat dressing)
- Cheese (low fat, if possible)
- Raisins or other dried fruits
- Peanut butter
- Yogurt and milk (low fat, if possible)
- Nuts
- Chicken (skinless)
- Sandwiches or half sandwiches made with lean meats

How much fat is okay?

The *Dietary Guidelines for Americans* recommends consuming no more than 30% of calories from total fat (saturated, unsaturated, and trans fat) with no more than 10% of calories from saturated fat. Individual foods may have more or less fat than this. Don't worry about occasional indulgences, but try to keep your average to no more than 30% for total fat and 10% for saturated fat. On average, fat intake should be limited to

- about 73 grams per day (24 or fewer grams saturated fat) for 11–14-year-old girls (based on a 2,200 calorie diet), and
- about 83 grams per day (28 or fewer grams saturated fat) for 11–14-year-old boys (based on a 2,500 calorie diet).

Not All Fat is Created Equal

The fat in foods contains a mixture of saturated and unsaturated (monounsaturated and polyunsaturated) fatty acids, commonly called fats. Many animal products, such as fatty meats, whole milk, butter, and lard, are high in saturated fat. This kind of fat is typically solid at room temperature. Eating too much saturated fat increases the risk of developing heart disease. Therefore, the *Dietary Guidelines for Americans* recommends a diet low in saturated fat. Most of the fat you eat should be unsaturated since substituting this type of fat for saturated fat in your diet decreases the risk of developing heart disease. Most plant fats or oils are high in unsaturated fats and generally are liquid at room temperature. Vegetable oils (olive, canola, corn, peanut), most nuts, olives, and avocados are good sources of unsaturated fat. However, eating a lot of any type of fat may not be healthy so try to get no more than 30% of your total calories from fat.

There is an exception to the rule. Not all plant fats are healthy. Through a commercial process called hydrogenation, the more healthy plant oils can be converted into solids called trans fats (also called partially hydrogenated vegetable oils). This is how some margarines are made. Not surprisingly, foods high in trans fats have been found to also increase the risk of heart disease. To avoid these fats, check the ingredient lists on packaged foods such as cookies and crackers. Avoid varieties made with partially hydrogenated vegetable oil. Also watch out for coconut oil and palm oil since these oils are naturally high in saturated fat.

Not all animal foods are high in saturated fat. Ocean fish (like salmon) is high in a polyunsaturated fat—called omega-3 fatty acid—that may protect you against heart disease. So choose to eat fish when you get the chance.

References

Cheung, L., Gortmaker, S., and Dart, H. 2001. *Eat well & keep moving.* Champaign, IL: Human Kinetics.

National Research Council. 1989. *Recommended dietary allowances.* 10th ed. Washington, D.C.: National Academy Press.

U.S. Department of Agriculture and U.S. Department of Health and Human Services. 2000. *Nutrition and your health: Dietary guidelines for Americans* 2000, 5th edition. **www.usda.gov/cnpp**

U.S. Department of Health and Human Services. 2000. Healthy People 2010, conference edition, vols. I and II.. **www.health.gov/healthypeople**

▶▶ Answer Key

Activity 1

Directions: In each group below, put an "X" next to food that has the greatest amount of fat. The grams of fat per serving are recorded next to each.

[X] Ice cream: 1/2 cup (5–14 grams)	[ ] Apple cereal bar: 1 (3 grams)
[ ] Low-fat frozen yogurt: 1/2 cup (2 grams)	[X] Apple pie: 1/8 of pie (12 grams)
[ ] Bagel: 1 (1 gram)	[ ] Salsa: 3 tablespoons (0 grams)
[X] Doughnut: 1 (10–15 grams)	[X] Guacamole: 1 avocado (30 grams)
[X] Potato chips: 1 oz. (9 grams)	[X] Bologna: 1 slice (6.6 grams)
[ ] Pretzels: 1 oz. (2 grams)	[ ] Roast turkey: 1 slice (< 1 gram)
[ ] Low-fat chocolate milk: 2% milk, 1 cup (5 grams)	[ ] Oatmeal cookie: 1 (8 grams)
[X] Chocolate milkshake: 10 oz. (11 grams)	[X] Croissant: 1 (12 grams)

Examine the list of healthy snack foods below. Based on the information, which food groups offer a variety of low-fat, healthy snack choices? (*Answer: Each of the five food groups offers low fat snack choices.*)

Snack	Serving size	Fat (grams)	Snack	Serving size	Fat (grams)
Bagel	1	1	Apple	1 medium	<1
Grapes	1 cup	1	Orange	1 medium	<1
Carrots	1/2 cup	<1	Banana	1 medium	<1
Fruit juices	1 cup	<1	Pretzels	1 oz.	2
Low-fat yogurt with fruit	1 cup	2	Low-fat milk	1 cup	2
Turkey breast	1 slice	<1	Light tuna (in spring water)	2 oz.	1

Adapted from the classroom lessons of *Eat Well & Keep Moving, 2001.*

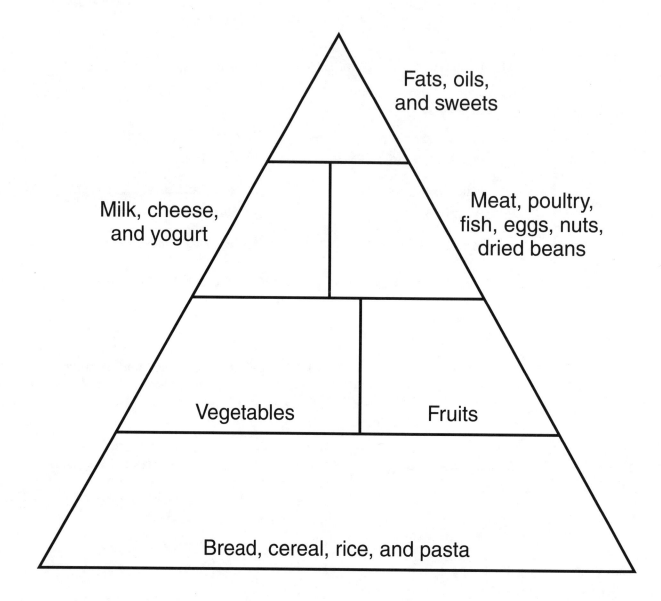

Fats, oils,
and sweets

Milk, cheese,
and yogurt

Meat, poultry,
fish, eggs, nuts,
dried beans

Vegetables

Fruits

Bread, cereal, rice, and pasta

Guidelines for Reading Food Labels

Food labels are a useful way to learn about the fat and other nutrients contained in the foods you eat.

1. Look at the statements or claims on the front of the packet. Labels often make claims like "bursting with energy," "high fiber," "lite," "lower in fat," or "oozing goodness." These statements can be misleading.

2. Read the nutrition facts:

   A. Check out how much of the product equals one serving size and how many servings the package contains.

   B. Examine the nutrient list to determine what percentage of the recommended daily value for fat, carbohydrates, proteins, and vitamins is provided by one serving of the food. For example, the product below provides 35 grams of carbohydrates, which is about 12% of your daily recommended carbohydrate intake.

   C. Examine the list of ingredients located near the label. Ingredients highest in weight are listed first.

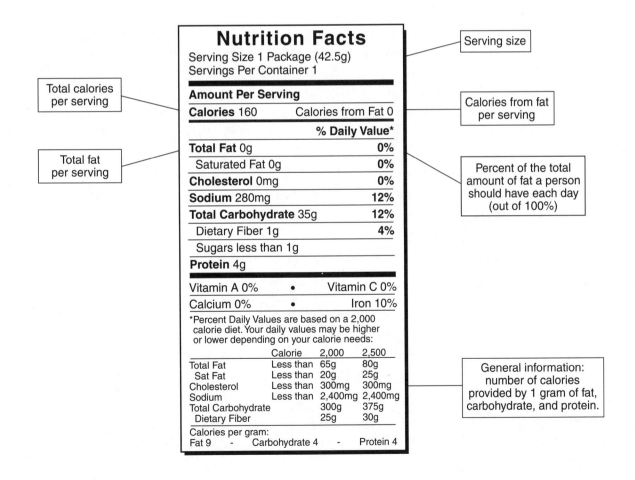

Total calories per serving

Total fat per serving

Serving size

Calories from fat per serving

Percent of the total amount of fat a person should have each day (out of 100%)

General information: number of calories provided by 1 gram of fat, carbohydrate, and protein.

Nutrition Facts

Serving Size 1 Package (42.5g)
Servings Per Container 1

Amount Per Serving

Calories 160   Calories from Fat 0

                                    % Daily Value*

Total Fat 0g	**0%**
Saturated Fat 0g	**0%**
Cholesterol 0mg	**0%**
Sodium 280mg	**12%**
Total Carbohydrate 35g	**12%**
Dietary Fiber 1g	**4%**
Sugars less than 1g	
Protein 4g	

Vitamin A 0%   •   Vitamin C 0%

Calcium 0%   •   Iron 10%

*Percent Daily Values are based on a 2,000 calorie diet. Your daily values may be higher or lower depending on your calorie needs:

	Calorie	2,000	2,500
Total Fat	Less than	65g	80g
Sat Fat	Less than	20g	25g
Cholesterol	Less than	300mg	300mg
Sodium	Less than	2,400mg	2,400mg
Total Carbohydrate		300g	375g
Dietary Fiber		25g	30g

Calories per gram:
Fat 9   -   Carbohydrate 4   -   Protein 4

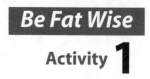

Directions: In each group below, put an "X" next to food that has the greatest amount of fat per serving.

❏ Ice cream		❏ Apple cereal bar	
❏ Low-fat frozen yogurt		❏ Apple pie	
❏ Bagel		❏ Salsa	
❏ Doughnut		❏ Guacamole	
❏ Potato chips		❏ Bologna	
❏ Pretzels		❏ Roast turkey	
❏ Low-fat chocolate milk		❏ Oatmeal cookie	
❏ Chocolate milkshake		❏ Croissant	

Examine the list of healthy snack foods below. Based on the information, which food groups offer a variety of low-fat, healthy snack choices?

Snack	Serving size	Fat (grams)	Snack	Serving size	Fat (grams)
Bagel	1	1	Apple	1 medium	<1
Grapes	1 cup	1	Orange	1 medium	<1
Carrots	1/2 cup	<1	Banana	1 medium	<1
Fruit juices	1 cup	<1	Pretzels	1 oz.	2
Low fat yogurt with fruit	1 cup	3	Low fat milk	1 cup	2
Turkey breast	1 slice	<1	Light tuna (in spring water)	2 oz.	1

Adapted from the classroom lessons of _Eat Well & Keep Moving_, 2001.

Directions: Examine the food labels provided to you by your teacher. Use the nutrient information provided on the label to complete the table.

Product name	Serving size	Servings per container	Total fat (grams)	Total fat (% daily value)	Saturated fat (grams)	Saturated fat (% daily value)

Analyzing the Data

1. Which three products have the most total grams of fat per serving? Do you usually eat more or less than a serving size of each of these snacks in one sitting?

Product name	Total fat (grams)	Typical amount eaten (more or less than serving size)

2. Which three products have the fewest total grams of fat per serving?

Product name	Total fat (grams)	Typical amount eaten (more or less than serving size)

3. Which three products have the fewest total grams of saturated fat per serving?

Product name	Total fat (grams)	Typical amount eaten (more or less than serving size)

Frozen pizza

Nutrition Facts

Serving Size 1 pizza (234g)
Servings Per Container 1

Amount Per Serving

Calories 540   Calories from Fat 260

                                                    % Daily Value*

Total Fat 29g	**45%**
Saturated Fat 10g	**50%**
Cholesterol 25mg	**8%**
Sodium 1.320mg	**55%**
Potassium 530mg	**15%**
Total Carbohydrate 53g	**18%**
Dietary Fiber 6g	**24%**
Sugars 7g	
Protein 21g	

Vitamin A 50%	•	Vitamin C 0%
Calcium 35%	•	Iron 10%

*Percent Daily Values are based on a 2,000 calorie diet.

Chicken nuggets

Nutrition Facts

Serving Size 4 Nuggets (76g)
Servings Per Container about 4

Amount Per Serving

Calories 210   Calories from Fat 130

                                                    % Daily Value*

Total Fat 15g	**23%**
Saturated Fat 3.5g	**18%**
Cholesterol 35mg	**12%**
Sodium 300mg	**13%**
Total Carbohydrate 9g	**3%**
Dietary Fiber 1g	**4%**
Sugars 0g	
Protein 11g	**22%**

Not a significant source of dietary fiber, sugars, vitamin A, vitamin C, calcium and iron.

*Percent Daily Values are based on a 2,000 calorie diet.

Spinach

Nutrition Facts

Serving Size 1/3 cup (83g)
Servings Per Container about 3.5

Amount Per Serving

Calories 20   Calories from Fat 0

                                                    % Daily Value*

Total Fat 0g	**0%**
Saturated Fat 0g	**0%**
Cholesterol 0mg	**0%**
Sodium 115mg	**5%**
Total Carbohydrate 2g	**1%**
Dietary Fiber 2g	**7%**
Sugars 1g	
Protein 2g	

Vitamin A 120%	•	Vitamin C 10%
Calcium 6%	•	Iron 2%

*Percent Daily Values are based on a 2,000 calorie diet.

Whole milk

Nutrition Facts

Serving Size 1 Cup (236mL)
Servings Per Container 4

Amount Per Serving

Calories 150   Calories from Fat 70

                                                    % Daily Value*

Total Fat 8g	**12%**
Saturated Fat 5g	**25%**
Cholesterol 35mg	**11%**
Sodium 125mg	**5%**
Total Carbohydrate 12g	**4%**
Dietary Fiber 0g	**0%**
Sugars 12g	
Protein 8g	**16%**

Vitamin A 6%	•	Vitamin C 4%
Calcium 30%	•	Iron 0%
Vitamin D 25%		

*Percent Daily Values are based on a 2,000 calorie diet.

Skim milk

Nutrition Facts

Serving Size 1 Cup (236mL)
Servings Per Container 8

Amount Per Serving

Calories 90   Calories from Fat 0

% Daily Value*

Total Fat 0g	**0%**
Saturated Fat 0g	**0%**
Cholesterol 5mg	**1%**
Sodium 125mg	**5%**
Total Carbohydrate 13g	**4%**
Dietary Fiber 0g	**0%**
Sugars 12g	
Protein 8g	

Vitamin A 10%   •   Vitamin C 4%

Calcium 30% • Iron 0% • Vitamin D 25%

*Percent Daily Values (DV) are based on a 2,000 calorie diet.

Fried chicken

Nutrition Facts

Serving Size 3oz. (84g)
Servings Per Container about 7

Amount Per Serving

Calories 270   Calories from Fat 160

% Daily Value*

Total Fat 18g	**27%**
Saturated Fat 5g	**23%**
Cholesterol 65mg	**22%**
Sodium 620mg	**26%**
Total Carbohydrate 13g	**4%**
Dietary Fiber 1g	**5%**
Sugars 1g	
Protein 14g	

Vitamin A 0%   •   Vitamin C 6%

Calcium 8%   •   Iron 4%

*Percent Daily Values are based on a 2,000 calorie diet.

Cheddar cheese

Nutrition Facts

Serving Size 1 oz. (30g)
Servings Per Container 4

Amount Per Serving

Calories 120   Calories from Fat 90

% Daily Value*

Total Fat 10g	**15%**
Saturated Fat 5.5g	**27%**
Cholesterol 30mg	**10%**
Sodium 190mg	**8%**
Total Carbohydrate 1g	**0%**
Dietary Fiber 0g	**0%**
Sugars 0g	
Protein 7g	

Vitamin A 8%   •   Vitamin C 0%

Calcium 25%   •   Iron 0%

*Percent Daily Values are based on a 2,000 calorie diet.

Orange juice

Nutrition Facts

Serving Size 8 fl oz. (237mL)
Servings Per Container 2

Amount Per Serving

Calories 100   Calories from Fat 0

% Daily Value*

Total Fat 0g	**0%**
Sodium 0mg	**0%**
Potassium 290mg	**8%**
Total Carbohydrate 24g	**8%**
Sugars 23g	
Protein 1g	

Vitamin C 90% • Thiamin 6% • Folate 2%

Phosphorus 2%   •   Magnesium 6%

Not a significant source of saturated fat, cholesterol, dietary fiber, vitamin A, calcium and iron.

*Percent Daily Values are based on a 2,000 calorie diet.

Reduced fat processed cheese

Nutrition Facts

Serv Size 1 slice (21g)
Servings 16
Calories 50
    Fat Cal 30

*Percent Daily Values (DV) are based on a 2,000 calorie diet.

Amount/serving	%DV*	Amount/serving	%DV*
Total Fat 3g	**5%**	**Total Carb** 2g	**1%**
Sat Fat 2g	**10%**	Fiber 0g	**0%**
Cholest 10mg	**3%**	Sugars 1g	
Sodium 330mg	**14%**	**Protein** 5g	

Vitamin A 4% • Vitamin C 0% • Calcium 15% • Iron 0%

Chocolate candy bar with almonds

Nutrition Facts

Serv Size 1 Bar
Calories 230
    Fat Cal 140

*Percent Daily Values (DV) are based on a 2,000 calorie diet.

Amount/serving	%DV*	Amount/serving	%DV*
Total Fat 14g	**22%**	**Total Carb** 20g	**7%**
Sat Fat 7g	**35%**	Fiber 1g	**5%**
Cholest 5mg	**2%**	Sugars 18g	
Sodium 35mg	**2%**	**Protein** 5g	

Vitamin A 0% • Vitamin C 0% • Calcium 8% • Iron 4%

Chocolate chip cookies

Nutrition Facts

Serving Size 1 Cookie (about 39g)
Servings Per Container 2

Amount Per Serving

Calories 190   Calories from Fat 80

% Daily Value*

Total Fat 9g	**14%**
Saturated Fat 2.5g	**13%**
Cholesterol less than 5mg	**1%**
Sodium 130mg	**5%**
Total Carbohydrate 25g	**8%**
Dietary Fiber 1g	**4%**
Sugars 11g	
Protein 2g	

Vitamin A 0%	•	Vitamin C 0%
Calcium 2%	•	Iron 6%

*Percent Daily Values are based on a 2,000 calorie diet.

Cheese flavored popcorn

Nutrition Facts

Serving Size 1 package
Servings Per Container 1

Amount Per Serving

Calories 160   Calories from Fat 90

% Daily Value*

Total Fat 10g	**15%**
Saturated Fat 2g	**11%**
Cholesterol 5mg	**2%**
Sodium 320mg	**14%**
Total Carbohydrate 14g	**5%**
Dietary Fiber 1g	**5%**
Sugars 2g	
Protein 3g	

Vitamin A 0%	•	Vitamin C 0%
Calcium 2%	•	Iron 0%

*Percent Daily Values are based on a 2,000 calorie diet.

Potato chips

Nutrition Facts

Serving Size 1 package
Servings Per Container 1

Amount Per Serving

Calories 150   Calories from Fat 90

% Daily Value*

Total Fat 10g	**16%**
Saturated Fat 3g	**14%**
Cholesterol 0mg	**0%**
Sodium 180mg	**8%**
Total Carbohydrate 15g	**5%**
Dietary Fiber 1g	**4%**
Sugars 0g	
Protein 2g	

Vitamin A 0%	•	Vitamin C 10%
Calcium 0%	•	Iron 0%

*Percent Daily Values are based on a 2,000 calorie diet.

Pretzels

Nutrition Facts

Serving Size 1 pkg. (45g/about 5 pretzels)
Servings Per Container 1

Amount Per Serving

Calories 180   Calories from Fat 15

% Daily Value*

Total Fat 1.5g	**2%**
Saturated Fat 0.5g	**3%**
Cholesterol 0mg	**0%**
Sodium 500mg	**21%**
Total Carbohydrate 36g	**12%**
Dietary Fiber less than 1g	**1%**
Sugars 1g	
Protein 5g	

Vitamin A 0%	•	Vitamin C 0%
Calcium 0%	•	Iron 3%

*Percent Daily Values are based on a 2,000 calorie diet.

Chocolate covered mints

Nutrition Facts

Serv Size 1 box (45g)
Calories 190
  Fat Cal 35
*Percent Daily Values (DV) are based on a 2,000 calorie diet.

Amount/serving	%DV*	Amount/serving	%DV*
Total Fat 4g	**6%**	**Total Carb** 38g	**13%**
Sat Fat 2.5g	**12%**	Fiber less than 1g	**3%**
Cholest 0mg	**0%**	Sugars 37g	
Sodium 10mg	**1%**	**Protein** less than 1g	

Vitamin A 0% • Vitamin C 0% • Calcium 0% • Iron 4%

Frosted donuts

Nutrition Facts

Serv Size 6 Donuts (85g)
Serv Per Container 1
Calories 390
  Fat Cal 210
*Percent Daily Values (DV) are based on a 2,000 calorie diet.

Amount/serving	%DV*	Amount/serving	%DV*
Total Fat 23g	**35%**	**Total Carb** 42g	**14%**
Sat Fat 15g	**75%**	Fiber 2g	**8%**
Cholest 10mg	**3%**	Sugars 21g	
Sodium 360mg	**15%**	**Protein** 5g	

Vitamin A 1% • Vitamin C 0% • Calcium 2% • Iron 15%
Thiamin 15% • Riboflavin 10% • Niacin 8%

The Plants We Eat

This lesson is designed to be incorporated into a unit on nutrition, plant structure, or plant classification. The goal of this lesson is for students to appreciate the importance of eating a variety of fruits and vegetables daily. Students classify foods as plant or animal products. They then examine the nutrient content of various plant products and classify them as roots, stems, leaves, or fruits.

The lesson also includes three extension activity options. Extension activity 1 provides students with the opportunity to examine the structural diversity of edible plant parts. Extension activity 2 familiarizes students with the functions of some vitamins. Extension activity 3 demonstrates the antioxidant role of vitamin C and provides the framework for discussing the rationale of increasing fruit and vegetable intake as a way of preventing cancer.

▶▶ Behavioral Objective

For students to eat a variety of fruits and vegetables.

▶▶ Learning Objectives

Students will be able to

1. identify the parts of a plant—roots, stems, leaves, and fruits—and define their function (extension activity 1),

2. classify foods as animal or plant products (activity 1),

3. classify plant products as roots, stems, leaves, or fruits (activity 1),

4. explain the importance of eating a variety of fruits and vegetables (activity 1 and extension activity 2),

5. accurately sketch and describe plant structures (extension activity 1),

6. use their observations to identify similarities and differences in plant structure and appreciate the diversity of plant forms (extension activity 1),

7. state examples of vitamin functions (extension activity 2), and

8. discuss the role of antioxidants in the body (extension activity 3).

▶▶ Materials

- Student resource 1 *Plant Parts*
- Activity 1 *The Plants We Eat*
- Extension activity 1 *Examining Plant Diversity*
- Extension activity 2 *Vitamin Function*
- Extension activity 3 *Vitamin C at Work*

- Optional supplies for activity 1: Small quantities of broccoli, romaine lettuce, celery, corn, tomatoes, spinach, carrots, peas, cauliflower, rhubarb, radishes, potatoes, peaches
- Supplies for extension activity 1: At least three types of edible roots, stems, leaves, and fruits; knives or scalpels.
- Supplies for extension activity 3: Apple, vitamin C tablet, knife

▶▶ Procedure

1. Point out the goals of this lesson:
   - To identify the parts of a plant (roots, stems, leaves and fruits) and define their function
   - To classify foods as animal or plant products
   - To classify plant products as roots, stems, leaves, or fruits
   - To explain the importance of eating a variety of fruits and vegetables

2. Ask students whether humans are herbivores, carnivores, or omnivores. *(Answer: Except for strict vegetarians, humans are omnivores.)*

3. (5 minutes) Hand out activity 1 *The Plants We Eat*. Have students complete part I and then go over the answers as a class. Although this activity seems very basic, students do not generally think of food in these terms (unless they live on a farm) and may have difficulty classifying some of the food items. (The Answer Key follow the References.)

4. (5-10 minutes) Hand out and discuss student resource 1 *Plant Parts*. Use diagrams, overhead transparencies, or actual plants to give examples of each of the plant parts.

5. (20-30 minutes) Have students complete parts II and III of activity 1. If possible, make some or all of the plant parts (fresh, frozen, or canned) listed in part II available for students to observe and handle. This will make it much easier for them to classify the edible plant parts.

6. (5-10 minutes) Go over parts II and III. Finish by asking students how many fruits and vegetables experts recommend they eat (5-A-Day recommendation).

▶▶ Extension Activities

Extension Activity 1 Examining Plant Diversity

Have students compare and contrast the structure of three roots, stems, leaves, or fruits.

Extension Activity 2 Vitamin Function

Completing this activity will introduce students to some of the functions of vitamins in the body.

Extension Activity 3 Vitamin C at Work

Use the browning apple demonstration to illustrate the antioxidant role of vitamin C. This demonstration provides the framework for discussing the rationale of increasing fruit and vegetable intake as a way of preventing cancer. See Teacher

Resources for a detailed description of the functions of vitamin C and the role of antioxidants.

▶▶ Teacher Resources

General Background Material

In preparing for this lesson, you may want to refer to *Time to Take Five*. See appendix A.

Specific Background Material

Definitions of the Plant Structures

Root: The underground part of the plant that stores food produced in the leaves, collects water and minerals, and anchors the plant to the soil. Examples of edible roots: carrots, radishes, turnips, parsnips, and sweet potatoes.

Stem: The stalk or trunk of the plant that supports the leaves and transports food, water, and minerals between the roots and the leaves. Examples of edible stems: asparagus and white potatoes (swollen end of stolon—underground stems).

Leaf: The green organ of a plant that produces food through photosynthesis. Leaves are made up of two parts: a leaf blade and a stalk (also called the petiole). The leaf blade is the flat, broad part. The stalk connects the blade to the stem. Examples of edible leaves: lettuce, spinach, cabbage, brussels sprouts, celery, and rhubarb. (The edible parts of these last two plants are leaf stalks, not stems as many people think.)

Flowers: The reproductive part of a seed plant. Examples of edible flowers: cauliflower, broccoli, and artichokes. (The edible part of cauliflower and broccoli is composed of the fleshy flower stalks and clusters of flower buds.)

Fruit: A structure that covers and protects the seeds of flowering plants. It develops from the maturing flower and is the plant's ripened ovary. Examples: apples, green beans, coconuts, avocados, pea pods, peanuts, acorns, cucumbers, rice, wheat, and corn. We don't usually think of grains like corn, wheat, and rice as fruits. However, each grain is a developed ovary. As the single seed inside the ovary grows, "the wall of the seed becomes joined to the ripening ovary wall and forms the grain or fruit" (Selsam 1981).

Seed: A plant embryo, surrounded by a food supply and a protective seed coat. Examples of edible seeds: sunflower seeds and peas.

Functions of Vitamin C (Ascorbic Acid)

- It has multiple functions in the body as either a coenzyme or cofactor.
- It has the ability to take on or lose hydrogen ions, giving it an important role in the metabolism of nutrients.
- It enhances the absorption of iron by changing it from the ferric form to the reduced or ferrous form, which is more readily absorbed.
- It is involved in the synthesis of collagen, a component of all fibrous tissue in the body, including cartilage, bone matrix, tooth dentin, skin, and tendons.
- It is involved in healing wounds, fractures, bruises, hemorrhages, and bleeding gums.
- It reduces the susceptibility of the body to infections.
- The value of vitamin C in preventing and curing the common cold has also been touted, but these findings remain controversial.
- It is believed to have a role as an antioxidant (refer to information below).

Good Sources of Vitamin C

- Broccoli
- Cantaloupe
- Grapefruit
- Oranges
- Limes
- Lemons
- Mangos
- Bell peppers
- Tomatoes

Preventing Food Browning (Oxidation)

Vitamin C prevents various food constituents from reacting with oxygen. This antioxidant action prevents the food from discoloring or spoiling.

Antioxidants

Nutrients such as vitamin C, vitamin E, vitamin B6, and folate are believed to protect the body with their antioxidant effects. Certain minerals such as iron, zinc, and selenium also are hypothesized to have important antioxidant roles.

In the aging process, free radicals (the by-products of normal oxidative chemical reactions) are thought to cause degeneration of the immune function by damaging DNA, perhaps leading to the formation of certain forms of cancer, as well as atherosclerotic damage and degenerative disease such as arthritis and Parkinson's disease. Free radicals are believed to damage chromosomes and thus cause mutations. Therefore, protection from DNA damage is believed to enhance the body's self-defense mechanisms. Vegetables and fruits and their relationship to good health and enhanced immunity have been studied extensively in recent years, as they are believed to help stop the damage to DNA caused by free radicals.

The American Cancer Society and the American Council on Science and Health have joined with other agencies to promote the consumption of adequate fruits and vegetables in campaigns such as "Strive for Five" and "5 A Day for Better Health." The hope is that by increasing our consumption of fruits and vegetables that contain antioxidants, we will be able to reduce our risks of developing several serious diseases.

References

Beck, B. 1970. *Vegetables.* New York: Franklin Watts.

Bierer, L., Warner, L., Lawson, S., and Cohen, T. 1991. *Life science: The challenge of discovery.* Lexington, MA: Heath.

Mahan, L.K., and Escott-Strump, S. 1996. *Krause's food, nutrition and diet therapy.* 9th ed. Philadelphia: Saunders.

Selsam, M. 1981. *The plants we eat.* New York: Morrow.

U.S. Department of Agriculture and U.S. Department of Health and Human Services. 2000. *Nutrition and your health: Dietary guidelines for Americans* 2000, 5th edition. **www.usda.gov/cnpp**

U.S. Department of Health and Human Services. 2000. Healthy People 2010, conference edition, vols. I and II. **www.health.gov/healthypeople**

Vander, A., Sherman, J., and Luciano, D. 1985. *Human physiology: The mechanisms of body functions.* 4th ed. New York: McGraw-Hill.

▶▶ Answer Key

Activity 1

Part I

Plant products	Animal products
Bread	Milk
Tomato	Margarine
Cereal	Yogurt
Peanut butter	Hamburger
Pasta	Eggs
Broccoli	Chicken
Apples	Cheese
	Butter
	Fish

Name one commonly eaten food that does not come from a plant or an animal. *(Answer: Mushrooms – fungi.)*

Part II

Amount per serving

Food	Vitamin A (RE)	Vitamin B_{12} (mcg)	Vitamin C (mg)	Folate (mcg)
Broccoli	68	0	41	31
Romaine lettuce	73	0	7	38
Celery	5	0	3	11
Strawberry	4	0	85	26
Tomato	77	0	24	18
Spinach	188	0	8	54
Carrot	2,025	0	7	10
Green beans	41	0	6	21
Cauliflower	1	0	36	33
Asparagus	48	0	15	132
Sweet potato	2,488	0	28	26
Orange	26	0	80	47
Squash	714	0	15	20
Peach	47	0	6	3
Cantaloupe	516	0	68	27

1. Are any of the foods good sources of *all* the nutrients listed? *(Answer: No.)*

2. Why is it important to eat a variety of fruits and vegetables? Explain. *(Answer: No one food can provide all of the vitamins and minerals our bodies need to be healthy.)*

Part III

Roots		Stems		Leaves	
Food	**Good source of vitamin(s)**	**Food**	**Good source of vitamin(s)**	**Food**	**Good source of vitamin(s)**
Carrot	A, C	Asparagus	C, Folate	Romaine lettuce	C, Folate
Radish	C			Celery	
Sweet potato	A, C, Folate			Spinach	A, C, Folate

Fruits		Flowers	
Food	**Good source of vitamin(s)**	**Food**	**Good source of vitamin(s)**
Strawberry	C, Folate	Broccoli	C, Folate
Tomato	C, Folate	Cauliflower	C, Folate
Green beans	C, Folate		
Orange	C, Folate		
Squash	A, C, Folate		
Peach	C		
Cantaloupe	A, C, Folate		

2. Which of the plant products in the table are classified as fruits in the Food Guide Pyramid? *(Answer: strawberries, peaches, oranges, cantaloupe.)*

3. What characteristics do these fruits have in common? *(Answer: They are fleshy or pulpy, often juicy, and usually sweet, with fragrant flavors. In addition, they all are ripened ovaries, so they generally contain seeds.)*

4. What characteristics do the vegetables have in common? *(Answer: A vegetable is the part of the plant usually eaten with the main portion of a meal. They include edible leaves, stems, roots, bulbs, fruits, and flowers. Vegetables are usually not as sweet as fruits.)*

5. You may have noticed that some plant products, like the tomato, are classified as vegetables in the Food Guide Pyramid and as fruits by plant scientists. What characteristics of the tomato, and other foods like it, enable them to be classified as vegetables? What characteristics make them fruits? *(Answer: The tomato, squash, and cucumber are examples of plant products that are technically fruits because they developed from flowers and contain seeds, but are typically called vegetables because they are not sweet and are usually eaten with the main portion of a meal.)*

6. Which are more nutritious: vegetables or the foods we commonly refer to as fruits? *(Answer: Foods from both groups are excellent sources of vitamin A, C, Folate, and fiber.)*

Extension Activity 2

Patient A: vitamin C deficiency
Patient B: vitamin A deficiency
Patient C: vitamin D deficiency
Patient D: vitamin K deficiency

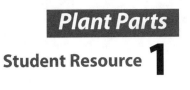
Roots: The underground part of the plant that stores food produced in the leaves. Roots collect water and minerals, and they anchor the plant to the soil.

Stem: The stalk or trunk of the plant that supports the leaves and transports food, water, and minerals between the roots and the leaves.

Leaves: The green organs of plants that grow out of the stem and produce food through photosynthesis. They are made up of two parts: a leaf blade and a stalk, the petiole. The leaf blade is the flat, broad part. The stalk connects the blade to the stem.

Flowers: The reproductive part of a seed plant. They are composed of petals, sepals, stamen, and pistils.

Fruit: A structure that covers and protects the seeds of flowering plants. It develops from the maturing flower and is actually the plant's ripened ovary.

Seed: A plant embryo surrounded by a food supply and a protective seed coat.

Name _____

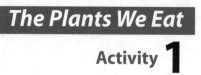

Part I

Most of the foods you eat come from plants or animals. Classify each of the foods below as a plant or animal product and record them in the appropriate column.

bread	cereal
cheese	butter
broccoli	yogurt
hamburger	apples
tomato	peanut butter
pasta	milk
margarine	fish
eggs	chicken

Plant products	Animal products

? Name one commonly eaten food that does not come from a plant or an animal.

Part II

Use the table below to compare the vitamin content of a typical serving of the various plant products listed. Indicate which three foods contain the largest quantity of each nutrient by circling the three largest values in each column.

Food	Vitamin A (RE)	Vitamin B$_{12}$ (mcg)	Vitamin C (mg)	Folate (mcg)
Broccoli	68	0	41	31
Romaine lettuce	73	0	7	38
Celery	5	0	3	11
Strawberry	4	0	85	26
Tomato	77	0	24	18
Spinach	188	0	8	54
Carrot	2,025	0	7	10
Green beans	41	0	6	21
Cauliflower	1	0	36	33
Asparagus	48	0	15	132
Radish	0	0	10	12
Sweet potato	2,488	0	28	26
Orange	26	0	80	47
Squash	714	0	15	20
Peach	47	0	6	3
Cantaloupe	516	0	68	27

1. Are any of the foods good sources of *all* the nutrients listed?

2. Why is it important to eat a variety of fruits and vegetables? Explain.

Part III

We eat many parts of plants. Leaves, stems, roots, fruits, seeds, and even some flowers are edible. Classify the plant products listed in part II as roots, stems, leaves, or fruits, and record them in the table on the next page. Be sure to classify the part of the plant that is most commonly eaten.

Foods are considered to be a good source of a nutrient if they provide at least 10% of the recommended daily allowance. Good sources of

- vitamin A provide greater than 80 RE per serving.

- vitamin B$_{12}$ provide greater than 0.2 mcg per serving.

- vitamin C provide greater than 5 mg per serving.

- folate provide greater than 15 mcg per serving.

→ Next to the foods classified below indicate for which vitamins they are a good source.

Roots		Stems		Leaves	
Food	Good source of vitamin(s)	Food	Good source of vitamin(s)	Food	Good source of vitamin(s)

Fruits		Flowers	
Food	Good source of vitamin(s)	Food	Good source of vitamin(s)

1. The Food Guide Pyramid contains a fruit food group (2-4 servings recommended per day) and a vegetable food group (3-5 servings per day). Circle the foods above that are classified as vegetables in the Food Guide Pyramid.

2. Which of the plant products in the table are classified as fruits in the Food Guide Pyramid?

3. What characteristics do these fruits have in common?

4. What characteristics do the vegetables have in common?

5. You may have notices that some plant products, like the tomato, are classified as vegetables in the Food Guide Pyramid and as fruits by plant scientist. What characteristics of the tomato, and other foods like it, enable them to be classified as vegetables? What characteristics make them fruits?

6. Which are more nutritious: vegetables or the foods we commonly refer to as fruits?

In this activity you will compare and contrast the structure of three commonly eaten roots, stems, leaves, *OR* fruits.

1. Decide which plant structure you will study: roots, stems, leaves, *OR* fruits.

2. Examine the structure in three different types of plants and sketch them below. Describe their color, texture, size, shape, and any defining characteristics below the drawing. Cut each food in half and sketch and describe what you see. (If possible, examine them with a magnifying glass or dissecting microscope.)

3. How were the structures of the three foods you observed similar?

4. How were the structures of the three foods you observed different?

5. How might the differences you observed affect the plant's function (how it works)?

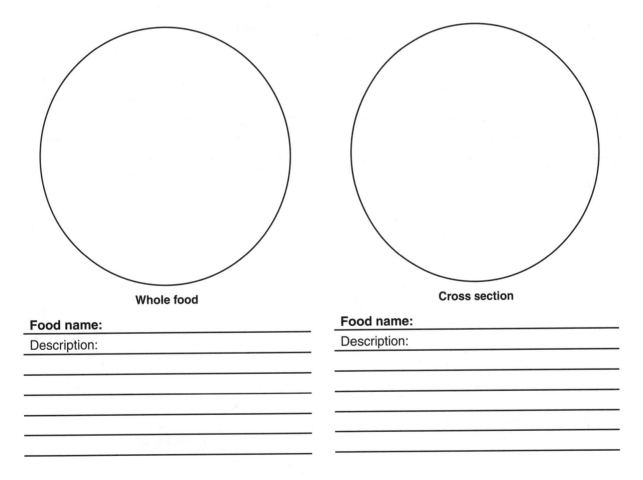

Whole food

Cross section

Food name: _____

Description: _____

_____

_____

_____

_____

Food name: _____

Description: _____

_____

_____

_____

_____

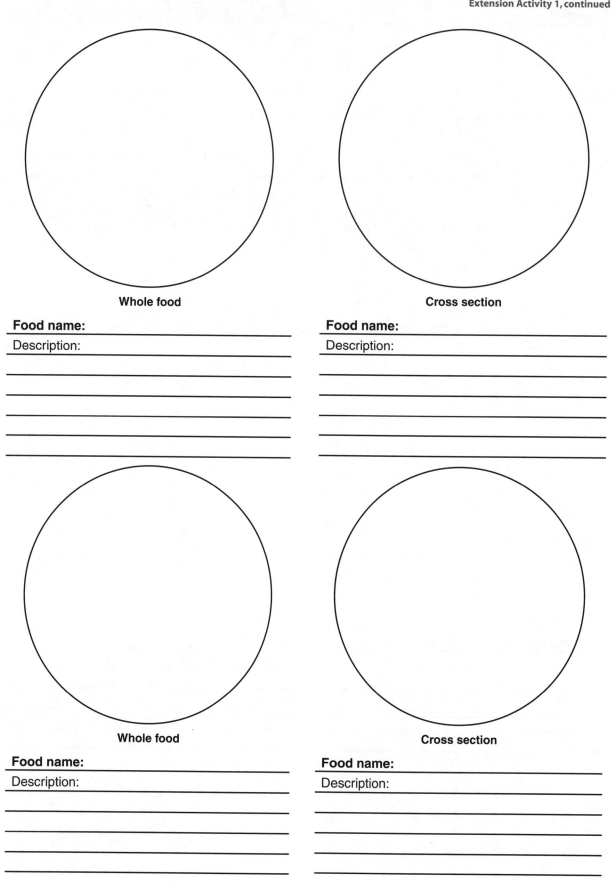

Whole food

Cross section

Food name: _____

Description: _____

_____

_____

_____

_____

Food name: _____

Description: _____

_____

_____

_____

_____

Whole food

Cross section

Food name: _____

Description: _____

_____

_____

_____

_____

Food name: _____

Description: _____

_____

_____

_____

_____

Vitamins are nutrients that assist with many chemical reactions in your body. The table below outlines some of the important functions of a few vitamins.

Vitamin	Function	Food source
A	Helps make eye pigments needed for sight; maintains healthy skin	Green vegetables, liver, milk, butter, cheese, fruits
C	Maintains healthy gums, teeth, blood vessels, and immune system*	Citrus fruits, tomatoes, green peppers, berries, melons, potatoes, green leafy vegetables
D	Helps build strong teeth and bones	Fortified milk products, cod-liver oil, eggs**
E	Protects cell membranes*	Seeds, green leafy vegetables, margarine, whole wheat
K	Aids blood clotting	Green leafy vegetables, whole wheat cereals, meat

*Vitamin C and E act as antioxidants. Antioxidants are substances that prevent cell damage that can lead to cancer.

**Sunlight stimulates the skin to produce vitamin D

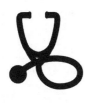

Imagine you are a doctor who specializes in nutrition disorders. You examined four patients and recorded their symptoms of illness. You drew a blood sample from each patient and sent it to the lab for analysis. Unfortunately, the lab technician mixed up the samples. Based on your knowledge of vitamin function, match the patients' symptoms to the vitamin deficiencies detected in the blood samples.

Write the letter of the vitamin that is deficient next to the patient's symptoms.

Patient symptoms	Lab results
_____ Patient A: bleeding gums, degenerating teeth, easily bruises	Vitamin A deficiency
_____ Patient B: night blindness	Vitamin C deficiency
_____ Patient C: bowed legs	Vitamin D deficiency
_____ Patient D: frequent nose bleeds, difficult to stop cuts from bleeding	Vitamin K deficiency

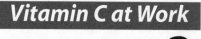

Materials: apple, vitamin C tablet, knife

Procedure

1. Cut the unpeeled apple in half.
2. Crush the vitamin C tablet and sprinkle the powder over the surface of one of the apple halves.
3. Allow both apple sections to set uncovered for at least 30 minutes.
4. Observe the color of each section.

Complete the following questions

1. Give a complete description of the apple before the experiment.

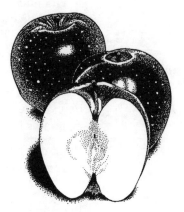

2. Predict how the color will change in both apple halves during the experiment.

3. At the end of the experiment, describe how the color actually changed in both apple halves.

4. What do you think caused the apple halves to change color?

5. How might eating fruits and vegetables high in vitamin C help us? (Hint: It doesn't keep us from changing color.)

Lesson 52

Foods for Energy

This lesson introduces the concept of physical endurance and the role carbohydrates play in fueling muscular activity. Students work in groups to design a food menu for a class hiking trip. This lesson reinforces concepts introduced in lesson 33.

▶▶ Behavioral Objective

For students to be more active and understand which foods provide them with the energy for activity.

▶▶ Learning Objectives

Students will be able to

1. define the term *endurance,*

2. state the primary function of carbohydrates in the body,

3. work with others to solve a problem,

4. plan food requirements for a situation requiring moderately intense to vigorous activity and understand why certain foods would be appropriate, and

5. discuss how physical fitness, carbohydrates, and fluids affect endurance for physical activity.

▶▶ Materials

- Activity 1 *Let's Take a Hike!*
- Student resource 1 *Foods for Energy*
- *Optional*: tennis balls, textbooks, or chairs (see optional activity in procedure)

▶▶ Procedure

1. Point out the goals of the lesson:
   - To discuss how physical fitness, carbohydrates, and fluids affect endurance for physical activity
   - To plan a menu of the food needed for a 10-mile hike

2. (5-10 minutes) *Optional activity:* If time allows, start this lesson by having students determine how much endurance they have for one of the following activities:
   - Squeeze a tennis ball firmly, then relax; repeat this as fast and as long as you can.
   - Perform biceps curls while grasping two textbooks.

- Step up and down on a chair.
- Perform push-ups.
- Perform sit-ups.

The experience of doing one of these activities for as long as they can will give students firsthand experience with endurance and fatigue and lots to say about the following questions. The first two activities are likely to be the least disruptive to your classroom. Have each student record her or his results. Ask students to list some factors that affect endurance.

3. (5 minutes) Ask students the following: What is endurance? What can you do to improve your endurance? Discuss student responses. Emphasize that endurance is dependent not only on physical fitness but also on adequate intake of carbohydrates and fluids. (See Teacher Resources for answers to these questions.)

4. (3-5 minutes) Ask students the following and record their responses on the board:

- What foods have you eaten today that are rich in carbohydrates?
- What is the primary job of carbohydrates in our body?

5. (10 minutes) Hand out and have students read student resource 1 *Foods for Energy*. Review

- what carbohydrates are,
- where they come from, and
- what they provide.

6. (15 minutes) Hand out activity 1 *Let's Take a Hike!* This activity requires students to plan the food supplies needed for a day hike. Have students work in groups of two to four to complete this activity. Be sure students understand the directions before they begin.

7. (10-15 minutes) Have each group exchange their menu plans with another group. Ask students to model constructive criticism by pointing out the pros and cons of their classmates' menu plans. Have each group share its critique.

▶▶ Extension Activities

1. Have students record their day hike menus on poster board and display them in the room.

2. Have the class decide which group's menu is the "best." Take a hiking field trip and have everyone bring the food on the "best" menu.

3. Have students make a list of everyone in their homes and list their weekly physical activities. Explain why the people in your home have endurance in different activities. Does anyone do moderately intense or vigorous physical activity on a regular basis? How are their activity patterns different from each other?

▶▶ Teacher Resources

General Background Information

In preparing for this lesson, you may want to refer to *Nutrition and Your Health: Dietary Guidelines for Americans*. See appendix A for information on how to obtain this resource.

Specific Background Information

Below are some definitions that may be useful for this lesson.

Nutrient: A substance that must be consumed as part of the diet to provide a source of energy, to provide material for growth, and to regulate growth or energy production. Nutrients include carbohydrates, fats, proteins, minerals, and vitamins.

Endurance: The time limit of a person's ability to maintain a specific muscular activity at a specific level of intensity. Endurance is a measure of how long a person can repeat an activity without getting tired. How many miles can an individual run? How many laps can a person swim? How many push-ups can she or he do?

Carbohydrates: Macronutrient molecules contain carbon, hydrogen, and oxygen. They are the primary fuel for muscle contraction. There are two types of carbohydrates: simple and complex. Simple carbohydrates are composed of one or two small molecules and are also called sugars (glucose, fructose, sucrose). Sweet foods such as cookies and candy tend to be high in simple sugars and low in vitamins and minerals; often they are high in fat as well. Sugars are easily absorbed into the blood from the digestive system and provide short bursts of energy. Unfortunately, this burst of energy sometimes is followed by a feeling of drowsiness or low energy. Sugars also are found naturally in fruits and other foods made from plants.

Complex carbohydrates, like starches and glycogen, are made up of long chains of glucose molecules linked together. These large molecules provide a longer lasting source of energy. Breads, cereals, pasta, rice, and other grain products are high in complex carbohydrates, as are many fruits and vegetables. Foods high in complex carbohydrates usually are low in fat and provide protein, some vitamins, and some minerals.

The starches in whole grains, found in foods such as whole wheat bread, raisin bran, popcorn, and brown rice, are surrounded by intact kernels of grain. They are broken down more slowly than starches found in foods made from refined grains such as white bread and white rice. Whole grain foods and some fruits and vegetables are high in fiber, a complex carbohydrate that helps the digestive system function properly. Fiber can't be broken down by the digestive juices, so it passes through the intestine, soaking up water and making it easier for waste to pass from the body. Eating plenty of fiber helps prevent heart disease and diabetes.

Carbohydrates (primarily complex carbohydrates) should make up the largest part (55-60%) of each day's total calorie intake. About 10-15% of daily calories should come from protein and no more than 30% from fat (only 10% from saturated fat). (For more information on dietary sources of carbohydrates, see student resource 1 in this lesson and transparency 2 in lesson 33).

What factors affect endurance?

- Physical fitness: aerobic fitness (the ability of the heart, lungs, and circulatory system to deliver oxygen and nutrients to all areas of the body), muscle strength, flexibility
- Nutrition
- Fluid balance

What activities help to improve endurance?

Endurance is improved progressively by doing activities that extend what you are normally used to doing. This can be done by increasing the frequency, intensity, or duration of exercise. Athletes have training programs that get progressively more demanding as time goes on. This slowly brings their bodies to higher capability levels. If you were to walk a half a mile further each day, walking long distances would become easier and more routine. How long, how hard, and how often you exercise will determine how fit you are.

How does nutrition affect endurance?

Only a small amount of carbohydrate is stored in the liver and muscles as glycogen (long chains of glucose molecules). Therefore, the best sports nutrition regime is one where a carbohydrate-rich diet is eaten *daily*. In most cases, this means following the same diet recommended for nonathletes. A daily calorie balance of 55-60% carbohydrates, 10-15% protein, and no more than 30% fat (10% saturated fat) will ensure that muscles remain loaded with glycogen and that energy and endurance levels remain high. Adolescent athletes who regularly compete in endurance events lasting longer than 60-90 minutes may benefit from increasing their carbohydrates to 60-65% (protein 10-15% and fat 20-30%). This pattern of intake can also be helpful in strenuous, long-lasting activities like lengthy hiking or biking trips.

Research has not yet shown a definitive difference between complex and simple carbohydrates and optimal sports performance. However, complex carbohydrates are preferable overall for good health, as they contain essential vitamins and minerals as well as fiber, and these contribute to a healthy diet. With the exception of fruits, foods rich in simple carbohydrates tend to be deficient in essential nutrients and fiber.

Carbohydrates are the primary fuel for muscle contraction and are stored only in limited amounts by the body. "After two to three hours of exercise, blood glucose concentration normally declines to relatively low levels" (Coyle 1988). Because an insufficient amount of blood glucose is available to compensate for depleted muscle glycogen stores, fatigue may result. Most athletes experience local muscular fatigue, not hypoglycemia (low blood glucose that causes symptoms such as light-headedness and nausea). Athletes in this state may have difficulty exercising intensely. "Sports such as soccer, while not played for more than two hours, can result in significant muscle glycogen depletion and fatigue" (Coyle 1988).

High-carbohydrate meals eaten within 6 hours of competition "top off" the glycogen stores in liver and muscle. "Consuming carbohydrate foods or beverages during exercise has been shown to delay fatigue (i.e., improve endurance and performance) for athletes involved in vigorous continuous or intermittent exercise lasting more than two hours. However, carbohydrate supplements are not necessary for non-fatiguing exercise" (Coyle 1988).

How important are drinks to endurance?

When you're active, you sweat. Sweat is largely made up of water and just a small amount of minerals and electrolytes (sodium, potassium, and magnesium). Not drinking enough water during exercise may lead to dehydration, which can result in cramps, exhaustion, and heat stroke. Prevention is easy: drink water when you exercise.

Water is the best and most economical drink for activities lasting less than an hour. Sports drinks are recommended for exercise that lasts longer than 1 hour and/or is performed in high temperature and humidity. They provide water and a carbohydrate supplement (20 g per 8 oz).

To avoid dehydration, drink one to two cups of water before exercising. When you work out, start drinking early and at regular intervals (4-8 oz every 10-15 min). Flavored drinks may encourage you to drink more. Avoid drinking soda and caffeinated drinks because caffeine increases water loss through urine, and large amounts of sugar (from soda) slow down stomach emptying and increase the time it takes for the fluid to reach your blood. Drink cool water, sports drinks, or *diluted* fruit juices (half juice/half water).

A common misconception that sweating depletes salt in the body leads some people to take salt tablets. However, they can make you sick to your stomach and can worsen dehydration since one salt tablet increases the amount of water you need by 1 pint. Never use salt tablets.

References

Cheung, L., Gortmaker, S., and Dart, H. 2001. *Eat well & keep moving.* Champaign, IL: Human Kinetics.

Coyle, E.F. 1988. Carbohydrates and athletic performance. *Sports Science Exchange* 1(7).

McArdle, E., Katch, F., and Katch, V. 1991. *Exercise physiology: Energy, nutrition, and human performance.* 3d ed. Philadelphia: Lea & Febiger.

National Dairy Council. 1994. *Leader's guide to the guide to good eating and daily food guide pyramid.* Rosemont, IL: Author.

National Research Council. 1989. *Recommended dietary allowances.* 10th ed. Washington, DC: National Academy Press.

U.S. Department of Agriculture and U.S. Department of Health and Human Services. 2000. *Nutrition and your health: Dietary guidelines for Americans* 2000, 5th edition. **www.usda.gov/cnpp**

U.S. Department of Health and Human Services. 2000. Healthy People 2010, conference edition, vols. I and II. **www.health.gov/healthypeople**

Willett, W. 2000. Got fat? Exploding nutrition myths. *World Health News* **www.worldhealthnews.harvard.edu**

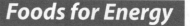
Carbohydrates

Carbohydrates are nutrients that are found in food and are our major source of energy. They are found in many foods and in all groups of the Food Guide Pyramid. However, the grain, fruit, and vegetable groups contain the greatest amount of carbohydrates. These foods generally are low in fat and provide protein, fiber, minerals, and vitamins as well. Eating a variety of grains, especially whole grains, fruits, and vegetables is the basis of healthy eating. Sweet foods such as soda, cookies, and candy that contain sugar also provide carbohydrates. Unfortunately, these foods usually contain very few vitamins and minerals, and some can be high in fat; therefore, these foods should be eaten only in small amounts.

Carbohydrates should make up the largest part (55-60%) of each day's total calorie intake. On a typical day, you should consume 300-375 grams of carbohydrates. However, if you participate in a moderate to vigorous activity lasting for **more than two hours,** you should eat additional carbohydrates during and after the activity. Carbohydrates are the primary fuel for muscle contraction and are stored in only limited amounts by the body; when depleted, athletes may feel fatigue and have difficulty exercising intensely. Riding your bike with friends, playing baseball all afternoon, hanging out at the pool, or jogging three miles can be fueled by the carbohydrates in a typical healthy diet. However, a 10-mile, all-day hike like the one described in activity 1 would require a lot more energy and about 65% of that energy should come from carbohydrates. You would need to eat about 150 additional grams of carbohydrates. (Your calorie and carbohydrate needs will vary depending on how hard you are working and your weight. The number 150 g approximates the carbohydrate needs of a 100-pound person hiking 10 miles at a speed of 1 mile every 20 minutes.)

Here's a list of foods to help you understand where carbohydrates come from in our diet. Mark the ones that are rich in carbohydrates (12 grams or more per serving). You may use this list to help you work on activity 1.

Food item	Serving size	Carbos (grams)	Fat (grams)	Food item	Serving size	Carbos (grams)	Fat (grams)
Grain				**Meat**			
Corn tortilla	6"	13	1	Bacon	3 slices	<1	9
Raisin bran	1 cup	37	1	Ham	1 slice	0	1
Spaghetti	1 cup, cooked	40	1	Chicken breast	1 piece	0	8
Rice, long grain	1 cup, cooked	58	1	Peanut butter	2 Tbsp	7	16
Bagel	1	36	1	**Vegetable**			
White bread	1 slice	12	1	Baked potato	1 large	32	0
Wheat bread	1 slice	12	1	Peas	1/2 cup	12	0

Food item	Serving size	Carbos (grams)	Fat (grams)	Food item	Serving size	Carbos (grams)	Fat (grams)
				Vegetables *(cont.)*			
Dairy foods				Corn	1/2 cup	21	0
Cheddar cheese	1 slice	<1	9	Beans	1 cup	41	1
Cottage cheese	1 oz.	6	10	**Fats and oils**			
Milk, whole	1 cup	11	8	Margarine (soft)	1 Tbsp.	1	11
Milk, 2%	1 cup	12	5	Butter	1 Tbsp.	<1	12
Yogurt, low fat, fruit flavored	1 cup	32	3	**Beverages**			
Egg (boiled)	1	1	5	Orange juice	1 cup	25	0.4
Fruits				Gatorade	3/4 cup	11.25	0
Apple	1	21	0.5	Water	1 cup	0	0
Banana	1	27	0.6	**Other**			
Orange	1	19.5	0.1	Pizza, cheese	2 of 12 slices	44	10
Grapes	1 cup	16	0.3	Milk chocolate	1 small bar, 1.5 oz.	23.7	12.5
Raisins	2/3 cup	79	0.5	Cheesecake	1 slice	23	21

Your science class is planning to explore a nearby mountain trail. The steep and demanding hike is 10 miles long, a day trip that will require a lot of energy. The class plans to eat breakfast together, walk for five miles in the morning, stop for lunch, and return in the afternoon by walking the remaining five miles.

You have been asked to plan the breakfast, snack, and lunch menu for the group. The teacher has asked you to include foods and beverages that will provide a lot of energy and replace the water students will lose exercising. Everyone in the group is active in sports on a regular basis, so fatigue should not be a problem. However, your typical diets won't cover your energy needs. Individuals your age typically consume 300-375 grams of carbohydrates in a day. Each hiker will require about 150 grams of additional carbohydrates to complete the hike. Since you won't be bringing dinner, aim for 350-400 g of carbohydrate.

Use the student resource sheet to help you plan the breakfast, snack, lunch, and beverage supplies that each member of the class should bring. You may include foods that are not on the student resource sheet in your menu. However, you will need to look at food labels at home or in a store to determine the number of carbohydrates these foods contain. Assume that everyone will carry a cold pack to keep food supplies cold. Remember to include some whole grain foods.

Food	Quantity	Carbos (grams)	Food	Quantity	Carbos (grams)
Breakfast			Lunch		
Snack			Beverages		

What is the total number of carbohydrates supplied by your menu for the day of your hike?

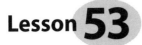

Muscle Mysteries

In this lesson, students perform prescribed motions, observe which muscles are involved, and make conclusions as to the type of fitness that the motions contribute to when done as exercise. The lesson reinforces the "three components of physical fitness" concept while giving students an opportunity to hone their anatomy skills and their powers of observation.

This lesson is designed to infuse into a classroom unit on the muscular system information about the many types of physical activity that are important to fitness.

▶▶ Behavioral Objectives

- For students to be physically active on a regular basis.
- For students to learn exercises that can be practiced regularly.

▶▶ Learning Objectives

Students will be able to

1. identify the major muscles of the body and the motions they produce when they contract, and
2. describe the three types of fitness: muscle strength and endurance (anaerobic fitness), cardiovascular (aerobic) fitness, and flexibility.

▶▶ Materials

- Student resource 1 *Muscles*
- Station cards
- Activity 1 *Solving the Muscle Mysteries*

▶▶ Procedure

Note: This is not a workout—it is a series of activities to show students how muscles are used in various ways. Think about how the classroom can be arranged into 12 workstations. Some stations require a wall; others need some floor space. Post the activity description and illustration (station card) at each station. Ideally, divide the class into pairs of students. Adjust group sizes as necessary. This activity may require more than one 45-minute period. Please note that moving through the workstations takes approximately 25 minutes. Procedures may be split between two periods.

1. (5 minutes) Distribute student resource 1 *Muscles* to the class. Discuss the function of the major muscle groups by generating discussion with students and writing answers on the board. Tell students that they do not need to memorize the muscle groups.

2. (3-5 minutes) Discuss the three types of fitness—muscle strength (anaerobic fitness), cardiovascular (aerobic) fitness, and flexibility—each of which uses muscles in a different way (see Teacher Resources).

3. (2-3 minutes) Distribute activity 1 *Solving the Muscle Mysteries* to students. On the worksheets, students are asked to identify

- which type of fitness the activity would improve if done regularly, and
- which muscles were used in the activity (using student resource 1 as a reference).

4. (10 minutes) Divide the class into pairs or small groups and move them to assigned areas. Review each activity with the class by having students at each station demonstrate the activity.

5. (25 minutes) Move students through the stations until each pair or group has completed all 10 activities. One student in each group will perform the activity at each station. Members of the group should take turns in this role. Have the students spend 45 seconds doing each activity. They have another minute to complete the worksheet. One student can act as a timer and can read the station card to assist the student doing the activity.

Note: Control time and move groups around the room in a clockwise fashion. The stations can be completed in any order. With 10 stations, the activity should be completed in approximately 25 minutes.

6. (5-7 minutes) Students return to seats. Review student experiences by drawing a chart similar to the worksheet on the board and filling in and discussing answers.

▸▸ Extension Activity

Have students come up with their own stretches and movements. Ask them to determine which muscles these movements work.

▸▸ Teacher Resources

General Background Material

In preparing for this lesson, you may want to refer to the following resources:

- *Healthy People 2010*
- *Centers for Disease Control and Prevention Fact Sheets on Physical Activity*

See appendix B for information on how to obtain these resources.

Specific Background Material

Planet Health's Activity Message

Physical activity promotes health and well-being and offers opportunities to socialize and have fun. Adolescents should be moderately active for at least 30 minutes every day or nearly every day as part of play, games, sports, chores, transportation, or planned exercise, *and* they should participate in at least three sessions per week of vigorous physical activity lasting 20 minutes or more. Adolescents should aim for a total of 60 minutes or more of activity on five to seven days a week.

The Three Components of Fitness

The three components of fitness are cardiovascular (aerobic) endurance, muscular strength (anaerobic fitness), and flexibility. If *Planet Health*'s physical education lessons are used, this lesson offers students another opportunity to learn these concepts:

1. Cardiovascular (aerobic) endurance:
   - The heart's ability to get enough oxygen to the muscles to let the body maintain a certain level of activity for a long period of time.
   - The ability to perform activities such as running, cycling, and swimming for long periods of time.
   - Aerobic endurance is the ability of the heart, lungs, and muscles to carry and use oxygen in order to perform continuous and rhythmic exercises.

2. Muscle strength (anaerobic fitness):
   - The ability to lift or move the body or objects.
   - The ability of muscles to produce force at high intensities over short intervals of time.
   - The ability to perform high-force exercises such as sit-ups for short periods of time (10-20 repetitions). Repetition means performing a movement without rest. Doing 10-20 reps means you did an activity such as sit-ups 10-20 times.

3. Flexibility:
   - The ability to bend, stretch, and twist with ease.
   - The ability to move muscles and joints through their range of motion.

4. Proper stretching technique.

This instruction is relevant to the flexibility stations in this lesson (stations 1, 2, 3, 10). Flexibility exercises are muscle specific and can be done for all the major muscles. Instruct students to stretch to the point where muscles are taut, not beyond. They should hold the stretch for at least 10 seconds in order to obtain any benefit from the stretch. Students also have an opportunity to learn this concept in the physical education lessons.

References

Cooper, K.H. 1991. *Kid fitness: A complete shape-up program from birth through high school.* New York: Bantam.

Hales, D., and Hales, R.E. 1985. *Be all you can be! The U.S. Army total fitness program.* New York: Crown.

Halper, M.S., and Neger, I. 1980. *Physical fitness: A preventive medicine institute/strong health clinic, health action plan.* New York: Holt, Rinehart & Winston.

Sallis, J.F., and Patrick, K. 1994. Physical activity guidelines for adolescents: Consensus statement. *Pediatric Exercise Science* 6: 302-314.

U.S. Department of Health and Human Services. 2000. Healthy People 2010, conference edition, vols. I and II. **www.health.gov/healthypeople**

▶▶ Answer Key

Activity 1

Station name	Type of fitness (flexibility, aerobic, or strength)	Muscles used
1. Up and Down Swings	Flexibility	Upper arm, shoulder, and upper back (deltoid group), and chest (pectoralis group)
2. Thigh Stretch	Flexibility	Quadriceps in thigh
3. Calf Stretch	Flexibility	Calf (gastrocnemius) and Achilles tendon
4. Wall Push	Strength	Upper arms, shoulders, and upper back (deltoid group, brachialis, trapezius), and chest (pectoralis group)
5. Side Hops	Aerobic	Calf (gastrocnemius and soleus) and Achilles tendon, thigh (quadriceps and hamstrings), and heart
6. Jogging in Place	Aerobic	Thigh (quadriceps and hamstrings), calf (gastrocnemius and soleus), and heart
7. Half Knee Bends	Strength	Thigh (quadriceps), calf (gastrocnemius and soleus), hips and buttocks (gluteus maximus), lower back (latissimus dorsi), and shoulders (pecs, deltoids, and trapezius)
8. Toe Raises	Strength	Calf (gastrocnemius and soleus)
9. Arm Curls	Strength	Upper arm (biceps)
10. Head Rotation	Flexibility	Neck and upper back (sterno-cleidomastoid and trapezius)

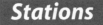

Station 1: Up and Down Swings

Stand erect with feet shoulder-width apart and arms hanging loosely at your sides. Raise and stretch arms over your head until your wrists touch. Move arms in a circle downward until wrists touch in front of your abdomen. Repeat for 45 seconds.

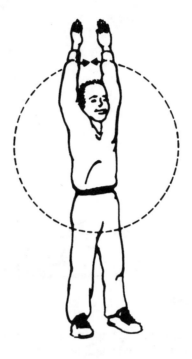

Planet Health: Muscle Mysteries

Station 2: Thigh Stretch

Lean against back of chair for balance. Bend forward and raise one foot up and back. Bend your knee and grasp your ankle with your hand. Pull gently until you feel tension. Hold for 20 seconds. Repeat with other leg.

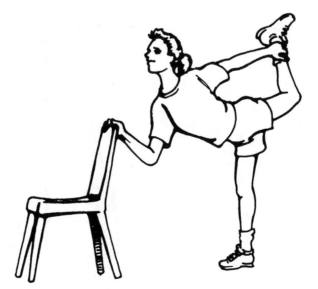

Station 3: Calf Stretch

Stand about 2 feet from a wall with both hands pressed flat on the wall at shoulder level. Press your heels to the ground. Keeping your knees and hips straight, lean into the wall until you feel a pull behind the knee or leg. Increase the tension gradually. Hold for 30 seconds. Repeat with other leg.

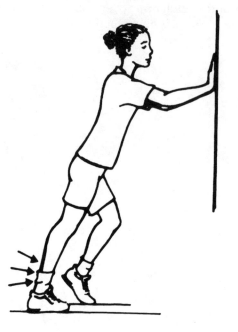

Planet Health: Muscle Mysteries

Station 4: Wall Push

Place your palms flat against the wall. Make sure your arms are straight with elbows locked and your back and legs are straight. Slowly bend your elbows until your nose and chest touch the surface. Slowly push back up and lock elbows again, making sure to keep your back and legs straight. Repeat continuously for 45 seconds.

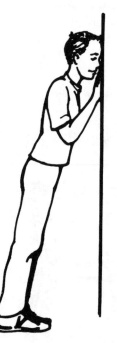

Planet Health: Muscle Mysteries

Station 5: Side Hops

Stand erect with feet together and hands on your hips. Hop about 12 inches to the left. Hop back to starting position. Repeat hopping from side to side for 45 seconds.

Planet Health: Muscle Mysteries

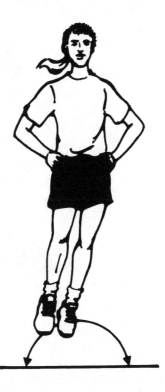

Station 6: Jogging in Place

Stand erect with feet a couple of inches apart. Jog in place, lifting your feet 4 to 6 inches off the floor. Hold your arms at your sides at a 90-degree angle. Continue for 45 seconds.

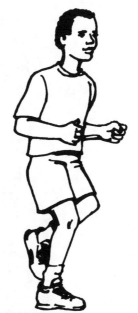

Planet Health: Muscle Mysteries

Station 7: Half Knee Bends

Stand erect with feet shoulder-width apart. Place hands on your hips. Bend knees halfway, bringing heels off the ground, while extending arms forward at shoulder level with palms down. Return to standing position. Repeat for 45 seconds.

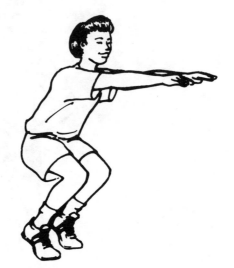

Planet Health: Muscle Mysteries

Station 8: Toe Raises

Stand straight with your weight on the balls of your feet. Lifting your heels, push your body toward the ceiling repeatedly, each time lowering your heels back to the ground. Continue for 45 seconds.

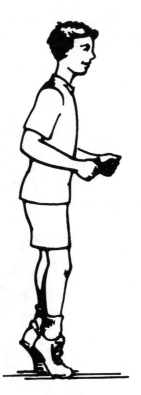

Planet Health: Muscle Mysteries

Station 9: Arm Curls

Stand straight with your arms hanging by your sides. Make a fist with fingers facing forward. Bending arms at the elbow, lift fists to nearly touch upper arm; lower slowly to starting position. Repeat for 45 seconds.

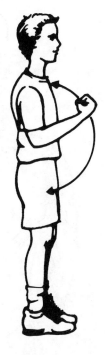

Planet Health: Muscle Mysteries

Station 10: Head Rotation

Stand erect but relaxed, with feet shoulder-width apart and arms behind your back. Look straight ahead. Let your head fall forward and then far to the right in one smooth motion until you can look at the floor behind your right shoulder. Reverse the motion and return to the starting position. Let your head fall forward and to the left in one smooth motion until you can look at the floor behind your left shoulder. Reverse the motion and return to starting position. Continue moving from right to left for 45 seconds.

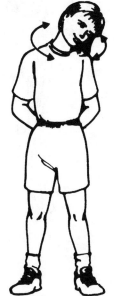

Name _____

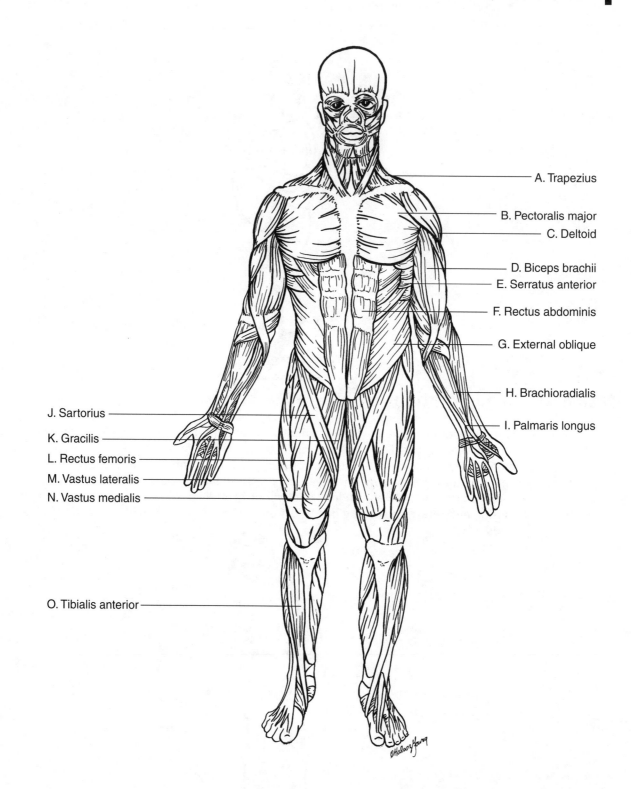

A. Trapezius

B. Pectoralis major

C. Deltoid

D. Biceps brachii

E. Serratus anterior

F. Rectus abdominis

G. External oblique

H. Brachioradialis

I. Palmaris longus

J. Sartorius

K. Gracilis

L. Rectus femoris

M. Vastus lateralis

N. Vastus medialis

O. Tibialis anterior

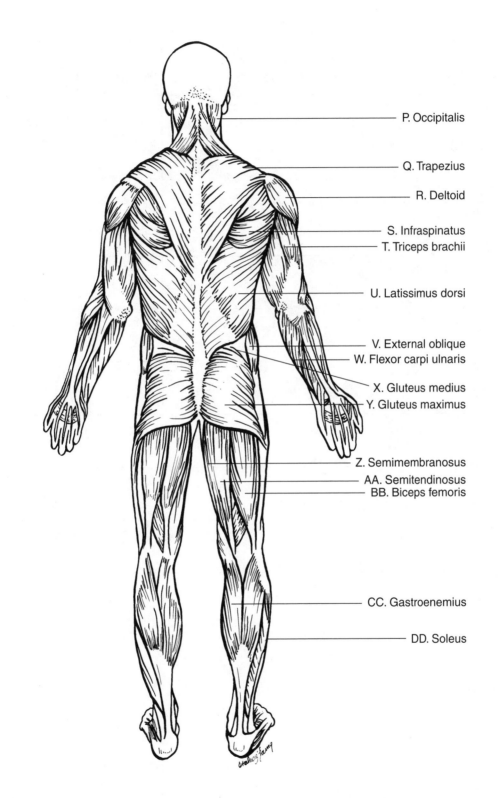

P. Occipitalis

Q. Trapezius

R. Deltoid

S. Infraspinatus
T. Triceps brachii

U. Latissimus dorsi

V. External oblique
W. Flexor carpi ulnaris

X. Gluteus medius
Y. Gluteus maximus

Z. Semimembranosus
AA. Semitendinosus
BB. Biceps femoris

CC. Gastroenemius

DD. Soleus

Station name	Type of fitness (flexibility, aerobic, or strength)	Muscles used
1.		
2.		
3.		
4.		
5.		
6.		
7.		
8.		
9.		
10.		

Lesson 54

The Human Heart

This lesson teaches students about the effect of exercise on the heart and the importance of exercise to general health. Students design and conduct an experiment to examine the effect of exercise, or another variable, on heart rate. This activity will probably require one and a half to two periods of class time.

▶▶ Behavioral Objective

For students to be more physically active.

▶▶ Learning Objectives

Students will be able to

1. describe the importance of activity to the health and strength of the heart,
2. measure their resting pulse rate,
3. make a hypothesis about the impact of exercise (or another variable of their choosing) on heart rate,
4. design and conduct an experiment to determine the impact of exercise (or another variable) on resting pulse rate, and
5. draw conclusions from their experimental findings.

▶▶ Materials

- Clock or watch with second hand
- Activity 1 ***How Much Do You Know About Your Heart?*** (handout, or overhead transparency, or use chalkboard)
- Copies of activity 2 *The Double-Barreled Pumper* and activity 3 *Designing an Experiment*
- *Optional:* tennis balls

▶▶ Procedure

1. Point out the goals of the lesson:
   - Describe the importance of activity to the health and strength of the heart.
   - Measure resting pulse rate.
   - Design and conduct an experiment to determine the impact of exercise (or another variable) on resting pulse rate.
2. (10 minutes) Hand out activity 1 to students (or display it as an overhead transparency, or use the chalkboard). Use this short introductory activity to spark stu-

dents' interest and to point out that the heart is an amazing organ. Ask students to record the answers to the fill-in-the-blank questions. Then call on students to share their responses. Review the answers (see the Answer Key, page 391). Next, discuss the critical thinking portion of the transparency. Give students time to formulate their own theories. Ask for their ideas before you discuss the conclusions.

3. (5 minute *optional* activity) To give students an idea of how hard the heart must work, even at rest, have them try to squeeze a tennis ball 70 times per minute. The force needed to squeeze a tennis ball is similar to the force needed to squeeze blood out of the heart. Can anyone do it?

4. (10 minutes) Have students read activity 2 *The Double-Barreled Pumper* and determine their resting pulse rate. Check for understanding by asking students: *How does exercise strengthen the heart and lower a person's resting pulse rate?*

5. (2-3 minutes) Ask students to brainstorm a list of conditions or variables that might increase or decrease a person's resting heart rate. *(Examples: exercise, body position (lying down vs. standing up), coffee, temperature, stress.)*

6. (5-10 minutes) Discuss activity 3 *Designing an Experiment* with students. In this activity, students choose one variable and test its impact on resting heart rate. They will work in pairs to make a hypothesis, write the procedure, record their heart rate under different conditions, record their results, and draw conclusions based on their findings. Ask them for some examples of experiments they might conduct or describe one of the examples below. Try not to provide too many ideas. *Encourage them to be creative and curious.* This is an opportunity to do what scientists do. *Be prepared:* this type of open-ended experiment will excite some students but frustrate others. You may wish to give students who seem frustrated possible questions to choose from, but let them design the experiment. Emphasize that they need to have you check their procedures before they begin the actual experiment.

Possible experimental questions and designs:

1. What effect does physical activity have on heart rate? There are many possible strategies for answering this question, but encourage students to try more than one intensity exercise. For example:
   - measure resting pulse rate;
   - jog in place for 2 minutes;
   - measure pulse rate;
   - run in place more energetically than before, raising your knees to your chest for 2 minutes; and
   - measure pulse rate.

2. Do different types of physical activity affect heart rate differently?
   - Measure resting pulse rate;
   - do 25 sit-ups;
   - measure pulse rate;
   - rest;
   - do 25 jumping jacks;
   - measure pulse rate;
   - rest;
   - run in place for 2 minutes (or about the same time it took you to do the other activities); and
   - measure pulse rate.

3. How does exercise duration affect heart rate? What happens to your heartbeat as you do more work?
   - Measure resting pulse rate,
     - step up and down on a chair for 1 minute,
     - measure pulse rate,
     - continue stepping up and down at the same rate for 3 more minutes, and
     - measure pulse rate.

4. How does body position affect heart rate? Is sitting, lying down, or standing more work?
   - Sit in chair for 2 minutes,
   - measure pulse rate,
   - lie down for 2 minutes,
   - measure pulse rate,
   - stand up, and
   - immediately measure pulse rate.

5. How does stress affect heart rate?
   - Measure resting pulse rate,
   - give someone a small amount of time to finish a written task or puzzle, and
   - measure pulse rate immediately after they finish racing through the task.

6. What happens to my heart rate when I am really cold and in pain?
   - Measure resting pulse rate,
   - stick hand in ice water for 1 minute, and
   - measure pulse rate at the end of the minute.

---

7. (30 minutes) Have students complete activity 3 *Designing an Experiment.*

8. (5-10 minutes) Ask several groups to share their results. Students are likely to have difficulty drawing conclusions and explaining *why* the observed results occurred. You may wish to have students record their results on the board and have the whole class interpret and discuss the results. Encourage all students to brainstorm possible explanations for why the results occurred. Place less emphasis on the "right" explanation. Emphasize the process of *thinking* like a scientist. (See Teacher Resourses for results you might expect.)

▶▶ Extension Activities

1. Determine the average resting heart rate for the students in your classes. What differences could explain variations in resting heart rate? *(Age, stress, caffeine, medication, active or sedentary lifestyle.)*

2. Ask students to take the resting pulse rates of each member of their families. What differences could explain variations in resting heart rate? *(Fitness level, stress, caffeine intake, age.)*

▶▶ Teacher Resources

General Background Material

In preparing for this lesson, you may want to refer to the following resources:

- *Centers for Disease Control and Prevention Fact Sheets on Physical Activity*
- *Healthy People 2010*

See appendix B for information on how to obtain these resources.

Specific Background Material

See activity 2 *The Double-Barreled Pumper*

How Strong Is the Heart?

The force needed to squeeze a tennis ball is similar to the force needed to squeeze blood out of the heart. "Although this four-chambered muscular organ weighs less than a pound, it beats so steadily and powerfully that the force generated during its 40 million beats per year could lift its owner 100 miles above the earth. Even for a person of average fitness, the maximum output of blood from this remarkable organ is greater than the fluid output from a household faucet turned wide open" (McArdle, Katch, and Katch, 1991).

Disorders of the Circulatory System

Heart attack: Artery carrying blood to heart becomes blocked by fatty deposits or blood clots. Area of heart muscle is deprived of oxygen and dies.

Stroke: Artery carrying blood to brain becomes blocked. Brain cells do not get enough oxygen and die.

Arteriosclerosis: Arteries become narrower due to a build-up of fatty deposits on walls.

Hypertension: Constant high blood pressure that can lead to a heart attack or stroke.

Varicose veins: Valves in the veins do not work properly. Veins become swollen due to accumulation of blood. Most common in leg veins.

What Effect Does _____ Have on Heart Rate?
(variable)

Possible experimental results for activity 3 *Designing an Experiment*.
Physical Activity: Increases heart rate. The more intense the exercise, the higher the heart rate. Exercise that utilizes large muscle groups and works against gravity results in the greatest increase in heart rate. Heart rate increases rapidly at the onset of exercise and levels off after 3-5 minutes of exercise at a steady rate. Through training (regular exercise), the heart increases in efficiency and pumps more blood per beat, so resting heart rate declines.

Stress: May increase heart rate. Stressful situations increase nerve impulses from the brain that stimulate the heart to beat faster.

Caffeine: May increase heart rate in some individuals. However, sensitivity to caffeine varies greatly. Individuals who consume caffeine regularly will likely notice less effect on heart rate.

Pain: Generally increases heart rate.

Temperature: Long-term exposure to the cold lowers heart rate.

Posture: Lying down lowers heart rate. Upright posture raises heart rate. The heart must work harder to pump blood against gravity from the lower extremities back to the heart and up to the brain. Standing perfectly still for an extended period of time results in blood pooling in the veins and can cause fainting due to insufficient cerebral blood supply.

References

Development of student activity 3 was influenced by laboratory activities created by Weston Public School Faculty (Weston, MA): Jill Carter, Patricia Corey, Janet Kresl Moffitt, and Joyce Schwartz.

Allison, L. 1976. *Blood and guts.* Boston: Little, Brown.

Bierer, L., Warner, L., Lawson, S., and Cohen, T. 1991. *Life science: The challenge of discovery.* Lexington, MA: Heath.

McArdle, W.D., Katch, F., and Katch, V. 1991. *Exercise physiology: Energy, nutrition, and human performance.* 3d ed. Philadelphia: Lea & Febiger.

Sallis, J.F., and Patrick, K. 1994. Physical activity guidelines for adolescents: Consensus statement. *Pediatric Exercise Science* 6: 302-314.

U.S. Department of Health and Human Services. 2000. Healthy People 2010, conference edition, vols. I and II. **www.health.gov/healthypeople**

▶▶ Answer Key

Activity 1

1. At rest your heart beats about **60–80** beats per minute.
2. Your heart weighs about **one** pound(s) and is the size of a **clenched fist.**
3. Heart disease is the leading cause of death in the United States (true or false). **True**
4. The maximum output of blood from your heart is greater than the water output from a household faucet turned wide open (true or false). **True**

5. An athlete's resting heart rate is higher than the resting heart rate of a person who does little exercise (true or false). **False (it's lower)**

Critical Thinking

Conclusion: Animals with **slower** pulse rates live **longer**.

So, what is one way that physical activity can help you live longer? Through regular physical activity the heart increases in efficiency and pumps more blood per beat (contraction), so resting heart rate declines.

1. At rest your heart beats about _____ beats per minute.

2. Your heart weighs about _____ pound(s) and is the size of a _____.

3. Heart disease is the leading cause of death in the United States (true or false). _____

4. The maximum output of blood from your heart is greater than the water output from a household faucet turned wide open (true or false). _____

5. An athlete's resting heart rate is higher than the resting heart rate of a person who does little exercise (true or false).

_____

Critical Thinking

What conclusions can you draw from the data below?

Animal	Heart rate (beats/minute)	Average life span
Shrew	1,000	Up to 1-1/2 years
Mouse	500	1–2 years
Rabbit	200	6 years
Elephant	25	60 years
Human	70	70 years

Conclusion: Animals with _____ pulse rates live _____.

- These mammals' hearts are good for about one billion beats, except for humans.
- Humans have a high-performance heart that averages about 2.5 billion beats per lifetime.
- If you could slow down your heart rate you would have a good chance of spreading those 2.5 billion beats over more years.

So, what is one way that physical activity can help you live longer?

What Is the Role of the Heart?

The heart is a muscular organ that controls the flow of the body's blood. It is the equivalent of an engine room, for it pumps blood through the body continuously, transporting **oxygen** to all the muscles of the body. The heart therefore controls the body's **circulatory system,** which includes arteries and veins, the tubes that carry the blood away from and back to the heart.

How Does Your Diet Affect the Heart?

In the United States, circulatory system disorders are the leading cause of death. There is good evidence to suggest that high saturated and trans fat consumption increases the risk of heart diseases. An excessive intake of these fats can lead to the build-up of fatty deposits in arteries—**arteriosclerosis.** As arteries narrow and harden, blood flow may be blocked to surrounding cells. If an artery supplying blood to the heart is blocked, some heart muscle may die from lack of oxygen; this is called a **heart attack.** For this reason, experts recommend that no more than 10% of our total calories come from saturated fat and that we avoid foods that contain trans fats (partially hydrogenated vegetable oil).

How Does Physical Activity Improve Your Heart?

With physical fitness and aerobic training, the heart will function more efficiently, beating at a slower rate and pumping more blood with each beat. It is only over time that good aerobic fitness can be developed, and training the body to function at more active levels makes it stronger and more productive during vigorous activity.

How Much Physical Activity Do I Need to Do to Make My Heart Stronger?

Do some moderate physical activity for at least 30 minutes every day, or nearly every day, as part of play, games, sports, chores, transportation, or planned exercise. Any activity that raises the heart rate above the resting heart rate can be beneficial to your overall health and can reduce the risk of heart disease. You should also participate in at least three sessions per week of vigorous physical activity lasting 20 minutes or more. This type of continuous exercise is best for strengthening your heart. Moderate physical activity includes walking, baseball, softball, dancing, heavy chores, skateboarding, bicycling, shooting baskets, and other activities of a similar level. Vigorous physical activity includes tennis, fast bicycling, jogging/running, lap swimming, hockey, roller skating/in-line skating, and other activities that make you breathe hard. How long, how hard, and how often you are active will determine how fit you are! Aim for a total of 60 minutes or more of activity nearly every day.

How Do You Measure Your Resting Pulse?

Each time the left side of the heart contracts (or beats) it forces blood into your arteries. Your pulse is caused by blood stopping and starting as it rushes through your arteries. Your pulse rate equals your heart rate. An average resting pulse is around 60-80 beats per minute. However, trained athletes can have resting pulse rates as low as 35 beats per minute. You can take a resting pulse at any time of the day, but the most accurate time to record it is when you first wake in the morning. The easiest way to find your pulse is either in your neck, to the left of the Adam's apple, or on your wrist below your thumb. Sit still for at least 1 minute, find your pulse, and record the number of times your heart beats in 15 seconds.

Number of beats in 15 seconds: _____

Multiply by 4 ($\times$ 4): _____

Resting heart rate beats per minute: _____

What effect does _____ (variable) have on heart rate?

Research Question

Come up with a research question that you hope to answer with this experiment.

Hypothesis

What effect do you think this variable will have on heart rate?

Procedure

Design an experiment to test your hypothesis. List and number the steps in your experiment. Have the teacher look over your procedure and sign this sheet *before* you do the experiment.

_____

(Teacher's signature)

Results

Record your results in the table.

Condition	Pulse rate: Student 1 (beats/minute)	Pulse rate: Student 2 (beats/minute)
Example: resting for 1 minute	*65*	*70*

Conclusions

What do your results tell you about pulse rate? Do your conclusions support your hypothesis? Explain why you think these results occurred.

Lesson **55**

How Far Can You Jump?

In this lesson, students are introduced to the classification of motor skills. They perform a hands-on laboratory activity that focuses on the improvement of a specific gross motor skill— the standing broad jump. Students form hypotheses and attempt to increase their jumping distances by analyzing performances. This lesson is designed to infuse information about the benefits of physical activity and the risks of inactivity into a classroom unit on growth and development or biomechanics.

▶▶ Behavioral Objectives

- To be physically active on a regular basis.
- To strive to evaluate and improve upon physical skills.

▶▶ Learning Objectives

Students will be able to

1. classify skills—gross motor versus fine motor;
2. develop hypotheses, take measurements, and make detailed observations;
3. complete an observation assessment of the standing broad jump; and
4. make effective group recommendations to promote individual skill improvement.

▶▶ Materials

- Activity 1 *How Far Can You Jump?*
- Six 6–7-foot tape measures and masking tape
- *Optional:* mats for students to land on

▶▶ Procedure

Planning

- Since students will be jumping and possibly falling, you might advise them to wear casual pants and sneakers or other shock-absorbing shoes. To save time, you may want to write the steps listed in #5 on the board before class.

- Tape measures should be taped on the floor ahead of time. You can improvise with masking tape by laying it down and marking in 6-inch increments.

1. (1 minute) Begin class by making a prediction: "By the end of this class, many of you will be able to jump farther than you can right now." Write this on the board.

2. (5-7 minutes) Using the Teacher Resources, present background material about motor development (you may have done this in another class):

- Define fundamental motor skills.
- List terms for the study of movement on the board (biomechanics and kinesiology).
- What do science and mathematics have to do with sports? *(Principles of physics guide the motions of bodies [and balls] through space; we measure and observe sports outcomes; trainers base their suggestions for improvement on hypotheses about what will change the outcome; then they test the hypotheses.)*
- Write *fine motor skill* and *gross motor skill* on the board and define with examples.
- Explain that fine motor activities are generally sedentary activities and gross motor activities are fitness and activity skills.

3. (5 minutes) Using the following questions, discuss the value of physical skill assessment: If you were really interested in a sport or activity, you'd want to get better at it. We're going to look closely at the process of improving gross motor skills using a kinesiology approach.

- How do physical fitness trainers (e.g., coaches) assess the skills of their athletes? *(Observation and measurement.)*
- How do people improve their performances? *(Practice [the right kind and type of practice]. This involves breaking down the motions, observing them objectively, forming a mental hypothesis [e.g., if I stretch out more, I will be able to run farther], and testing the hypothesis.)*

4. (3-5 minutes) Have the class participate in formulating a hypothesis to the effect that "athletes can increase their standing broad jumps by x inches when coaches advise them of the skill components they need to improve." To do this, begin with the statement on the board (see #1). Tell the students you are going to recreate the prediction as a *scientific hypothesis*.

A *scientific hypothesis*

- is predictive or explanatory,
- is based on a rational theory,
- can be tested, and
- yields measurable results.

5. (5-10 minutes) Write the steps below on the board. Explain to the class that they are about to become athletes and coaches who will attempt to improve gross motor skills through the standing broad jump (a simple gross motor skill). While using a student to demonstrate this jump, generate a group discussion on the steps involved:

- Start in a crouch (with knees bent and feet together).
- Arms reach backward.
- Arms swing forward.
- Arms extend overhead at takeoff.
- Knees flex or bend to propel body through space.
- Push off with both feet (two-foot takeoff).
- Body tips forward during flight (head in front of hips).
- Land on both feet (two-foot landing).
- Arms are extended forward on landing (at shoulder level).

6. (3 minutes) Divide the class into small groups with approximately five students per group. Pass out one copy of the activity to each group. Each group will pick one student to be the athlete, while all the other students will be coaches. One of the coaches will hold onto the worksheets and is responsible for recording data.

7. (15 minutes) *Group activity*: Students have 15 minutes to complete the activity.

- The recorder will note the measurement goal and the actual measurement for each jump. The measurement goal is the athlete's estimate of how far he or she will jump. The athlete will guess at the first jump goal and work to improve the actual jump in the following two jumps using the observations and hypotheses of the coaches.

- The student chosen as the athlete will perform three standing long jumps while the coaches observe and evaluate the jump using the Coaches' Checklist (activity 1) as a guide, noting each action that happened or did not happen.

- Between each jump, the group should discuss what parts of the jump did or did not happen and then make recommendations for how to improve the jump. The recorder should note the recommendations in the results section of the activity sheet.

- During this time the teacher should circulate among groups to answer questions as they come up. In addition, the teacher should gather data from each group, record the data on the Class Data sheet, and calculate averages for the first, second, and third jumps for presentation to the class during the discussion.

8. (5-10 minutes) Students return to seats. Use the following discussion questions to generate a class discussion of the evaluation and assessment process:

- Evaluate the class's starting hypothesis using the averages calculated by the teacher:

  A. Did the athletes' jumps improve with observation and coaching?

  B. How far was the average starting jump? Average second jump? Average third jump?

- Was any single component of the standing broad jump more important to do right than others?

- Was this a gross motor or fine motor skill?

- Have you ever worked hard to get better at a skill or sport? How did it make you feel?

▶▶ Extension Activity

Select a skill from any sport or physical activity that you do and break it down into different parts or components as we did with the standing broad jump. Select anything that involves motion, including playing an instrument, painting, drawing, pottery making, gardening, carpentry (fine motor skills), or walking, kicking, running, catching, throwing (gross motor skills).

▶▶ Teacher Resources

General Background Material

In preparing for the lesson, you may want to refer to the following resources:

- *Healthy People 2010*
- *Television Viewing as a Cause of Increasing Obesity Among Children in the United States, 1986–1990*

See appendix B for information on how to obtain these resources.

Specific Background Material

Fundamental Motor Skills or Basic Motor Skills

Fundamental or basic motor skills are common motor activities with specific movement patterns. Walking, running, jumping, and throwing are fundamental motor skills. These basic skills form the basis for more advanced and specific movement activities.

Proficiency in movements or motor skills are described in terms of immature (initial) form to minimal form to sport skill form. Generally, children two to three years of age show immature forms of motor skills. By the sixth year, most children acquire some features of *mature* movement patterns. Mature movement patterns are then adapted to special requirements for a particular movement activity, such as pitching in baseball (from a basic throw) or running hurdles (from a basic leap). These skills can be refined for stronger and better performance.

Analysis of Movement

Definition of terms for the study of movement:

- *Biomechanics:* The physics of human motion or the study of forces produced by and acting on the body.
- *Kinesiology:* Often used synonymously with biomechanics but means "the science of motion."

Classification of Motor Skills

A motor skill is an action or task with a goal that requires voluntary body movement to achieve the goal. Playing the piano and kicking a soccer ball are motor skills, but they can be further classified into *fine motor skills* and *gross motor skills* (see the table).

- *Fine motor skill:* A skill performed by the smaller muscles of the body, particularly the hands and fingers.
- *Gross motor skill:* A motor skill requiring large musculature of the body or the larger muscles.

Examples of fine motor skills	Examples of gross motor skills
Playing the piano	Kicking a soccer ball
Keyboarding on the computer	Throwing a baseball
Writing with a pen	Walking to school
Sewing a button on a shirt	Playing basketball
Opening a combination lock	Climbing stairs
Using video game controls	Ballet dancing

Fine and gross motor skills are performance-based movements. Individuals can improve their performances through the right practice. Experts, teachers, and coaches assist people in refining their fine and gross motor skills. A piano teacher helps students with finger placement and touch of the piano keys, whereas a coach breaks down a gross motor skill into parts to help athletes improve their performances.

Both fine and gross motor skills can be important components in a person's life. Activities involving gross motor skills, when performed regularly, improve physical fitness, reduce stress, and appear to contribute to good health throughout the life span. From a health standpoint, finding a gross motor skill that one enjoys and can keep doing for many years is quite important. Sedentary activities that involve fine motor skills can be relaxing, satisfying, and can form the basis of a lifelong career or vocation. These are wonderful alternatives to TV viewing. In contrast, TV viewing is a sedentary activity that requires no skill, offers no room for improvement, and provides none of the benefits of fine and gross motor skills.

References

Gabbard, C. 1992. *Lifelong motor development.* Dubuque, IA: Brown.

Haywood, K. 1993. *Life span motor development.* Champaign, IL: Human Kinetics.

Magill, R.A. 1993. *Motor learning: Concepts and applications.* Dubuque, IA: Brown.

Ontario Science Center. 1989. *Sportworks.* Reading, MA: Addison-Wesley.

Sallis, J.F., and Patrick, K. 1994. Physical activity guidelines for adolescents: Consensus statement. *Pediatric Exercise Science* 6: 302-314.

U.S. Department of Health and Human Services. 2000. Healthy People 2010, conference edition, vols. I and II. **www.health.gov/healthypeople**

Purpose

To improve _____'s ability to do the standing long jump.
(name)

Hypothesis

Procedure (time limit: 15 minutes):

1. Choose one student to be the athlete. The other students will act as coaches.
2. Choose one coach to record everyone's observations.
3. Have the athlete warm up by stretching his or her legs and rotating his or her ankles.
4. Have the athlete set a distance goal and record it below.
5. Coaches should observe the athlete's jump, measure and record the length of the actual jump, and then use the Coaches' Checklist to analyze the jump. Put a ✓ in the box next to the action(s) the athlete did and a Ø in the box if an action did not happen.
6. The coaches and athlete work together to think about how to improve the performance of the jump. Write your hypothesis (recommendation) below.
7. Have the athlete complete three jumps. (Repeat steps 4-6 three times.)

Results

Name of recording coach: _____

Names of coaches: _____

Name of athlete: _____

First Jump

Goal: I will jump _____ (measurement in feet and inches).

Actual jump: _____

Coaches' hypothesis (recommendation) for next jump: If you_____,
you will improve your jump by going farther.

Second Jump

Goal: I will jump _____ (measurement in feet and inches).

Actual jump: _____

Coaches' hypothesis (recommendation) for next jump: If you_____,
you will improve your jump by going farther.

Third Jump

Goal: I will jump_____ (measurement in feet and inches).

Actual jump: _____

Coaches' hypothesis (recommendation) for next jump: If you_____, you will
improve your jump by going farther.

Coaches' Checklist

Put a ✓ in the box if an action happened. Put a ø in the box if an action did not happen.

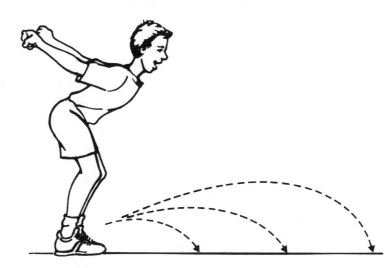

List of skills to observe	Jump 1	Jump 2	Jump 3
Starts in a crouch			
Two-foot takeoff			
Arms start backward			
Legs straighten after takeoff			
Arms extend overhead during jump			
Body tips forward during flight (head in front of hips)			
Arms extend forward at landing			
Landing is in control			
Two-foot landing			

Conclusions

Did the athlete use your recommendations to improve his or her technique? Explain.

Did the athlete improve his or her jump?

What skills should the athlete continue to work on?

How Far Can You Jump?

Class Data Sheet

Group	Jump 1	Jump 2	Jump 3
Class average			

Social Studies

This unit contains eight lessons. Use the At A Glance chart below to help you select the lessons that best fit your curriculum objectives. Some of the lessons offer a choice of activities. Adapt the lesson procedures to fit your teaching style, students' skills, and time constraints.

Lessons in this unit meet many Massachusetts learning standards that may be similar to standards in your state. Refer to appendix E (page 508) to see which of the 1996-1999 Massachusetts Curriculum Frameworks (MCFW) each lesson incorporates.

Social Studies At A Glance

Theme	Lesson	Level of difficulty (grade)*			Subject-specific skills	Materials needed
		6th	7th	8th		
Balanced diet	56 Food Through the Ages	M	M	L	Eating patterns of ancient people	Overhead transparency
Balanced diet	57 Democracy and Diet	H	M-H	M	Government decision-making, debate process	
Fruits and vegetables	58 Global Foods	M	M	L	Cultural comparison, geography	World map, overhead transparencies
Fruits and vegetables	59 Around the World With Five a Day	M	M	L	Agriculture, geography, group research and presentation	Overhead transparency
Activity	60 Map Maker	M	L	L	Map skills	Large town map, colored thumbtacks or markers, overhead transparency
Activity	61 Free to Be Fit	H	M-H	M	Constitutional rights, law making	
Lifestyle	62 Impact of Technology	H	M	M	Industrial Revolution, 19th- and 20th-century technology	Social studies textbook
Lifestyle	63 Food Rituals and Society	M	M	L	Religious and ethnic tradition	

* Level of difficulty: L = low, M = medium, H = high

Balanced Diet Theme

Food Through the Ages

This lesson reinforces the importance of eating a balanced diet based on the Food Guide Pyramid (FGP). It also explains that these food recommendations were developed and modified over time as our knowledge of nutrition and diseases associated with poor nutrition grew. Students are asked to compare and contrast the foods eaten by ancient and historical populations (early Hominids, St. Benedictine monks [530 AD], English peasants and knights [1200s], and English mill workers [1800s]) with the FGP recommendations, and to determine whether these people were likely to have suffered from certain diseases as a result of deficiencies in their diets. Students are encouraged to discuss the economic, trade, food production, and knowledge changes that have decreased undernutrition in industrialized countries and that might help solve the problem of undernutrition in developing countries.

▶▶ Behavioral Objective

To improve student knowledge of the Food Guide Pyramid.

▶▶ Learning Objectives

Students will be able to

1. compare and contrast the foods eaten by ancient people with the Food Guide Pyramid recommendations;

2. discuss some of the nutritional disorders associated with vitamin and mineral deficiencies;

3. discuss the economic, trade, food production, and knowledge changes that have led to a decrease in disorders associated with undernutrition in industrialized countries and that might help solve the problem of undernutrition in developing countries;

4. classify food items into the five food groups;

5. use the Food Guide Pyramid to design balanced meals (extension activity 1); and

6. conduct oral surveys of adults to determine changes in eating patterns during the last 50 years (extension activity 2).

▶▶ Materials

- Activity 1 *Food Through the Ages*
- Student resource 1 *Vitamins and Minerals* (1 copy for each pair of students)
- Overhead transparency 1 blank Food Guide Pyramid (or handout, or use chalkboard)
- *Optional:* Extension activity 1 *Designing a Menu* or extension activity 2 *Food Survey*

▶▶ Procedure

1. Point out the goals of this lesson:

- Review the Food Guide Pyramid recommendations for eating a balanced diet.

- Compare and contrast the foods eaten by ancient people with the Food Guide Pyramid recommendations.

- Discuss the economic, trade, food production, and knowledge changes that have decreased undernutrition in industrialized countries and that might decrease undernutrition in developing countries.

2. (3-5 minutes) Display the overhead transparency of the blank Food Guide Pyramid. Have students recall the names of the food groups and the number of servings recommended each day. (See the Answer Key on page 412.)

3. (3-5 minutes) Ask some of the students to name foods they ate yesterday. Ask other students to classify these foods in the appropriate food groups.

4. (3 minutes) Briefly review the three principles of the Food Guide Pyramid:

- Eat a *variety* of foods from each of the food groups.

- Eat the *appropriate number of servings* from each food group.

- Eat sweets and high-fat foods only *occasionally*.

5. (5 minutes) Introduce the student activity by discussing the following:

- As scientists have become more knowledgeable about nutrition and diseases associated with poor nutrition, diet recommendations have changed. Your parents probably learned about the Basic Four food recommendations when they were your age. The Food Guide Pyramid recommendations that we use today were finalized in 1992.

- For most of history, poor, working-class individuals, and even some wealthy individuals, have been undernourished. The original dietary recommendations were designed to decrease the symptoms and disorders associated with vitamin, mineral, and protein deficiencies.

- In this activity we will compare the diets of ancient people with the diet recommended by the Food Guide Pyramid.

6. (30 minutes) Hand out activity 1 and student resource 1. Have students work in pairs to complete the activity. (See page 413 for answers to selected questions.)

7. (5 minutes) Discuss the following questions:

- Why did many of these ancient people eat diets that do not meet the Food Guide Pyramid recommendations? *(Answer: They did not have access to the variety and quantity of food needed for a balanced diet. They also lacked knowledge of what foods were needed for good health. Food availability, income, and, in some cases, myths or religious beliefs determined their diet.)*

- Why are most people in industrialized countries today better fed than these ancient people? *(Answer: Improved transportation, food production, international trade and economy, and advances in knowledge of what makes up a healthy diet.)*

- Why are many people in developing countries still undernourished? (It may be better to use a specific country as an example.) *(Answer: It depends on the country. Government instability and war can disrupt transportation, food production, trade, education, and public health.)*

- Currently, many people in the United States eat too much food. Therefore, there has been a rise in the diseases associated with obesity. What is responsible for this new nutritional problem? *(Answer: People in industrial societies live more sedentary lifestyles than did people in other times in history and eat high-calorie diets rich in saturated fats and partially hydrogenated vegetable oils [trans fats].)*

▶▶ Extension Activities

1. Imagine you were able to use your knowledge to improve the nutrition of children living during one of the time periods discussed in the class activity. Use extension activity 1 to design five lunch menus that would provide them with a balanced diet.

2. How are your eating habits different from those of children living 50 years ago? Interview a grandparent, great aunt, neighbor, teacher, or friend of the family who was 11 to 14 years old during the 1920s, 1930s, or 1940s. Ask them the questions listed in extension activity 2.

3. Can you think of another way to organize the pyramid? Use some other shapes to design another food guide using the same food groups. (Different-sized circles for each group may be another way.)

4. Visit the school cafeteria and talk to the food manager to find out how the menu is designed. Does she or he use the Food Guide Pyramid?

▶▶ Teacher Resources

General Background Material

In preparing for this lesson, you may want to refer to the following resources:

- *Nutrition and Your Health: Dietary Guidelines for Americans*
- *Daily Food Guide Pyramid*

See appendix A.

Specific Background Material

What Is the Food Guide Pyramid?

The Food Guide Pyramid (FGP) is an educational tool designed by the U.S. Department of Agriculture (USDA) and released in 1992. The FGP promotes moderation, variety, and balance in the diet and helps individuals choose what and how much to eat from each of the five food groups. Following the FGP recommendations ensures consuming essential nutrients sufficient to meet the dietary needs of most people.

The position of the food groups in the FGP reflects the number of daily servings people should eat from each food group. The pyramid has a wide base and a small tip, showing that the food group requiring the most daily servings is at the bottom and the group requiring the least is at the top. Specifically, the grain group takes up the most space on the pyramid and forms its base, indicating we should eat more servings of grain products (especially whole grains) than of any other food group. The tip includes foods such as fats, oils, and sweets. Individuals should limit their consumption of these foods.

The FGP encourages three basic principles:

- *Proportionality (balance):* Eat the recommended number of servings from each food group. Your age, sex, and physical activity level make a difference in the number of servings you need to maintain a well-balanced diet.

- *Variety:* Choose a variety of foods within each of the five food groups. For example, while selecting from the grains food group, select bread, rice, pasta, and other grains (especially whole grains) rather than just bread. No single food supplies all the nutrients you need and foods within the same food group have different amounts of nutrients. Eating many different foods will ensure that you meet the nutritional recommendations.

- *Moderation:* Eat the appropriate number of servings from each food group using the FGP serving sizes as a guide. Eat fats, oils, and sweets, the foods in the tip of the pyramid, sparingly. These "sometimes" foods are low in essential vitamins and minerals and high in calories from fat or sugar. Limiting one's intake of animal fats, trans fats, and sweets can lower a person's risk of developing many health problems in adulthood. Animal fats, which are found in foods such as meat, butter, and whole milk, are the major source of the saturated fats listed on food labels. Snack foods and baked goods are the major source of trans fats, or partially hydrogenated vegetable oils as they are more commonly called.

The FGP applies to diets around the world. For example, 3/4 cup of mango juice from Brazil is a serving of juice.

How Have Dietary Recommendations Changed?

The *Basic Seven* (1943) specified a foundation diet that was designed to help people consume adequate diets to optimize health. It was meant to address issues of undernutrition more than overnutrition. This plan was developed in 1943 because one-third of the men who applied to join the armed services for World War II were rejected because their growth had been affected by a poor diet. The seven groups were:

- milk and dairy (2 cups/day),
- meats, poultry, fish, eggs, dried beans, peas, nuts (1–2 servings/day),
- leafy green or yellow vegetables (1 ser ving/day),
- citrus fruits (1 ser ving/day),
- potatoes and other fruits or vegetables (2 ser vings/day),
- bread, flour, cereal—enriched or whole grain (every day), and
- butter-fortified margarine (some daily).

The *Basic Four* (1956) was a simplified version of the Basic Seven. It also specified serving size and frequency of daily consumption from each food group. Again, it was intended to address issues of dietary deficiency more than overconsumption of foods from specific food groups. The four groups were:

- milk group (2 cups/day),
- fruits and vegetables (4 ser vings, dark-green leafy or yellow vegetables, citrus daily),
- meat group (2 ser vings, with 1 serving equal to 2–3 oz), and
- breads and cereals (4 ser vings where 1 serving is equal to 1 oz dry cereal, 1 slice bread, or 1/2 to 3/4 cup cooked cereal).

By the 1970s, research was showing that the overconsumption of certain nutrients in food—such as fat, saturated fat, cholesterol, sodium, and processed sugar—was related to increased risk of heart disease, some cancers, and diabetes. Research also showed that a higher intake of fruits and vegetables rich in vitamins A, C, and E decreased risk for heart disease and some cancers. Taking these findings into consideration, the USDA revised its nutrition recommendations in 1980. The basic educational message changed from "variety" to "variety and moderation." Recommended serving size in each of the four groups was reduced, and a fifth group (fats, sweets, and alcohol; no serving size recommended but moderation encouraged) was added.

To promote the need for moderation and variety in the diet, the USDA designed the *Food Guide Pyramid* (1992). The pyramid translates the Food and Drug Administration's recommended daily allowances (RDA) and the USDA's dietary guidelines into the kinds and amounts of foods to eat every day. It highlights grains, fruits, and vegetables as the foundation of healthy eating.

The USDA updated the *Dietary Guidelines for Americans* in 2000. Although the principles of proportionality, variety, and moderation remain essentially the same, there are a few changes in the recommendations. The new guidelines place a greater emphasis on increasing intake of whole grain foods, as evidence continues to show that eating a diet high in fiber reduces the risk of heart disease and diabetes. The new guidelines also place a greater emphasis on eating a diet low in saturated fat and cholesterol and limiting consumption of trans fats (partially hydrogenated vegetable oils). Nutrition experts recommend replacing saturated fat (found primarily in animal products such as meat, butter, and whole milk) and trans fat (found in some margarines and many convenience snack foods such as crackers and cookies) primarily with unsaturated fats (safflower, sunflower, corn, canola, soybean, and olive oils). Unsaturated fats lower blood cholesterol and substituting this type of fat for saturated and trans fat can reduce the risk of heart disease. While the recommendations for total fat* (30% of total caloric intake) and saturated fat (10%) did not change, the new guidelines tell us to choose a diet that is moderate in total fat, not low in total fat, as the 1992 guidelines suggested. This change in wording emphasizes that not all fats have the same health effects, and we need to watch our intake of saturated and trans fats most closely.

* Total fat includes saturated, unsaturated, and trans fats

References

Hu, F.B., Stampfer, M.J., Manson, J.E., Rimm, E., Colditz, G.A., Rosner, B.A., Hennekens, C.H., and Willett, W.C. 1997. Dietary fat intake and the risk of coronary heart disease in women. *New England Journal of Medicine* 337(21): 1491-1499.

Knutson, R.D., Penn, J.B., and Boehm, W.T. 1983. *Agricultural and food policy.* Englewood Cliffs, NJ: Prentice Hall.

National Research Council. 1980. *Recommended dietary allowances.* 10th ed. Washington, D.C.: National Academy Press.

Park, R. 1992. Human energy expenditure from *Australopithecus afarensis* to 4-minute mile: Exemplars and case studies. *Exercise Science and Sports Medicine Review* 20: 185-220.

Shils, M.E., and Young, V.R. 1988. *Modern nutrition in health and disease.* 7th ed. Philadelphia: Lea & Febiger.

U.S. Department of Agriculture and U.S. Department of Health and Human Services. Food Guide Pyramid.

U.S. Department of Agriculture and U.S. Department of Health and Human Services. 2000. *Nutrition and your health: Dietary guidelines for Americans* 2000, 5th edition. **www.usda.gov/cnpp**

Willett, W. 2000. Got fat? Exploding nutrition myths. *World Health News.* **www.worldhealthnews. harvard.edu**

The Food Guide Pyramid
A Guide to Daily Food Choices

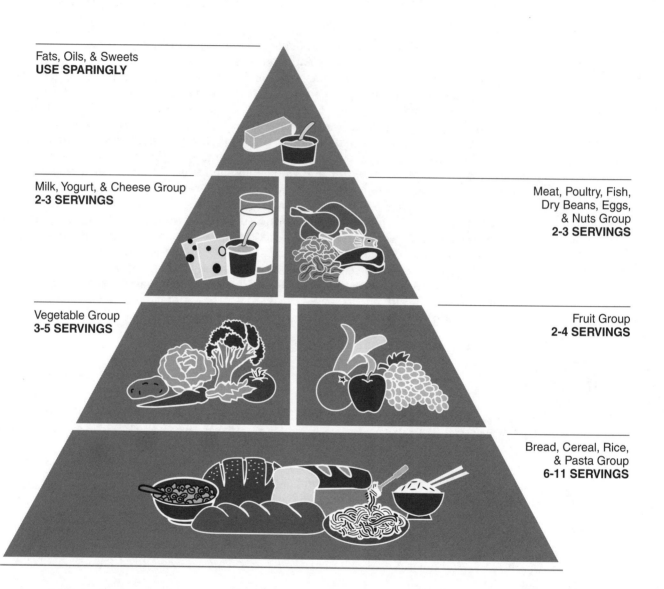

Fats, Oils, & Sweets
USE SPARINGLY

Milk, Yogurt, & Cheese Group
2-3 SERVINGS

Meat, Poultry, Fish,
Dry Beans, Eggs,
& Nuts Group
2-3 SERVINGS

Vegetable Group
3-5 SERVINGS

Fruit Group
2-4 SERVINGS

Bread, Cereal, Rice,
& Pasta Group
6-11 SERVINGS

Looking at the Pieces of the Pyramid

The Food Guide Pyramid emphasizes foods from the five major food groups shown in the three lower tiers of the Pyramid. Each of these food groups provides some, but not all, of the nutrients you need. Foods in one group can't replace those in another. No one of these major food groups is more important than another—for good health, you need them all (USDA and DHHS).

▶▶ __Answer Key__

Selected Answers to Activity 1

Ancient people	Grain	Fruits	Vegetables	Meats	Dairy	Other
Monks	1 pound bread		2 cooked veggie dishes, salad	Occasionally fish or chicken		1/2 pint wine
Peasants	5.25 pounds rye bread, 2.75 oz oats		Beans, peas	Beans; occasionally eggs, herrings, eels, cod, meat (bacon, chicken, pigeon, sheep, beef)	Cheese; occasionally sour or sweet milk	Butter
Knights	Grains, white bread, wheat bread	Preserved fruit	Legumes, onions, leeks, garlic, cabbage, smallage	Pork, veal, swans, cranes, herons, peacocks, eels, trout, salmon, haddock, etc., nuts		Fennel, parsley, salt, saffron, lard, suet, tallow, beer, ale, wine
Urban dwellers	Oatmeal porridge, bread		Potatoes	Rarely meat	Rancid milk	

Park 1992

The Food Guide Pyramid

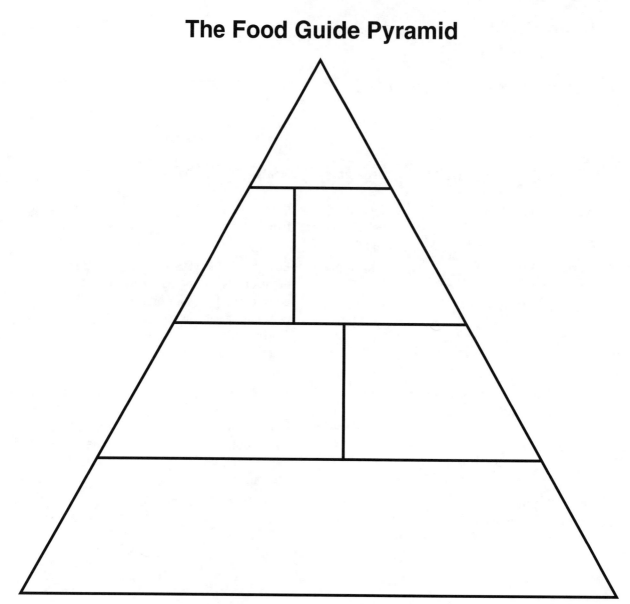

Throughout history poor nutrition (diet) has been the cause of poor health in a large number of people. Examine the following list of vitamins and minerals and the types of foods they are found in. Compare the diet of the ancient people you are examining to this list and determine whether they were susceptible to these disorders.

Vitamins and minerals	Good dietary sources	Function in the body	Disorder associated with deficiency
Vitamin A	Liver, fish liver oil, carrots, eggs, dark green leafy vegetables, fortified milk*	Essential for vision, growth, reproduction, a properly working immune system.	**Night blindness:** partial or total loss of vision, weakened immune system
Vitamin D	Exposure of the skin to sunlight, eggs, butter, fortified milk*	Essential for proper bone development	**Rickets:** deformed skeleton. For example bowed legs.
Vitamin B_1 (Thiamin)	Unrefined cereal grains, brewer's yeast, organ meats, (liver, heart, kidney), legumes, seeds/nuts, fortified grains and cereals*	Essential for breaking down carbohydrates.	**Beri beri:** mental confusion, loss of appetite, muscle wasting and weakness, inability to move arms or legs, irregular heartbeat
Vitamin C	Oranges, lemons, limes, green and red peppers, broccoli, spinach, tomatoes, potatoes, strawberries, and other citrus fruits	Essential component of collagen, a connective tissue. Important for wound healing and a proper functioning immune system	**Scurvy:** bleeding gums, bleeding in the skin, sore muscles and joints, fatigue
Iron	Beef, poultry, fish, eggs, vegetables, fortified cereal*	Essential component of hemoglobin, the oxygen-carrying pigment in red blood cells.	**Anemia:** loss of red blood cells results in fatigue.
Calcium	Milk, yogurt, cheese, broccoli, kale, collards, lime-processed tortillas	Essential for making bones.	**Osteoporosis:** loss of calcium from the bones makes them weak and more likely to break. Most common in elderly.

*Fortified means that the vitamins or minerals are added to the food during processing. Fortified products did not exist during the time periods of the people being discussed in this lesson.

Part I

Directions:

1. Read the accounts of diets eaten by people living at different time periods.
2. Complete the table below each paragraph by writing the foods eaten by the people in the boxes under the appropriate food group.

Example

Australopithecus afarensis (early hominids, 3–1.75 million years ago): "Most scientists now agree that australopithecines, human ancestors, gathered and scavenged for food rather than hunting. Some evidence of meat-eating extends as far back as 1.75 million years. Early humans probably scavenged the kills of large carnivores and fed on birds, reptiles, fruits, grasses, seeds, grubs, and roots" (Park 1992).

Grains	Fruits	Vegetables	Meats	Dairy	Other
Grasses, seeds	Fruits (no detail)	Roots	Birds, reptiles, grubs		

St. Benedictine Monks (AD 530)

The one winter meal, served at 2:00 PM, consisted of two cooked vegetable dishes, eggs, salad, bread, wine, and possibly fish or chicken. Beef was strictly prohibited. They were allowed 1 pound of bread and a half pint of wine daily. In the summer, they had two meals (Park 1992).

Grains	Fruits	Vegetables	Meats	Dairy	Other

English Peasants (13ᵗʰ Century)

At Peterborough Abbey, the average servant daily consumed about 5.25 pounds of rye bread, 2.75 ounces of oats, and small portions of beans, peas, cheese, and butter. At harvest time, these protein-deficient diets were enhanced by additional amounts of cheese, butter, sour and sweet milk, eggs, herring, eel, cod, and a bit of fresh or salted meat. Only on special occasions might they get bacon, chicken, pigeon, sheep, or a piece of beef (Park 1992).

Grains	Fruits	Vegetables	Meats	Dairy	Other

Knights (13ᵗʰ Century)

The daily diet of most knights was probably quite simple, but tournaments and other celebrations were occasions for eating and drinking large quantities. The wealthy ate large quantities of meat: pork, veal, swan, crane, heron, peacock, eel, trout, salmon, haddock, shark, dried fish, and more. They also ate grains, legumes, onions, garlic, leeks, and cabbage. Fennel, parsley, smallage (wild celery), and herbs were used to flavor dishes. Soup and broth contained vegetables, marrow bones, saffron, salt, and boiled bacon. When fruit was eaten, it was usually cooked or preserved as fresh fruit was thought to be unhealthy or poisonous. Bread was eaten at all meals. Ground white bread (manchet) was preferred by those who could afford it; cheat (wheat bread) was second quality. They flavored their foods with lard, beef suet, and mutton tallow. Nuts were popular. Barley was used to make ale. Beer, cider, and wine were also available for drinking (Park 1992).

Grains	Fruits	Vegetables	Meats	Dairy	Other

English Mill Workers (Early 19ᵗʰ Century)

Their year-long diet consisted of potatoes, oatmeal porridge, bread, and rarely, a bit of meat. Meat and milk were often rancid (Park 1992).

Grains	Fruits	Vegetables	Meats	Dairy	Other

Part II

Directions: Choose **one** of the diets described to compare to the recommendations of the Food Guide Pyramid. Answer the questions below.

Diet of the _____.

1. Did they eat foods from each of the food groups? _____ If not, which food groups were missing?

2. Did their diets contain a variety of foods in each of the food groups? _____ If not, which food groups lacked variety?

3. Use student resource 1 to determine whether these people were likely to have suffered from certain diseases as a result of deficiencies in their diet. Remember, if they ate a food only on rare occasions, they probably were not getting enough of the nutrients they needed.

Type of food missing	Vitamin or mineral deficiency	Disease
Example: fruit	Vitamin C	Scurvy

4. Why do you suppose these people did not eat a well-balanced diet? There are probably several contributing factors.

Name _____

To eat a balanced diet, you need a variety of foods. The Food Guide Pyramid divides the foods we eat into six categories and helps us to know how much of each category we need to eat to stay healthy.

Directions

Imagine you could help children from ancient times learn about eating foods that would benefit their health. Using the Food Guide Pyramid, plan a week of lunch menus for a 12- year-old from one of the ancient peoples discussed in the class activity. Take into consideration the deficiencies in the child's normal diet and the recommended number of servings for each food group. Assume that the child has access to all types of foods.

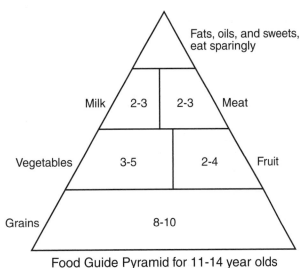

Food Guide Pyramid for 11-14 year olds

Diet for: _____

	Lunch menu
Monday	
Tuesday	
Wednesday	
Thursday	
Friday	

Name _____

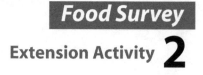
How are your eating habits different from those of children living 50 years ago?

Directions

Interview a grandparent, great aunt, neighbor, teacher, or friend of the family who was 11–14 years old during the 1920s, 1930s, or 1940s. Ask him or her the following questions. Record his or her answers and your answers to the same questions in the table.

Question: When you were 11–14 years old . . .	Adult response	Your response
Did you eat all three meals with your family? If no, explain.		
If you ate lunch at school, did you bring or buy your lunch?		
Did your family produce any of its own food?		
Describe the size of the store (corner store? supermarket?) where your family did most of its shopping.		
How often did you eat at a restaurant?		
What kind of bread did you eat (white, wheat, rye, etc.)?		
What kind of milk did you drink (whole, skim, etc.)		
Did you use butter, margarine, oleo, or something else to flavor your foods?		
How often did you eat dessert or what might be considered "junk foods" (2 times a day, weekly, monthly, etc.)?		
How often did you drink soda?		

Question: When you were 11–14 years old . . .	Adult response	Your response
Which of these fruits were commonly available to you: bananas, oranges, plums, kiwi, mango, apples, melon, pineapple, pears, strawberries, plantains, tangerines?		
How often did you usually eat fruit (once a day, twice a day, three times a day, once a week, once a month, never)?		
How often did you eat meat?		
What kind of meat did you eat?		
How often did you eat vegetables?		
What vegetables were your favorites?		

Compare your responses to those of the adult you interviewed. How do you explain the major differences?

Democracy and Diet

In this lesson, students will use nutrition survey data to learn about how decisions that affect public health policy can be made. A group activity in which students role-play key groups in a legislative public hearing enables students to practice skills of participation and persuasion. The individual activity is homework that requires students to articulate their own responses to the arguments they hear in class and to think about their personal nutrition actions.

This lesson is designed to infuse information about choosing healthy snacks into a classroom unit on the democratic process. It is best taught after you have spent a class learning about how laws are made and how citizens can get involved in that process.

▶▶ Behavioral Objective

For students to learn how to replace snacks high in saturated and trans fat with healthy alternatives, including fruits and vegetables.

▶▶ Learning Objectives

Students will be able to

1. use information (data) to guide their actions and decisions;
2. describe the role that public participation and legislative debate play in making health policy decisions; and
3. explain how legislatures, public health agencies, and special interest groups interact.

▶▶ Materials

- Student resource 1 *Making a Public Health Decision* (handout or chalkboard)
- Findings from a nutrition study (handout, overhead, or chalkboard)
- Activity 1 *Group A: Students for Healthy Snacks*
- Activity 1 *Group B: CHIP (Choice Is Personal)*
- Activity 1 *Group C: State Legislature*
- *Optional:* Student resource 1 *What's the Rap on Fat* from lesson 49 (page 335)

▶▶ Procedure

1. (5 minutes) Review lawmaking in a democratic system (time estimate assumes students are already familiar with this topic). Legislators make laws following specific procedures. Ask students, "Where do ideas for laws come from?" List students' ideas on the chalkboard.

Many times ideas come from citizens. If interested citizens can get a legislator (representative or senator elected to represent a district comprising one or more cities or towns) to sponsor their idea (introduce it to the legislature), the idea can be written up as a bill that is voted on by the legislature (all the legislators). If the bill passes the vote, it becomes legislation, or law. List students' examples of laws they know on chalkboard.

Then the appropriate government agency (like a public health agency) needs to carry out or enforce the legislation. Organized citizens have been successful in getting laws passed concerning many issues such as the environment and child care as well as public health.

2. (5 minutes) *Read the following situation:* Nutrition scientists are very interested in what students eat. In a recent study, scientists asked, "What kinds of snacks do middle school students eat? Do their snacks fit into a healthy diet?" After doing a survey of almost 2,000 middle school students, they found out that

- middle school students eat an average of 3.5 fruits and vegetables per day,

- only about 25% of middle school students eat five or more fruits and vegetables per day, and

- on average, they get about 34% of their daily calories from fat and about 12% from saturated fat.

Nutrition experts recommend eating at least five fruits and vegetables every day and eating high-fat foods in moderation (occasionally), so that you get no more than 30% of your total calories from fat and no more than 10% of your calories from saturated fat.

When the results of this survey came out in newspapers and on TV, students banded together to form Students for Healthy Snacks. They realized there are plenty of healthy snacks around (see Teacher Resources). These include fruits, vegetables, low-fat yogurt, low-fat milk, and pretzels. You can also have small portions of other, higher-fat foods, especially foods high in unsaturated fat, a healthier fat, like peanut butter and nuts. But when students want snacks, the easiest and cheapest things they can buy are candy, cookies, and fast food from vending machines and local restaurants, foods that often are not very nutritious and may be very high in saturated fat, trans fat, or sugar. The group Students for Healthy Snacks wants the state government to help make healthy snack foods more available to them by passing legislation (a law) to fund a healthy snack campaign. The idea for this new law is contained in a bill that legislators (elected representatives or senators from towns and cities) need to vote on.

Another student group tried to block the action. They call themselves CHIP, or *CH*oice *Is P*ersonal, because they felt that government should not get involved in telling people what to eat.

During a public hearing, the legislature listened to testimony (oral presentations) from both sides before deciding whether to fund the campaign.

3. (30 minutes) Have a public hearing. Assign/recruit students into three groups of equal size. (Group C, the state legislature, has to have an odd number of students in it. This will avoid a tie vote.) Distribute student resource 1 *Making a Public Health Decision* to all students so they understand how the legislature votes. (This student resource is intended to supplement, not replace, other materials and textbooks on lawmaking that you may already be using.) *Optional:* You also may wish to distribute student resource 1 *What's the Rap on Fat?* from lesson 49 (page 335). This resource describes the different kinds of fat and may help students form their arguments.

- Group A receives activity 1 *Group A: Students for Healthy Snacks.*
- Group B receives activity 1 *Group B: CHIP (CHoice Is Personal).*
- Group C receives activity 1 *Group C: State Legislature*
- Review the worksheet procedures with students.
- Give the groups 10-15 minutes to prepare 5 minutes of *testimony,* oral presentations in support of or against a particular action.
- Listen to the testimony. You should cut off testimony at 5 minutes. Likewise, you should give a 2-minute and 1-minute warning. (You may want to schedule presentations for another day.)
- After listening to the testimony, allow the legislature to ask a few questions and vote on what they have heard.
- Discuss the outcome. Why do you think the vote came out the way it did? What could each side do differently to improve its position next time? If the bill passed, what would happen now?

▶▶ Extension Activities

Choose one of the following and write a paragraph addressing the issue.

1. In this debate you heard arguments for and against a proposal. Members of the legislature had to decide whether to vote yea or nay. Pretend the vote was a tie. You are a legislator and you offer to negotiate a compromise in order to break the tie. Write a paragraph describing the compromise. Try to think of a compromise that addresses elements of each side's arguments.

2. CHIP argued that if the campaign worked, people would stop eating the "less healthy" snack foods completely, causing the businesses that made or sold them to close and forcing people out of work. Critique this argument. Was it supported by facts? Did it appeal to emotions, to reason, or to both? Also, is it necessary to stop eating high-fat foods completely in order to have a balanced diet?

3. The industry group also argued that an advantage of typical snack foods over fruits and vegetables is that they have more of the calories that growing, active teens need. Critique this argument. What's missing from most high-fat snacks? Why is it unhealthy to eat foods that are high in saturated and trans fat? To make your point, read some labels! Find a snack that provides more than 20% of the daily value of saturated fat and compare it to a snack with the same number of calories but less saturated fat. Check the ingredient list for partially hydrogenated vegetable oil (trans fat). Can you find a variety or brand of the high-saturated fat food made with healthier unsaturated fat?

▶▶ Teacher Resources

General Background Material

In preparing for this lesson, you may want to refer to the following resources:

- *Time to Take Five* (appendix A)
- *Fat: Where It's At* (page 252)
- *Nutrition and Your Health: Dietary Guidelines for Americans*
- *Lawmaking in Massachusetts* (appendix C)
- *The Ladybug Story: A Story About Lawmaking* (appendix C)

Specific Background Material

How Laws Are Made

The resource listed in appendix C will assist you with teaching about citizen participation in developing legislation. *Lawmaking in Massachusetts* describes the legislative process in Massachusetts. You might wish to send for a resource that describes the legislative process in your state. However, this is not necessary if you are already aware of the process and can discuss it with your students.

Healthy Snacking

The health message in this lesson is that healthy snacks are part of a balanced diet. Snacking is an important component of adolescent nutrient intake, constituting a quarter or more of daily calorie intake. Because of adolescents' increasing independence in making food choices, as well as their growing ability to earn money on their own, it is important for them to learn how to select snacks that are enjoyable and that are healthy. They need tools to help them be responsible for their own nutritional well-being. Unfortunately, many of the snacks they choose (like ice cream, cookies, chips, and candy) are high in saturated fat and trans fat. Eating too many of these fats increases the risk of developing heart disease. Unsaturated fats found in vegetable oils, nuts, olives, and avocados do not contribute to heart disease. It is important for adolescents to understand that, while lots of any kind of fat can provide excess calories, the type of fat is more important than the absolute number of calories from fat. Encourage students to choose a diet low in saturated and trans fat and moderate in total fat.

Snack Choices

Quick, simple-to-prepare, or easy-to-buy foods that are low in saturated and trans fat and high in nutrients make good snacks. These include

- many breakfast cereals;
- savory baked goods like bagels, pretzels, and breads;
- unbuttered popcorn;
- fruits (fresh, dried, or juice) and vegetables;
- low-fat yogurt or milk; and
- sandwiches made with lean meats.

Other foods that are good snacks when consumed in moderation are those that are not low-fat but pack lots of other nutrients, too, like peanut butter, nuts, and cheese. Peanut butter and nuts are high in unsaturated fat, a healthier type of fat; substituting this type of fat for saturated and trans fats in the diet lowers the risk of developing heart disease. Finally, students should know that it is all right to eat an occasional serving of potato chips, french fries, or ice cream; look for varieties that substitute healthier fats for saturated and trans fat. The *Fat: Where It's At* resource described in appendix A can help students identify lower-fat snack choices (see also lesson 42, page 252).

Name ______________________________

Making a Public Health Decision

Student Resource 1

There are many paths to the creation of public health legislation, or laws. One such path is shown below.

Research	Media	Citizen advocacy	Legislation	Action
A nutrition study shows that on average middle school students eat fewer vegetables and fruits and more fat than experts recommend.	Local newspapers and TV newscasters make a fuss about the results.	Students campaign to get the state to carry out a Healthy Snacks campaign. They ask Representative Smith to sponsor their legislation. A second student disagrees with the legislation.	1. Representative Smith agrees to sponsor a bill funding a Healthy Snacks campaign to be run by the state public health agency. 2. The legislature listens to testimony for and against the bill 3. The legislature votes on the bill. 4. Will the bill pass?	If the bill passes, the state public health agency now has to run the campaign. The agency may work with local community groups to do this.

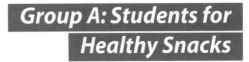

Why the State Legislature Should Fund a Healthy Snacks Campaign

Instructions

You have 10 minutes to plan and 5 minutes to present. Use the resources below to develop your testimony. Work as a group to build on the statements, adding to them to make solid arguments. Select one or more speakers to present each of the arguments. Feel free to be creative.

1. Speaker(s)

Read this at the beginning of your testimony: Students for Healthy Snacks believes the state legislature should fund the State Public Health Agency to run a Healthy Snacks Campaign because _____.
(Fill in using results from the nutrition study that your teacher presented.)

2. Speaker(s)

Many snack foods currently available to students are high in saturated and/or trans fats, which can increase the risk of developing heart disease. There are two parts of the campaign. The first part is: Encourage students to eat more fruits and vegetables and fewer high-fat or non-nutritious foods by making fruits and vegetables available where students buy food. For example, _____.
(Think of two places where students your age buy food. Think of two healthy foods these places could (or already do) offer that students your age like to eat.)

3. Speaker(s)

The second part of the campaign is: Run an ad campaign that teaches healthy snack alternatives. For example, _____.
(Think of two high-fat foods and alternatives to them.)

4. Speaker(s)

This legislation makes sense for several health reasons. Experts think everyone should eat at least _____ *(how many?)* fruits and vegetables a day to keep them healthy now and throughout their lives. Examples of fruits and vegetables students our age like are

_____.
(Name five.)

5. Speaker(s)

High-fat diets, where more fat is eaten than is needed, can include foods that are only high in calories, not in vitamins, and can make you feel full so you don't feel like eating foods that are better for you. Examples of high-fat foods that students our age like to buy are _____.
(Name three.)

6. Speaker(s)

Active, growing teens need lots of calories, but it is best to get calories from eating nutritious foods instead of foods high in unhealthy fats that have calories but few nutrients. For example, instead of eating a chocolate-caramel-cookie bar, you could eat an apple or a bag of _____ *(pretzels or potato chips—which has less saturated and trans fat?)* and drink a small carton of _____ *(whole milk or 2% milk—which has less fat?).*

Why the State Legislature Should Not Fund a Healthy Snacks Campaign

Instructions

You have 10 minutes to plan and 5 minutes to present. Use the resources below to develop your testimony. Work as a group to build on the statements, adding to them to make solid arguments. Select one or more speakers to present each of the arguments. Feel free to be creative.

1. Speaker(s)

Read this at the beginning of your testimony: CHIP believes the state legislature should not fund the State Public Health Agency to run a Healthy Snacks Campaign for several reasons. First, active, growing teenagers need lots of calories. Fruits and vegetables are typically very low in calories. Fat, however, has plenty of calories, and students love high-fat foods. Three examples of high-fat foods we love are_____

_____.

(Identify three high-fat foods.)

2. Speaker(s)

The main danger from sugar in sweet snacks is cavities, which occur when people do not brush their teeth regularly. If you brush your teeth _____ *(at least how many times?)* per day and floss your teeth _____ *(how many times?)* per day and brush your teeth every time you have cookies, candy, or other sticky snacks, there's no problem!

3. Speaker(s)

Students like fast foods, cookies, candy, and other similar foods because they are

_____.

(Name two or three reasons; for example, think about price, whether it is easy to find them, flavor, etc.)

4. Speaker(s)

Food choices are personal! If people want to eat diets that are _____ *(high or low?)* in fat, even though it might harm their health in the long run, that's their choice. Besides, how can teens learn to make healthy choices if the range of foods available to them is limited?

5. Speaker(s)

A Healthy Snacks Campaign could prove bad for local businesses that make or sell high-fat snack foods, like _____
(name three kinds of businesses). If such a campaign worked, people would stop buying the foods made or sold at these places. Businesses would shut down, and people would be out of work.

How Shall I Vote?

1. Listen to the testimony of the two groups.

2. Ask questions of each group. You can ask the groups to clarify points or to respond to one another's points.

3. When you are done asking questions, vote on the proposal to fund the State Public Health Agency to run a Healthy Snacks Campaign. Base your vote on your beliefs and on the arguments you heard. Your teacher will conduct the voting by asking all those in favor of funding the Healthy Snacks Campaign to raise their hands. After counting the "Yeas," your teacher will then ask all of those opposed to (against) funding the Healthy Snacks Campaign to raise their hands. After counting the "Nays," your teacher will determine which side has convinced legislators.

Lesson 58

Fruits and Vegetables Theme

Global Foods

This lesson asks students to discover the differences in foods regularly consumed in different countries and cultures. The student resource provides general information about different countries and the diets they currently and traditionally maintain. The comparison of any two countries will make the student aware of the differences in food patterns across countries and the variety of fruits and vegetables available worldwide. The goal of the lesson is to encourage students to eat a variety of fruits and vegetables. Some previous knowledge or discussion of world climates may be helpful in preparing students for this lesson.

▶▶ Behavioral Objective

For students to eat a variety of fruits and vegetables.

▶▶ Learning Objectives

Students will be able to

1. explain why it is important to eat a variety of fruits and vegetables;
2. compare and contrast the types of foods and methods of food preparation used by different countries and cultural groups;
3. list some of the factors that determine which foods are commonly produced by a country; and
4. locate Haiti, Puerto Rico, Cambodia, Brazil, and the United States on a map.

▶▶ Materials

- Activity 1 *Discover Foods of the World*
- Student resource 1 *Fruits and Vegetables of the World* (one copy per group of two)
- Map of the world
- Overhead transparencies 1 and 2 (or handout, or use chalkboard)

▶▶ Procedure

Some previous knowledge or discussion of world climates would be helpful in preparing students for this lesson.

1. Point out the goals of the lesson:
   - To discuss why it is important to eat a variety of fruits or vegetables
   - To compare and contrast the types of fruits and vegetables consumed and cooking methods used in different countries around the world
2. Ask students, "What vegetables does your family eat most often?"

3. (5 minutes) Display overhead transparency 1. Have students study the vitamin and mineral content of the fruits and vegetables listed. What do they notice? How are the foods different? Based on the information, why do they think it's important to eat a variety of fruits and vegetables? Remind them that they should eat at least 2 fruit and 3 vegetable servings a day. (See Teacher Resources for help with this discussion.)

4. (5 minutes) Have students locate Haiti, Cambodia, Brazil, Puerto Rico, and the United States on a map of the world.

5. (5-10 minutes) Discuss the climates and the size of these countries. How are they different? How are they the same? How would this affect the variety and quantity of fruits and vegetables grown in each country? (You also might want to discuss the fact that many fruits and vegetables grown in the other countries are imported to the United States and are available at some local supermarkets, ethnic markets, and specialty stores.)

6. (20 minutes) Hand out activity 1 and student resource 1. Have students work in pairs to complete the activity. You may wish to display overhead transparency 2 *Methods of Food Preparation* as a reference to students while they work on the activity.

7. (5-10 minutes) To wrap up the lesson, ask students to share their answers to the last two questions of activity 1.

▶▶ Extension Activities

1. Teach this lesson on Friday and have students prepare a traditional dish over the weekend to be brought to school and shared.

2. Complete extension activity 1 *Hidden Foods.*

3. What are the international restaurants in your area? Discuss the types of foods that are available in each of the restaurants. Which cuisines include dishes that are high in vegetables and/or fruits? Which include dishes that are high in saturated fat or partially hydrogenated vegetable oils (trans fat)? Have students who don't eat out pick up take-out menus to do the assignment.

4. Choose a country, maybe one that your ancestors emigrated from, and make a collage of the foods eaten in that country.

▶▶ Teacher Resources

General Background Material

In preparing for this lesson, you may want to refer to *Time to Take Five*. See appendix A.

Specific Background Material

What can we learn from studying the commonly consumed foods of a country?

The study of food can enhance understanding about cultural and climatic differences. People in different countries eat different foods, prepare foods differently, and maintain different traditions related to food. Foods from many countries exist in some form in the United States. Restaurants now serve the foods of many ethnic groups. For example, Chinese, Italian, and Mexican cuisines have become an integral part of the American diet, although dishes are often prepared differently in this country than they are in the countries of origin.

What determines the commonly produced foods of a country?

Climate is a major determinant of a nation's ability to grow and harvest foods. Natural resources, amount of arable land, landscape, economics, and political factors also affect food production.

How many fruits and vegetables should we eat daily?

The 5-A-Day campaign promotes eating at least five fruits and vegetables every day. This is consistent with the Food Guide Pyramid, which recommends consuming 2-4 servings of fruits and 3-5 servings of vegetables every day. Encourage students to eat at least 2 servings of fruit and at least 3 servings of vegetables (with at least 1 serving of a dark green or orange vegetable) for a total of 5 servings each day.

What are the benefits of fruits and vegetables?

- Many are good sources of vitamin C: oranges, lemons, grapefruit, cantaloupe, raspberries, strawberries, tomatoes, cabbage, potatoes, spinach, cauliflower, peppers, radishes, and green leafy vegetables such as kale and spinach.
- Many are good sources of vitamin A: bright orange vegetables like carrots, sweet potatoes, and pumpkin; bright orange fruits like mango, cantaloupe, and apricots; dark green leafy vegetables like spinach, collards, and turnip greens.
- Many are important sources of B vitamins: green leafy vegetables, legumes (beans and peas), nuts, and oranges.
- They are an important source of potassium and fiber.
- They are low in fat.
- They reduce the risk of certain forms of cancer.
- They provide nutrients important for healthy skin and eyes and immunity, healing, and other functions.

Why is it important to eat a variety of fruits and vegetables?

No single food supplies all the nutrients one needs to grow, repair, and maintain a healthy body. Eating a variety of fruits and vegetables as part of an overall healthy diet helps ensure that a person will meet the daily recommended allowances of vitamins and minerals.

How should vegetables be prepared?

Because chopping, dicing, grating, mincing, or mashing vegetables can destroy some of the vitamins in the food, whenever possible, chop or slice vegetables just prior to serving or cooking.

Does cooking vegetables also affect their nutritional value?

Yes. Over-boiling or over-cooking vegetables can greatly reduce the amount of vitamins; therefore, steaming vegetables is preferable. The less water involved in the cooking process, the better.

Are frozen vegetables nutritious?

Yes. In fact, frozen vegetables can be just as nutritious as fresh. However, don't buy frozen vegetable packets that have ice crystals on the outside; it usually means they have been thawed and refrozen. Use thawed vegetables as soon as possible.

Are all vegetables the same nutritionally?

All vegetables are good for you, but some are "better" because some have a lot more nutrients that can help you stay healthy. Dark green leafy vegetables (spinach, kale, collard greens), as well as yellow or orange vegetables (pumpkin, carrots, tomato, butternut squash) have many more nutrients than corn, peas, or potatoes, which are very popular vegetables in the United States. In general, brighter color vegetables contain more vitamins and minerals.

What about canned vegetables?

Canned vegetables can still provide many important nutrients even though they may have lost a lot of their nutrients in the high-heat process involved in canning foods. Canned tomatoes, beets, and spinach still have a lot of vitamin A and carotenoids. Avoid canned vegetables that have a lot of added salt or sodium and sugar. Vegetables canned in water or their own juices are best.

How can we include plenty of different fruits and vegetables in meals and snacks?

The *Dietary Guidelines for Americans* recommends the following:

- Keep ready-to-eat vegetables handy in a clear container in the front of your refrigerator for snacks or on-the-go meals.
- Keep a day's supply of fresh or dried fruit handy on the table or counter.
- Enjoy fruit as a naturally sweet end to a meal.
- When eating out, choose a variety of vegetables at a salad bar.
- Serve raw vegetables with dip.
- Mix fruit or vegetables with other foods in salads, casseroles, soups, and sauces. For example, add shredded vegetables to pasta sauces.

Are ketchup, french fries, and potato chips considered vegetables?

Technically yes, but we say no! They are all derived from vegetable sources, but because of the way they have been prepared, the beneficial nutritional content of those foods is masked by excessive amounts of fat, salt, or sugar. For example, when you deep-fry vegetables in oil, like french fries and potato chips, they become high-fat foods that should be consumed infrequently and in small quantities. While ketchup is not high in fat, it is high in sodium. Americans tend to consume too much sodium, and it mainly comes in the form of added salt. The recommendation for sodium intake is no more than 2,400 milligrams per day (which is about 1 tsp of salt). Some other foods in the vegetable group that are high in sodium include relish and pickles. You should use these foods sparingly!

What about spaghetti sauce?

Tomato sauce is a great source of vitamins A and C. Eating tomatoes and tomato products may help men reduce the risk of prostate cancer. Lycopene, the red pigment in tomatoes, seems to be responsible for this effect. Interestingly, lycopene is more available to the body when tomatoes have been cooked and are in the presence of small amounts of fat. (Lycopene is a fat-soluble nutrient and, therefore, needs a small amount of fat to be better absorbed.) So apply spaghetti sauce liberally to pasta, skinless chicken, pizza, and anything else you want to. When choosing a store-bought sauce, select one low to moderate in sodium and oil. For homemade sauce, add a small amount of olive oil to the sauce to help with lycopene absorption and throw in some grated carrots or peppers for extra nutrition. It's a great way to add vegetables to your diet.

References

Brigham and Women's Hospital. 2000. Health matters: Nutrition news for you to use. **www.brighamandwomens.org**

National Cancer Institute and National Institutes of Health. 1999. *Time to take five: Eat 5 fruits and vegetables a day.* NIH Publication No. 95-3862.

U.S. Department of Agriculture and U.S. Department of Health and Human Services. 2000. *Nutrition and your health: Dietary guidelines for Americans* 2000, 5th edition. **www.usda.gov/cnpp**

▶▶ Answer Key

Extension Activity 1

Find the Hidden Foods

```
P  N  M  N  R  T  H  P  D  H  N  U  Q  W  R  T  Y  U  I
U  C  F  T  M  C  L  A  L  O  X  S  E  L  E  T  S  A  P
E  F  H  H  N  B  V  C  X  Z  L  K  J  H  P  O  I  U  U
R  Q  W  I  R  H  S  T  I  R  G  Y  N  I  M  O  H  T  M
T  C  N  G  T  A  A  V  Y  A  S  T  Q  A  Z  X  E  E  P
O  S  U  N  H  T  O  I  T  Y  U  B  E  G  H  J  T  K  K
R  E  T  R  G  Y  E  V  T  R  B  R  A  Z  I  L  A  I  I
I  T  T  Y  R  V  T  R  K  I  Q  Y  I  O  B  N  N  C  N
C  A  V  B  V  Y  R  E  C  A  M  B  O  D  I  A  A  V  S
O  T  V  A  P  S  Y  O  O  H  O  O  B  M  A  B  R  Q  O
A  S  A  A  B  S  O  F  R  I  T  O  N  J  Q  A  G  C  U
W  D  P  B  N  S  E  F  G  T  Y  J  J  U  K  B  E  H  P
T  E  A  N  Q  W  E  R  T  Y  U  I  O  P  H  M  M  N  X
A  T  S  S  T  O  O  H  S  O  O  B  M  A  B  O  O  Z  X
G  I  T  Q  C  H  I  T  T  E  R  L  I  N  G  S  P  B  Y
N  N  A  X  P  L  M  O  K  N  I  J  B  U  H  B  Y  G  V
M  U  A  T  E  L  P  M  O  C  A  D  A  O  J  I  E  F  C
```

Find and circle the four countries and the one US commonwealth and some foods specific to each place. Some words are written top to bottom. Other words are written bottom to top. Finally, there are even words written left to right and right to left. The words are listed below.

Haiti: Pumpkin soup, Lalo
United States: Pasta, Turkey, Hominy grits, Chitterlings
Cambodia: Bamboo shoots, Curry
Puerto Rico: Sofrito, Pasteles
Brazil: Feijoada completa, Pomegranate

Examine the list of foods below. Which two foods offer the most vitamin A? vitamin C? folate? calcium?

Food	Vitamin A (RE)	Vitamin C (mg)	Folate (mcg)	Calcium (mg)
Banana	9	10	22	7
Orange	26	80	47	56
Apple	7	8	4	10
Corn	18	5	38	2
Tomato	139	22	12	8
Carrot	2,025	7	10	19
Cantaloupe	516	68	27	17

*Units: RE = Retinol equivalents; mg = milligrams; mcg = micrograms

Why is it important to eat a variety of fruits and vegetables?

Methods of Food Preparation

Stove-top cooking	Boil	To cook in water at 220˚ until bubbles rise continuously and break on the surface.
	Stew	To simmer food in a small quantity of liquid.
	Simmer	To cook in liquid that is maintained just below the boiling point, with bubbles forming slowly.
	Blanch	To preheat in boiling water or steam. Done to inactivate enzymes and to shrink food for canning, freezing, or drying; also to aid the removal of skins from nuts, fruits, and some vegetables.
	Steam	To cook in steam, with or without pressure.
	Fry	To cook in fat.
	Pan-broil	To cook uncovered on a hot surface, usually a fry-pan. Fat is poured off as it accumulates.
Oven cooking	Bake	To cook by dry heat in an oven or oven-type appliance. Covered or uncovered containers may be used, although uncovered baking can be considered roasting.
	Roast	To cook uncovered by dry heat. Usually done in an oven, cooking meats and vegetables.
	Broil	To cook by direct heat.

Country	Fruits	Vegetables	General preparation of vegetables	Traditional diet	National dish
Cambodia Capital: Phnom Penh Location: Indochina Population: 6.6 million Pop. density: 121/sq. mi. Land area: 70,238 sq. mi. Arable land: 16% Native lang.: Khmer	Grapes, pears, melon, pineapple, fruit juices, coconut, apples, and varieties of mangoes and bananas	Green leafy vegetables prepared in soups and sautéed with tofu; bamboo shoots, bean sprouts, celery, eggplant, leeks, spinach, watercress, squash, broccoli, carrots, and celery	Often sautéed with tofu and served with rice or noodles or prepared in soups. For example, in a chicken noodle salad, vinegar, sugar, and garlic are added to shredded cabbage, carrots, and cucumbers	Rice is the primary source of energy, and diets usually contain adequate vegetables and fruits, with small amounts of meat (fish is plentiful) and dairy products	A curry that includes coconut milk, potatoes, and onions. It can be made with a variety of meats including chicken, duck, pork, beef, or quail
Haiti Capital: Port-au-Prince Location: West Indies Population: 5.8 million Pop. density: 544/sq. mi. Land area: 10,579 sq. mi. Arable land: 20% Native lang.: French, Creole	Mangoes (15 varieties) are the most popular fruit. Bananas, oranges, tangerines, grapefruit, and pineapple	Green vegetables are plentiful in Haiti, including lalo, which is a small leafy vegetable high in iron. Green peppers, garlic, and tomatoes are widely used. Starchy vegetables include yuca, yams, and taro. Other types include green peas, watercress, spinach, carrots, and okra	Beans are prepared similarly throughout the Caribbean with salt and lard. Haitians enjoy spicing their food with celery, garlic, hot pepper, black pepper, scallions, and parsley. Vegetables are prepared in soups, stews, and sautéed as side dishes	The Haitian diet is high in carbohydrates such as rice, tubers, millet, and corn. Corn is incorporated into many dishes such as breakfast porridge, bread, and dessert. The traditional diet includes lots of soups and stews made with vegetables, meat, and/or beans. Meats such as pork and fish are often salted and dried	A pumpkin soup called joumou with cabbage, carrots, celery, pasta, and oxtail. It is traditionally eaten on New Year's Day or for Sunday dinner.

	Fruits	Vegetables	Cooking methods	Traditional diet notes	Special dishes
Puerto Rico Capital: San Juan Location: Eastern West Indies Population: 3.4 million Pop. density: 944.1/sq. mi. Land area: 3,421 sq. mi. Arable land: 20% Native lang.: English, Spanish	Oranges, grapefruits, papayas, pineapples, mangoes, and guavas	Corn, okra, eggplant, green beans, onion, green peppers, garlic, tomatoes, sweet potatoes, and beets are popular. Starchy vegetables dominate such as cassavas and yucas	Often combined into a dish known as sofrito, a mixture of vegetables and pork. Lard and olive oil are commonly used in cooking. Starchy vegetables are often boiled and served with boiled dry codfish	Beans and rice are emphasized in the traditional diet. Few green leafy vegetables are consumed. Fish, such as codfish, is usually dried and salted	A snack or dessert called pasteles is prepared with meat that is mixed with cornmeal and mashed plantains, and then wrapped in plantain leaves and steamed. Pasteles are traditionally eaten at Christmas.
Brazil Capital: Brasilia Location: South America Population: 154 million Pop. density: 47/sq. mi. Land area: 3,286,470 sq. mi. Arable land: 8% Native lang.: Portuguese	Mangoes, acerola, oranges, pineapple, passion fruit, guava, papaya, grapes, bananas, and strawberries	Green collards, pumpkin, cabbage, green beans, tomatoes, lettuce, mustard greens, butternut squash, zucchini, carrots, sweet potatoes, yuca, and tubers, such as mandioca. The type of beans consumed varies by region. For example, in Rio de Janeiro, black beans are most common, whereas in the southeastern region, red and brown beans are preferred.	Frying and stewing are common methods of preparation. Chilies, garlic, parsley, and onions are often added to vegetable dishes	Coconuts, bananas, and hot peppers are prevalent in the spicy delicacies of Brazil. Brazilians add a lot of salt to their food as well as a lot of white sugar to their coffee. Beans are emphasized in the traditional diet. A popular traditional dish is farofa, which is mandioca flour, fried with a little oil	Feijoada completa is prepared with black beans, bacon, pork, beef, dried beef, smoked tongue, and sausage. It is accompanied by sliced oranges, seasoned rice, toasted cassava meal, and vegetables such as kale

(continued)

(continued)

Country	Fruits	Vegetables	General preparation of vegetables	Traditional diet	National dish
United States Capital: Washington, D.C. Location: North America Population: 250 million Pop. density: 68/sq. mi. Land area: 3,618,770 sq. mi. Arable land: 21% Native lang.: English	Apples, bananas, cantaloupe, cherries, grapes, honeydew melon, plums, strawberries, blueberries, blackberries, pears, peaches, pineapple, tangerines, oranges, nectarines, raspberries, watermelon, dried fruits, and fruit juices	Asparagus, artichokes, broccoli, cauliflower, green cabbage, red cabbage, beets, peas, string beans, carrots, tomato, cucumber, lettuce, mustard greens, turnip greens, kale, collards, spinach, scallions, pumpkin, summer and winter squash, corn, snap beans, bell peppers (green, red, and yellow), eggplant, mushrooms, celery, radish, and zucchini	Steaming, boiling, sautéing, frying, broiling, grilling, and roasting	Greatly influenced by northern European cooking. Traditionally, meals have been centered around a meat dish. As a consequence, meals have a lot of saturated fat. A variety of vegetables including potatoes, cabbage, and carrots are common in most American diets, as well as a wide variety of yellow and dark green leafy vegetables. Common meats are beef, pork, and poultry.	Thanksgiving dinner: roast turkey, pumpkin pie, mashed potatoes, and cranberry sauce

Directions: Choose two countries to compare. Use student resource 1 to help you complete the table below.

Country		
Climate		
Commonly consumed fruits You have tried		
You have not tried		
Commonly consumed vegetables You have tried		
You have not tried		
Methods of cooking vegetables *Example: boiling*		
National dish: Which of the five food groups are represented in this dish?		

1. If you had the opportunity to go to a restaurant that served food from one of these countries, which restaurant would you go to and why?

2. What would you order? Be sure to include some fruits and vegetables and a description of how the food would be prepared.

Find the Hidden Foods

```
P  N  M  N  R  T  H  P  D  H  N  U  Q  W  R  T  Y  U  I
U  C  F  T  M  C  L  A  L  O  X  S  E  L  E  T  S  A  P
E  F  H  H  N  B  V  C  X  Z  L  K  J  H  P  O  I  U  U
R  Q  W  I  R  H  S  T  I  R  G  Y  N  I  M  O  H  T  M
T  C  N  G  T  A  A  V  Y  A  S  T  Q  A  Z  X  E  E  P
O  S  U  N  H  T  O  I  T  Y  U  B  E  G  H  J  T  K  K
R  E  T  R  G  Y  E  V  T  R  B  R  A  Z  I  L  A  I  I
I  T  T  Y  R  V  T  R  K  I  Q  Y  I  O  B  N  N  C  N
C  A  V  B  V  Y  R  E  C  A  M  B  O  D  I  A  A  V  S
O  T  V  A  P  S  Y  O  O  H  O  O  B  M  A  B  R  Q  O
A  S  A  A  B  S  O  F  R  I  T  O  N  J  Q  A  G  C  U
W  D  P  B  N  S  E  F  G  T  Y  J  J  U  K  B  E  H  P
T  E  A  N  Q  W  E  R  T  Y  U  I  O  P  H  M  M  N  X
A  T  S  S  T  O  O  H  S  O  O  B  M  A  B  O  O  Z  X
G  I  T  Q  C  H  I  T  T  E  R  L  I  N  G  S  P  B  Y
N  N  A  X  P  L  M  O  K  N  I  J  B  U  H  B  Y  G  V
M  U  A  T  E  L  P  M  O  C  A  D  A  O  J  I  E  F  C
```

Find and circle the four countries and the one US commonwealth and some foods specific to each place. Some words are written top to bottom. Other words are written bottom to top. Finally, there are even words written left to right and right to left. The words are listed below.

Haiti: Pumpkin soup, Lalo
United States: Pasta, Turkey, Hominy grits, Chitterlings
Cambodia: Bamboo shoots, Curry
Puerto Rico: Sofrito, Pasteles
Brazil: Feijoada completa, Pomegranate

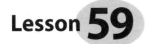
Around the World With Five a Day

In this lesson, students will learn about growing conditions for some fruits and vegetables in different parts of the world, as well as where they were first cultivated. Working in groups, students will do library research, design a poster, and use the poster to present their assigned fruit or vegetable to the class.

▶▶ Behavioral Objective

For students to eat at least five fruits and vegetables per day.

▶▶ Learning Objectives

Students will be able to

1. state the growing conditions for some fruits and vegetables,
2. state where some fruits and vegetables were first cultivated,
3. work in groups to investigate fruits and vegetables from different countries,
4. design a poster that clearly presents information, and
5. make an oral presentation of a group research project.

▶▶ Materials

- Activity 1 *Around the World With Fruits and Vegetables*
- Recipes
- Overhead transparency of world climates (or handout; see Teacher Resources)
- Student resource 1 *Foods and Their Origins*
- Student resource 2 *Sample Recipes* (optional)
- *Optional:* Samples of cole (Brassica) crops (cabbage, cauliflower, turnips, etc.), potato, apple, citrus fruit

▶▶ Procedure

Day 1

1. (10 minutes) Using an overhead transparency or handout, discuss climates as they relate to certain latitudes.

2. (2-3 minutes) Review the 5-A-Day recommendation, making sure students understand that eating at least five a day refers to fruits and vegetables combined, not 5 servings each of fruits and vegetables. Encourage students to eat at least 2 servings of fruit and at least 3 servings of vegetables (with at least 1 serving of a dark green or orange vegetable) for a total of at least five each day.

3. (5 minutes) Hand out student resource 1 *Foods and Their Origins* and activity 1 *Around the World With Fruits and Vegetables*. Explain the purpose of the student resource. It provides background information about a sample of foods. To better connect this lesson to your curriculum, you may choose to assign fruits and vegetables specific to the region of the world your class is currently studying. This would allow them to find the climate, map, and countries that produce the food in their textbooks. However, they would need to do library research to determine the family name, nutrient value, and location of first cultivation of these foods. (Most encyclopedias would be good sources for this information.)

4. (15-20 minutes) Divide the class into groups of five to begin designing their posters and dividing up the research tasks. If possible, have students use class time to begin their library research at the school library.

Day 2

1. (15-20 minutes) Give students time to complete their posters, design their quiz questions (see activity 1), and plan their presentations.

2. Collect the quiz questions prepared by each group.

3. (20 minutes) Have students give their 2–3-minute presentations. Prior to the presentations, remind students that they will be quizzed on the material presented. This will encourage students to pay attention to the presentations.

4. (10 minutes) Give students the quizzes on another day.

▶▶ Extension Activity

Have students bring in food dishes that include the fruits or vegetables they researched.

▶▶ Teacher Resources

General Background Material

In preparing for this lesson, you may want to refer to *Time to Take Five*. See appendix A.

Specific Background Material

About 11 billion acres of land—almost one-third of the earth's total land area—is used for farming. Crops are grown on about a third of this land, and the rest is used for raising livestock. In this unit, we will focus on root crops (e.g., potatoes and cassava) and fruits and vegetables.

Climate determines the ability of a nation to grow and harvest foods. Most crops need a *frost-free* period, a growing season of at least 90 days, in order to develop from seeds into mature plants. Most parts of the world, except the far north and Antarctica, have growing seasons of at least 90 days. However, many regions receive less than 10 inches of rain per year. Few crops can grow under these conditions without irrigation. Bananas and potatoes require a lot of moisture, while wheat grows best in a fairly dry climate.

Examples of climates include tropical, temperate with mild and rainy winters, temperate with cold and snowy winters, dry, and polar (see figure).

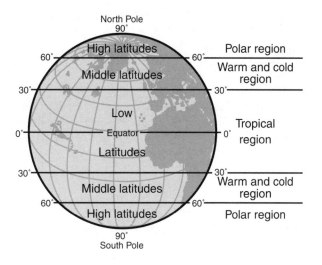

References

Albyn, C., and Webb, L. 1993. *The multicultural cookbook for students.* Phoenix: Oryx Press.

Arntzen, C., ed. 1994. *Encyclopedia of agriculture.* Vols. 1 and 3. San Diego: Academic Press.

Burton Brown, E. 1981. *Vegetables: An illustrated history with recipes.* Englewood Cliffs, NJ: Prentice-Hall.

Gross, H. 1986. *World geography.* Newton, MA: Allyn & Bacon.

Limburg, P. 1972. *What's in the names of fruit?* New York: Coward-McCann & Geoghegan.

U.S. Department of Agriculture and U.S. Department of Health and Human Services. 2000. *Nutrition and your health: Dietary guidelines for Americans* 2000, 5th edition. **www.usda.gov/cnpp**

Cabbage and Cole Crops

- **Family:** Belongs to the *Cruciferae* family (examples include: cabbage, cauliflower, broccoli, turnips, and radishes)
- **Nutritional value:** High in fiber and vitamin C.
- **Origin:** Along Mediterranean coast but now the widest production of cole crops is in California.
- **Other facts:** Modern names for cabbage, *cabus* (French), and *cabbage* (English), come from the Celtic word for head (cole). The cabbage is the most treasured vegetable in the Korean diet. Pickled cabbage is Korea's national dish and is consumed at every meal.

Potato

- **Family:** Belongs to the *Solanaceae* family which includes eggplant and pepper and is high in vitamin C.
- **Nutritional value:** Starch content varies between 10-25% of fresh weight.
- **Origin:** In the Andes and domesticated by native South Americans (cultivated since pre-Incan times).
- **Other facts:** Largest potato production in former Soviet Union, Poland, and China. Discovered by Spanish conquerors and brought to Spain about 1570.

Apple

- **Family:** Belongs to the *Rose* family which includes peaches, plums, pears, cherries, and strawberries.
- **Nutritional value:** Provides small amounts of vitamins and minerals and is a good source of fiber.
- **Origin:** In southwestern Asia (between Caspian and Black Seas). More than 4,000 years old.
- **Other facts:** Appears in ancient Greek myths and legends, e.g., Hercules was sent to pick golden apples that grew in a tree guarded by a hundred-headed dragon. The giant Atlas protected Hercules from the dragon so that he could pick the apples. In Germany, apples are often cooked and blended with vegetables such as cabbage and potatoes.

Citrus Fruits

- **Family:** Citrus is from the *Rutaceae* family.
- **Nutritional value:** Citrus fruits are high in vitamin C and potassium.
- **Origin:** Most species have their origins in tropical regions, Southeast Asia, and the Pacific, particularly China and India. Grapefruit comes from the West Indies. Some records indicate citrus cultivation in Asia dating back 4,000 years.
- **Other facts:** Mainly eaten fresh, but also processed into jams, juices, and sweets. Grown in warm, moist, subtropical or Mediterranean environments.

Kimchi (Korea) (pickled cabbage)

Yield

About 4 cups.
Kimchi can be varied by adding different vegetables. The longer *kimchi* ferments, the stronger and spicier it gets. Serve as a relish with other dishes or add to meat, soups, or stews.

Ingredients

2 cups chopped Chinese cabbage (also called Napa cabbage), washed and drained
1/2 cup coarse (kosher) salt
4 green onions (including tops), finely chopped
1 cup finely shredded carrots
1 Tbsp peeled, grated fresh ginger or 1/2 tsp ground ginger
3 cloves garlic, finely chopped or 1 tsp garlic granules
1 tsp sugar
4 Tbsp dried red pepper flakes

Equipment

Large-size mixing bowl, colander or strainer, 2-quart crock or glass jar with cover

1. Toss cabbage with salt in large mixing bowl to coat evenly. Set aside for 30 minutes; toss frequently.

2. Transfer cabbage to colander or strainer, rinse under cold water, and drain well. Return to large bowl and add green onions, carrots, ginger, garlic, sugar, red pepper flakes, and mix well to blend.

3. Pack mixture in crock or jar, cover, and keep at room temperature for about 2 days, then refrigerate.

Bata Ne Tameta (Bangladesh) (potatoes with gravy)

Yield

Serves 4-6.
This gravy is simply seasoned potato water. Serve as condiment with rice and curried fish or meat.

Ingredients

2-4 Tbsp vegetable oil
4 potatoes, peeled and cubed
4 cups water
1 Tbsp vinegar
1 tomato, cubed
1/2 tsp each dry ground mustard, ground coriander, crushed red pepper flakes, ground ginger, and ground turmeric
Touch of salt and pepper
1 tsp sugar

Equipment

Large-size skillet with cover, mixing spoon

1. Heat oil in skillet over medium heat, add potatoes, and fry for 3 minutes stirring continually to coat potatoes with oil. Add water and vinegar, cover, and cook for about 15 minutes.
2. Add tomato, mustard, coriander, red pepper, ginger, turmeric, sugar, and salt and pepper to taste, mix well, and cook until potatoes are tender (about 5 more minutes).

Himmel und Erde (Germany) ("Heaven and Earth"; cooked potatoes and apple)

Yield

Serves 6-8.
This recipe, blending fruit and vegetables, is typical of German country cooking. Perhaps it is named *himmel und erde* (heaven and earth) because apples grow on trees toward the heavens and potatoes grow in the earth.

Ingredients

2 pounds new potatoes, washed and quartered
6 cups water
1 Tbsp vinegar
2 pounds cooking apples, peeled and cut into chunks
6 slices bacon, finely diced
1/2 cup bread crumbs
Salt and pepper to taste

Equipment

Medium-size saucepan with cover, medium-size skillet, mixing spoon

1. Put potatoes in saucepan and cover with water. Add vinegar and bring to a boil over high heat. Reduce heat to simmer, cover, and cook for 10 minutes. Add apple chunks, mix well, and continue cooking until potatoes are tender but not mushy, about 10 more minutes. Drain well.
2. While the potatoes and apples are cooking, fry bacon in skillet over medium-high heat until crisp. Reduce heat to medium, add bread crumbs, and mix well to coat crumbs. Fry for about 2 more minutes to heat through.
3. Add bacon mixture and salt and pepper to taste to potatoes and apples, toss gently, and transfer to serving bowl. Serve *himmel und erde* hot as a side dish with meat, poultry, or fish.

Laranjas (Brazil) (orange salad)

Yield

Serves 6.

Ingredients

6 oranges, peeled with pith removed, cut in slices
1 tsp ginger
Salt and pepper to taste

Equipment

Serrated-edge knife, medium-size platter

1. Arrange orange slices, slightly overlapping, on a platter.

2. Sprinkle with ginger and salt and pepper to taste.

3. Refrigerate until ready to serve. Serve as a side dish with feijoada.

Around the World
With Fruits and Vegetables

Activity **1**

Student names _____

_____

Food _____

1. Make a poster that includes the following information about the fruit or vegetable your group has been assigned. Items D, E, and F require library research.

   A. The scientific name of the food.

   B. A map with the part of the world where the fruit/vegetable was first cultivated. (Draw or find a map and point to the region when you make your presentation.) Draw an arrow pointing to the region.

   C. A listing of the nutrient value of the food.

   D. A recipe which includes your food as an ingredient. Put the recipe on the poster.

   E. A listing of several countries that currently grow this food.

   F. The characteristics of the climate best suited for growing the food.

   G. Pictures of the food. Use drawings or pictures from magazines.

2. Write five multiple choice quiz questions that your teacher can use to test the class's knowledge of your food.

3. You are the experts! Use your poster to make a *clear, concise,* and *creative* oral presentation to the class about your food. Each member of your group should have a role in explaining some aspect of the poster.

Lesson 60

Map Maker

This lesson is a mapping exercise that encourages students to be aware of the facilities and opportunities for recreation in their school and community. Often adolescents are not familiar with the area in which they live, and this can restrict the amount of physical activity in which they participate. As adolescents develop into adults, they will realize that being physically fit and healthy requires more of a commitment of time and effort.

▶▶ Behavioral Objective

For students to be more active in recreation, leisure activities, sports, and fitness.

▶▶ Learning Objectives

Students will be able to

1. locate places on city or town maps,
2. give directions to recreation facilities in their neighborhoods,
3. discuss the distribution of recreation facilities in their town,
4. state the physical activity recommendations for adolescents, and
5. discuss the importance of physical activity to individuals and the community.

▶▶ Materials

- Large map of the town or city in which the school is located (one for each of your classes). These can be obtained for free from your city government, tourism board, or many real estate agencies.
- Colored thumbtacks or markers
- Activity 1 *Exploring Your Neighborhood*
- Activity 2 *Designing a Fitness Program*
- Overhead transparency 1 (or use chalkboard)

▶▶ Procedure

Activity 1 should be introduced on day 1; students must complete a homework assignment before completing the activity on day 2.

Day 1

1. (5 minutes) Display overhead transparency 1. Point out the goals of the lesson and the physical activity recommendations for adolescents. Discuss the benefits of physical activity. (See overhead transparency 1.)

2. (5 minutes) Have students brainstorm answers to the following questions:

- What are some reasons people your age give for not doing enough physical activity?
- What are some reasons adults give for not doing enough physical activity?
- What suggestions would you make to someone who gave these reasons for not doing enough physical activity? Why should they try to be fit?

Record their responses on the board or overhead transparency.

3. (2 minutes) Make the following points:

- Physical activity doesn't necessarily have to be done at the gym. Going for walks, riding bikes, swimming, and/or visiting the park all benefit health.
- Accessibility to recreational facilities can impact the amount of physical activity a person participates in.

4. (1-2 minutes) Hand out activity 1 and provide this overview: *In this activity each of you will determine the location of recreational facilities in your neighborhood. In class, we will plot the location of the recreational facilities on a map of the city/town and discuss the distribution of facilities in your neighborhood/community. We'll also identify safe places to be physically active and discuss improvements that could be made to the local exercise facilities. What facilities are needed, or could be improved?*

5. (5 minutes) Put students into groups of three or four and ask them to discuss the following questions:

- Are there a number of recreational facilities within walking or biking distance from your house?
- Do you think that recreational facilities are evenly distributed (spread out) in your community? (You may wish to discuss the school neighborhood or the whole town/city). Make an assumption.

6. Students should record their assumptions on the sheet for activity 1.

7. Have students complete activity 1 for homework.

Day 2

1. Hang a copy of your town/city map on the wall.

2. (5 minutes) Explain how to find locations on the town map using the lettered and numbered grid system. (You might prefer to do this step on day 1.)

3. (5 minutes) Ask students to name different types of recreational facilities they found in their neighborhood and town. Make a list of these categories on the chalkboard and assign a color to each category. This legend should be listed next to the map. *(Examples: basketball courts, tennis courts, tracks, parks, playgrounds, swimming pools, health clubs, bike paths, ponds.)*

4. (10-15 minutes) Have students take turns (two at a time) locating on the map the recreational facilities they identified in activity 1. They should use the appropriate colored marker or thumbtack to plot the location of the facility on the map. Each facility should be identified by only *one* thumbtack. Tell students that if someone else has already identified one of the facilities on their list, they should not put a second identifying mark on the map.

5. (25 minutes) While students are taking turns completing the step above, the rest of the class should be working individually or in pairs to complete activity 2.

6. (10 minutes) Discuss the distribution of recreational facilities on the map. Ask students:

- Are the recreational facilities evenly distributed throughout town, or are they clustered in certain neighborhoods?
- Is there a good variety of facilities to choose from?
- Discuss improvements that could increase access to the exercise facilities for youth in your community. What facilities are needed, or could be improved?

7. Ask students to implement the fitness programs they designed in activity 2 this week.

8. Ask students to share their experiences. Did they meet their goals? What were the barriers to success?

▶▶ Extension Activities

Write a letter to the local newspaper or mayor, suggesting ideas to improve the opportunities for recreation in the area, and why that would improve everyone's health.

▶▶ Teacher Resources

General Background Materials

In preparing for this lesson, you may want to refer to the following resources:

- *Centers for Disease Control and Prevention Fact Sheets on Physical Activity*
- *Healthy People 2010*

See appendix B for more information on how to obtain these resources.

Specific Background Materials

Why Do People Become Less Active as They Get Older?

You often hear people talking about their lives and why they're not physically active. Here are some reasons they give:

- "I don't have time for fitness. All I do is work and sleep."
- "There's always something else to do. My family is a full-time job."
- "It's too expensive to do sports once you leave school."
- "I'd rather spend time with my friends."
- "I don't enjoy hard fitness work."

Some of these statements have some truth—as one gets older, life is more demanding in many ways, you have more responsibilities, and it takes a lot more discipline to remain active and fit once you are studying at a high school or college, working, or raising a family. It can be expensive to play sports or join a gym, but there are always inexpensive ways to be active. Lastly, fitness programs can be difficult if they're not appropriate to someone's fitness level.

All these problems can be overcome once you realize the value and importance of being active and eating well. Just half an hour of moderate activity a day can keep you physically fit. The message here is simple: fitness and health takes some effort, time, and organization—but we don't need to be fitness "freaks" to be fit.

What Is a Fitness Program?

For worksheet and introduction activities.

A fitness program doesn't have to mean going to the gym to work out. Some people like to do team sports or run. However, that's not what everyone enjoys doing. You don't need to do strenuous exercise to achieve a minimum level of fitness. You can stay fit by simply being active in everyday activities—for instance, walking briskly to school each day or cycling to a friend's house. Baby-sitting can be a fitness program in itself! *All* active time helps fitness and health.

What Are Some Ways to Stay Active and Healthy?

Here are several steps toward achieving a more active and healthy lifestyle:

1. Understand the importance of fitness, activity, and nutrition. Many people just don't realize how important good eating and activity are in their lives. Being fit and eating right will make you feel good about yourself and will give you energy to be active. Also, getting into the habit of fitness as adolescents will make life easier in years to come, and will lower the risk of developing some diseases. In adult life and old age, the benefits of fitness can be dramatic, including decreasing the risk of injury, increasing the ease of daily tasks, reducing stress, and preventing chronic disease.

2. Identify your needs and make some goals. *(For worksheet.)* Some people would just like to be able to walk to the local store; others want to run marathons. You need to decide what you want to achieve or how you would like to feel, and build up your health progressively toward that goal. Different goals may be appropriate at different stages in life. To increase fitness, create your goals around increasing

- endurance,
- strength, and
- flexibility.

Keeping muscles moving is important for growth, development, and overall health. This doesn't mean you have to do bodybuilding at a gym. Participating in a variety of sports and other interests keeps the muscles of the body active and moving.

3. Decide what is realistic with your daily schedule. Everyone has different schedules, and some have more free time than others. Some may have to prioritize activities to be fit, depending on their goals. For many people, better organization of their time will be enough to create space to do regular exercise. People with many responsibilities may have a hard time believing that taking time out for fitness is valid. Keep in mind that your health and well-being is important to you, your family, and your friends. Start by just making a small space for fitness in your life.

4. Try to do a variety of activities. Variety is important to keeping up your interest in any part of your life, and fitness is no exception. A variety of activities also works a wide range of muscles and joints.

5. Design a schedule that keeps you challenged and motivated. A schedule should keep you active on a regular basis and possibly become more demanding over time. This keeps it challenging and often motivates you to keep going.

6. Encourage friends to join you. Doing active things with friends is an excellent way to stay motivated and involved. People often need the help of others to keep their interest and enjoyment up. Many people prefer team sports for this reason.

Lesson goals:

- Discuss the importance of physical activity.

- Research the location of recreational facilities in your neighborhood and plot them on a classroom map.

- Discuss the distribution of recreation facilities in town.

Physical activity recommendations:

- Be moderately active for at least 30 minutes every day or nearly every day as part of play, games, chores, work, transportation, or planned exercise.

- Participate in at least three sessions per week of vigorous physical activity lasting 20 minutes or more.

- Aim for a total of 60 minutes or more of activity nearly every day.

What are the benefits of an active lifestyle?

- Develop cardiovascular fitness, muscle strength, confidence in physical ability.

- Maintains a healthy body weight and reduce fat.

- Reduces stress and brightens a person's mood.

- Lowers the risk of developing heart disease, diabetes, high blood pressure, and colon cancer, which can lead to premature DEATH.

Make a Prediction

Do you think recreational facilities are evenly distributed in your community (yes or no)?

What is there to do in your neighborhood that would increase your level of fitness?

1. In the table below, make a list of three to five recreational facilities that are within walking or biking distance of your home. *(Examples: basketball courts, tennis courts, tracks, parks, playgrounds, swimming pools, health clubs, bike paths, ponds).*

2. List the street address for each facility and the nearest cross streets. *(Example: Skyline Park is located at 100 Eastern Avenue between Park Street and Highland Avenue. Park Street and Highland Avenue are the cross streets and will help you locate the park on a map.)*

3. Give directions to each location from your home.

Facility name	Types of activities	Address and cross streets	Directions from your home
Example: Skyline Park	*Basketball, tennis, playground, soccer, baseball*	*Eastern Ave. between Park Street and Highland Ave.*	*Walk west on Gray St. to Highland Ave., turn right on Highland, walk 3 blocks and take left on Eastern Ave.*

Here are several suggestions that will help you design a fitness program:

1. Set a fitness goal. Why do you want to be more fit?
2. Decide what activities will realistically fit into your daily schedule.
3. Try to do a variety of activities.
4. Design a program that keeps you challenged.
5. Encourage friends to join you.

List some fitness goals that will help you stay healthy:

1.

2.

3.

4.

Design an activity schedule for one week. Of course, you have school Monday to Friday, but after school and the weekends are good times to be active! You can include sports and other activities that you already do.

Make sure the schedule

- includes a variety of activities that you like to do, and
- keeps you challenged.

Day of week	Activity	Location	Duration	Time of day
Sunday				
Monday				
Tuesday				
Wednesday				
Thursday				
Friday				
Saturday				

Lesson 61

Free to Be Fit

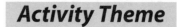

In this lesson, students think about the rights and freedoms guaranteed by the Constitution of the United States. They discuss the possible actions (recommendations, laws, education, etc.) that the federal or state governments might take to encourage an increase in physical activity and a decrease in inactivity. In small groups, students consider several laws and discuss whether the laws would be effective at increasing physical activity and whether they would interfere with individual rights protected by the Constitution. They try to reach a consensus to support or oppose the laws and defend their positions.

▶▶ Behavioral Objective

For students to participate regularly in physical activity or sports.

▶▶ Learning Objectives

Students will be able to

1. define the term **freedom,**
2. give examples of freedoms and rights guaranteed by the U.S. Constitution,
3. discuss whether federal or state governments have the power to pass laws that deprive us of personal choice in order to promote physical activity and healthier lifestyles,
4. listen carefully to the thinking of others,
5. explain the difference between a government recommendation and a mandate or law, and
6. state the physical activity and inactivity recommendations for adolescents.

▶▶ Materials

• Activity 1 *Free to be Fit*

▶▶ Procedure

1. Point out the goals of the activity:
   • To discuss the concept of freedom
   • To discuss the freedoms and rights guaranteed by the U.S. Constitution
   • To discuss whether federal or state governments have the power to pass laws that deprive us of personal choice in order to promote physical activity and healthier lifestyles

- To brainstorm actions the government might take (other than passing laws) to promote physical activity and decrease inactivity

2. Distribute activity 1 *Free to Be Fit.*

3. Have the class brainstorm answers to the first two questions on the worksheet. *(Possible answers for question 2 concerning freedoms and rights guaranteed by the Constitution: free speech, right to assemble, religious freedom, right to bear arms, right to vote, right to privacy, trial by jury, no unwarranted searches, right to an appeal, due process, equal protection under the law.)*

4. Divide the class into groups of three or four students. Have each group complete questions 3, 4, and 5 as follows: Discuss question 3, and try to develop a group consensus (opinion) that the group can defend; assign each group *one* or *two* of the laws listed in question 4 to discuss; brainstorm answers to question 5. One person should record the group responses to each question. Emphasize the importance of taking turns speaking and listening carefully to one anothers' ideas. You may wish to walk around the room and point out incidences where students are not following these recommendations.

5. Conduct a class discussion of questions 3, 4, and 5. Ask one person (not the recorder) from each group to report their group's answers. During this discussion, make sure students understand the difference between government recommendations and a mandate or law. Encourage students to be creative in their response to question 5 and to really *think* about possible actions the government might take to encourage an increase in physical activity. *(Possible answers to question 5: fund education programs; offer grants of money to schools, towns, or cities interested in improving their physical activity facilities or sports programs; develop a media campaign to advertise the recommendations; encourage health insurance companies to provide cash credits to people who join health clubs or other physical activity programs.)*

6. Conclude by asking a volunteer to state the physical activity and inactivity recommendations.

▶▶ Extension Activities

Activity 1

Analyze community resources and examine sports in your society to determine why certain sports are played in your neighborhood. Do unsafe parks or recreation facilities influence what kinds of activities are available? Do you have a right to a safe place to play? How can a community overcome a lack of resources to offer different sports to its residents?

Activity 2

Think about sports and democracy for different ages. Are there opportunities for younger children to play on soccer or basketball teams? Interview 10 children of different ages and ask them what sports they participate in and what sports they would like to learn. Analyze the results and write a letter to the local newspaper, the mayor, or a local town official.

Activity 3

Write an essay about why sports and physical activity are important to you and to our society. Focus on the positive benefits and the different reasons people participate in different sports or activities.

Activity 4

Establish a pen pal, by e-mail or letter, in a country of your choice. What type of government does this country have? Is it a democracy? If so, what type of democracy? Find out about the opportunities to participate in sports in this country. In what sports does your pen pal participate? How much physical activity does your pen pal get? Does your pen pal walk to school? How many hours per day does your pen pal watch TV or sit in front of a computer?

Activity 5

Pick a sport to research. Is everyone in our democratic society "free" to participate in this sport? Why or why not? Is everyone "free" to compete in this sport at both the amateur and professional levels? Why or why not? Is the sport you picked an Olympic sport? If so, are there limitations in terms of age, sex, ability, and/or politics that affect who competes in this sport at the Olympic level, not only in this country but in other countries as well?

Activity 6

Choose a country and find a newspaper from this country at the library. Is there a sports section in this newspaper? What sports are represented in the reports? Do any of the sports make the front page of the paper? What type of government does the country have? Is the country a democracy? If so, what type of democracy? Does the type of government seem to affect the newspaper reporting of the sport? Why or why not?

▶▶ Teacher Resources

General Background Material

In preparing this lesson, you may want to refer to the following resources:

- *Television Viewing as a Cause of Increasing Obesity Among Children in the United States, 1986-1990*
- *Healthy People 2010*
- *Centers for Disease Control and Prevention Fact Sheets on Physical Activity*

See appendix B for information on how to obtain these resources.

Specific Background Material

1. *Planet Health*'s Activity Message: Physical activity promotes health and well-being, and offers opportunities to socialize and have fun. Adolescents should be moderately active for at least 30 minutes every day or nearly every day as part of play, games, sports, chores, transportation, or planned exercise, AND they should participate in at least three sessions per week of vigorous physical activity lasting 20 minutes or more. Adolescents should aim for 60 minutes or more of activity on five to seven days per week.

Adult recommendations are for a minimum of 30 minutes of moderately intense activity per day, not necessarily continuous, with more time and intensity required to achieve higher fitness levels.

2. *Planet Health*'s Inactivity Message: We endorse the American Academy of Pediatrics' recommendation that leisure time spent watching TV (or at a computer) should total no more than 2 hours per day.

3. *Recommendations versus mandates or laws.* In this lesson, students are asked to debate the pros and cons of a statement that ties the abstract concepts of freedom and democracy to the concrete notion of requiring people to be physically active because it is good for their health. Students should be made aware that in this country, governments at all levels address many behaviors associated with health through recommendations to the public (e.g., quit smoking, drink more milk, eat less salt, etc.). They do not mandate or require people to behave in a certain way. In our culture, mandates or laws of that type would be considered intrusive and a violation of our freedom.

4. *Sport* is mentioned in the lesson extensions. This term denotes competitive organized team or individual physical activities like basketball, soccer, or competitive figure skating. *Physical activity* refers more broadly to a wide variety of gross motor activities carried out for recreation or with a purpose, including bicycling, raking leaves, walking, dancing, and cleaning.

References

Edlin, G., and Golanty, E. 1992. *Health and wellness: A holistic approach.* Boston: Jones and Bartlett.

The new Grolier multimedia encyclopedia for Macintosh, CD-ROM. 1996.

Sallis, J.F., and Patrick, K. 1994. Physical activity guidelines for adolescents: Consensus statement. *Pediatric Exercise Science* 6:302-314.

Unger, I. 1994. *Instant American history.* New York: Byron Press.

U.S. Department of Health and Human Services. 2000. Healthy People 2010, conference edition, vols. I and II. **www.health.gov/healthypeople**

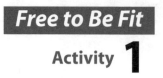
1. Define the word *freedom*.

2. The *Declaration of Independence* states the following:

   "We hold these truths to be self-evident, that all men are created equal, that they are endowed by their creator with certain unalienable rights, that among these are life, liberty [the state of being free; the power to do as one pleases], and the pursuit of happiness."

   The *Constitution of the United States* protects certain individual rights and prohibits state governments from, "depriving any person of life, liberty, or property without due process of law; nor deny to any person . . . equal protection under the law . . . "

   What individual freedoms and rights are we guaranteed by the *Constitution of the United States*?

3. Research has shown that physical activity helps children develop and retain cardiovascular fitness, muscle strength, and confidence in their physical ability. Regular activity helps individuals maintain a healthy weight, build muscle, and reduce fat. It can reduce stress and brighten a person's mood. Active adults have a lower risk of developing heart disease, diabetes, high blood pressure, and colon cancer and of dying prematurely. Scientists recommend that adolescents be moderately active for at least 30 minutes every day or nearly every day, AND they should participate in at least three sessions per week of vigorous physical activity lasting for 20 minutes or more. They encourage them to aim for a total of 60 minutes or more of activity nearly every day. They also recommend that youth spend no more than 2 hours per day watching TV (or on computer games).

   Based on these findings and recommendations, do you think the federal or state government could pass laws that would **require** people to follow these physical activity and TV guidelines? Would these laws interfere with individual rights protected by the Constitution? (Consider other health-related laws that have been passed: laws requiring seat belts, car seats, helmets.)

4. Below are a list of some laws that the federal (or state) government might consider passing to increase physical activity and improve the health of people in the United States. Read the law assigned to your group, and discuss the following questions:

- Would the proposed law increase physical activity (or decrease TV watching) in a large number of people?
- Would the law interfere with individual rights protected by the Constitution?
- Would your group recommend that this law be passed? Why?

Summarize and justify your opinions below the law.

Possible federal (or state) laws aimed at increasing physical activity and improving the health of people in the United States:

A. School districts are required to offer physical education daily.

B. In order to get health insurance, individuals must meet the physical activity recommendations.

C. Individuals under the age of 18 are prohibited from logging onto the Internet for more than 2 hours each day.

D. All towns and cities must spend 10 percent of their budgets on recreation facilities (pools, parks, bike paths) and physical activity programs.

E. Girls must be allowed to participate on male sports teams if comparable female sports teams are not available at the school.

F. All students must pass a physical fitness test in order to graduate from high school.

5. What might the government do (besides passing laws) to encourage people to follow the activity and TV viewing recommendations?

Lifestyle Theme

Impact of Technology

This lesson is designed to be used while teaching a unit on the Industrial Revolution. It asks students to examine the impact of technological advances on the lifestyles of people living in the 19th century and the present. For much of the world, everyday existence now requires far less physical energy because modes of transportation and food gathering have generally improved. Similarly, new technologies, such as TV, computers, and VCRs, encourage inactive leisure-time interests. Physical fitness now requires people to set aside time for physical pursuits. An understanding of the historical developments in technology generates an awareness of this phenomenon.

▶▶ Behavioral Objective

For students to be more physically active.

▶▶ Learning Objectives

Students will be able to

1. list several important inventions (and the inventor) that led to the Industrial Revolution and describe why they were important;
2. discuss the influence of technology and inventions on society (the economy, geography, transportation, education, communication, medicine, politics, food production, social changes) and daily life in the United States during the Industrial Revolution and the present;
3. discuss the effects of technology on the availability and uses of free time;
4. give examples of inventions that have brought world advances, but resulted in unintended health consequences; and
5. discuss the importance of making time for physical activity.

▶▶ Materials

- Activity 1 *Inventions and Discoveries*
- Extension activity 1 *Relating the Past to the Present*
- Social studies textbook

▶▶ Procedure

1 Point out the goals of the activity:

- To discuss the influence of technology and inventions on society and daily life in the United States during the Industrial Revolution and the present
- To discuss the effects of technology on the availability and uses of free time, and its unintended health consequences
- To discuss the importance of making time for physical activity

2. (5 minutes) To introduce the activity, ask students to think about and discuss the following: Compare your lifestyle to that of children living on farms in the early 1800s. Why do you need to *make* time for physical activity, while they did not have to think about this? *(Possible answer: Lack of machines for food and clothing production and transportation required the children in the 1800s to be more active.)*

3. Put students into groups of three.

4. Hand out activity 1 to all students.

5. (5 minutes) Assign each group *one* of the seven inventions in part I of the activity. Make sure students understand that they are to discuss the invention—what it does, why it is/was important, and its impact—on *only one* of the many factors in society. Encourage them to refer to their textbooks and any other available classroom resources.

6. (10 minutes) Ask one person in each group to report the group's findings orally or by writing them on the chalkboard. The other individuals should record the information in their tables. (See Teacher Resources for possible answers.)

7. (10 minutes) Have students work in their groups to complete the rest of part I.

8. (20 minutes) Assign each group *one* of the inventions in part II and have the groups exchange information, or have each student complete part II for homework.

9. (5-10 minutes) Summary discussion. This activity will likely generate a lot of discussion and various responses. You will want to direct the discussion to emphasize the impact of technology on our decreased physical activity during work and leisure time and its unintended health consequences. End by reminding students of *Planet Health*'s Activity Message and encouraging them to reduce their TV watching. (See Teacher Resources.)

▶▶ Extension Activities

1. Imagine if you had no TV—how would your life be different? Explain.

2. Describe areas of the world that have the least and the most technology. Which countries often have insufficient money for education, health care, and food? Are the people in these countries less or more active than people in industrialized nations? Which countries have health problems related to eating too much and being too sedentary?

3. How much technology is there in your school and community? Make a list of the inventions that have helped your city, school, or home.

4. Write a story or essay explaining why technology has brought the world many advances, but has not necessarily been good for health. Give examples.

5. Complete extension activity 1. How is your lifestyle different from that of your grandparents when they were your age? Interview a grandparent, great aunt/uncle, neighbor, or friend of the family who was 11-14 years old during the 1920s, 1930s, or 1940s. What were their lives like as children? How did they spend their free time? Did they spend more of it on self-improvement or amusement? What kind of

jobs did they do? (Another option would be to have students prepare their own interview questions.)

►► Teacher Resources

General Background Materials

In preparing for this lesson, you may want to refer to the following resources:

- *Centers for Disease Control and Prevention Fact Sheets on Physical Activity*
- *Healthy People 2010*

See appendix B for information on how to obtain these resources.

Specific Background Materials

Planet Health's activity message: Physical activity promotes health and well-being, and offers opportunities to socialize and have fun. Adolescents should be moderately active for at least 30 minutes every day or nearly every day, as part of play, games, sports, chores, transportation, or planned exercise, and should participate in at least three sessions per week of vigorous physical activity lasting 20 minutes or more. Adolescents should aim for a total of 60 minutes or more of physical activity on five to seven days per week.

Planet Health's inactivity message: We endorse the *Healthy People 2010 Goals* for TV viewing by the U.S. Department of Health and Human Services, which encourages children to watch no more than 2 hours of TV per day. The American Academy of Pediatrics also makes this recommendation.

Why is it important for adolescents to understand the changing lifestyles of the world?

Technology is greatly affecting the play and leisure interests of youth, and many studies have shown that the young are less active today than ever before. If they become aware that their parents' and grandparents' lives were probably very different in their youth, then they may better appreciate the need for activity. Inactivity is dangerous to health. It increases the risk of developing cardiovascular disease, diabetes, colon cancer, obesity, and osteoporosis.

How have leisure pursuits changed so much?

Studies suggest that there is a difference between playtime now and in the past. Today, TV and computers hold great fascination and interest for most children. Currently, 43% of adolescents watch 5 or more hours of TV daily. These new technologies, along with a rise in crime, a dramatic decline in the number of park keepers, parents' changing work patterns, more single-parent families, and an erosion of the sense of community, have all been cited as reasons for a decline in outdoor play. This is unfortunate since outdoor play is something that has been a part of growing up since the beginning of time. Children are less active now than in the past. Those that are active spend more of their activity time in supervised, structured school and community programs.

What has been the progression of occupations and lifestyles?

When hunting, gathering, and farming were required for food, activity was a central part of life. Adults and even children were required to work 12 to 16 hours a day during certain times of the year. Before motorized transportation, people also expended more energy walking and running from place to place. Even early factory, mill, and mining jobs required long hours of moderately intense to vigorous activity. Working 12 to 13+ hours a day, 6 days a week (72-81 hr/wk), was common for even women and children in New England mills in the early 1800s. At that time, there was a movement in England and the United States to reduce the length of the workday. However, many of the workers were not in favor of these early legislative efforts because they reduced wages. In 1840, a 10-hour workday was approved for government employees (Davidson and Batchelor 1986). "In 1903, Macmillan and Company published a revised edition of Volume 9 of Charles Booth's *Life and Labour of the People in London* (1897). Investigators reported that, of the 206 occupations surveyed, 6% required 48 (or fewer) hr/week, 25% required 48-54 hr, 41% required 54-60 hr, and 14% required over 72 hr/wk" (Park 1992). Use the table to compare the intensity, type, and hours per day of the activities of various groups.

Workers	Intensity	Type	Hours/day
Benedictine Monks ca. AD 600	Light to moderate	Cerebral, light muscular	5.25 (winter), 6.5 (Lent), 9 (summer)
Medieval knights ca. 1100-1400	Moderate to heavy	Muscular and endurance	2-6?
Medieval peasants	Moderate to very heavy	Muscular and endurance	15-16 (harvest), 10-14 (winter)
Lincolnshire farm laborers mid-1800s	Heavy to very heavy Moderate to heavy	Muscular and endurance	15-16 (harvest) 10-14 (winter)
Cotton mill workers 1830s (men and women)	Moderate	More endurance than muscular	12-16
Females in coal mining 1840s	Heavy to very heavy	Muscular and endurance	11-18
Victorian middle-class females	None to light	Sewing, needlework, walking at slow pace	NA
American college women (1985 survey)	Light to moderate	Very limited muscular and/or endurance	>0.5-1
1960-1975 survey of 16–29-year-olds	Light to moderate	Cerebral, moderate to moderately heavy	8-10 (professional; clerical, skilled/semi-skilled; service labor) 12 (managerial)

Park 1992.

As we developed machinery and technology, occupational work, housework, and transportation have required less overall physical activity. Jobs that used to require moving around now can be accomplished by sitting in front of a computer. Even many construction and farming jobs have become less active because machinery is available that achieves higher rates of production and efficiency than manual labor. Children likewise spend less time in physical activity, particularly in urban areas where there are often limited facilities for recreation.

"Even when the average number of [hours per] week spent in voluntary participation in sports, exercise, and other active leisure pursuits is added to those consumed in an 'average' work week of 40 hours, very few individuals in the United States or other industrialized countries today can approach the daily energy expenditure levels of medieval or 19th century farmers, 'pit brow lasses', or the men, women, and children who toiled up to 16 hours per day in the cotton mills or the Caribbean sugar industry. In many non-industrialized societies, however, daily work patterns differ little from those of labor intensive occupations in past eras" (Park 1992).

How have these changes affected lifestyle and health in the United States?

Jobs and leisure-time activities have both become less active. Inactivity in adolescents and adults has increased, and as a result, obesity is on the rise in both groups. For many people being physically fit means making an effort each day to be active and moving. The gymnasium and fitness boom has led many adolescents to misunderstand the requirements of fitness and health. Many have been discouraged from exercising because they think they need to be athletes to be fit. Excessive exercise is not required to maintain good health—merely regular movement and muscular use is sufficient. Of course, higher levels of fitness will result only from more rigorous training.

What are the recreational opportunities for adolescents in urban settings?

Seemingly, there are never enough. Funding for recreation both in schools and towns may be inadequate. The expense of joining or using many facilities is also a hindrance to participation for many. Youth clubs, sports clubs and gyms, however, are great ways for children to get regular activity. Local parks are underused for recreation, as are swimming pools and the seaside.

How do we encourage adolescents to be active?

Organized sports teams and recreation help some adolescents become involved in physical activity. Moderating TV viewing to a maximum of 2 hours a day, as recommended by the American Academy of Pediatrics, will encourage other more physically active uses of their free time. Moving TVs out of the main activity areas and/or bedrooms helps children forget about the TV. If students are surrounded by educators and families who are active themselves, they will also develop an understanding of the benefits of movement and fitness, and seek ways to be active. Role modeling at school and home are both important to students.

"Providing opportunity and encouragement for unstructured play outside, where possible, is also important. Psychologists and others say unstructured outdoor play fosters a deep appreciation for nature and a sense of independence, creativity, and serenity. According to Robin C. Moore—professor of landscape architecture and president of the International Association for Children's Right to Play—neighborhoods, schools, and governments must also take a role in providing adequate outdoor play space for children. She has examined how improving the physical diversity of schoolyards can encourage a broader range of activities among children. In England, it has become popular to break up portions of blacktop with planted areas, streams or other types of water, creating areas appropriate for small groups" (van Dam 1997).

Additional Facts About Technology Development in the 20th Century

Computers

- 1890: First punch card tabulator developed by Hollerith (his company becomes IBM)
- 1941: First programmable computer designed to solve complex engineering equations

- 1946: First high-speed electronics digital computer (ENIAC)
- 1950s: Mainframes first available commercially
- 1975: First mini-computer retailed for $397. It had to be assembled by the owner and manually programmed
- 1983: First machine with a mouse and a graphical user interface

Internet

- 1965: First computers linked for military defense reasons
- 1969: Four host computers connected (university and military)
- 1976: First e-mail sent
- 1992: Term "surfing the Internet" coined by Jean Armour Polly
- 1997: 19,540,000 host computers linked

Portable Music

- 1980: Walkman (portable cassette player) introduced by Sony
- 1985: Portable CD player introduced by Sony

Other Technological Advancements

- DNA fingerprinting: "A lab technique that compares the patterns of bands of analogous DNA fragments from two or more separate individuals; this is done to find out how closely related DNA are to each other" (*BioTech Life Science Dictionary* 1995-97.) This technique can be used to compare a suspect's DNA with evidence left at the scene of a crime.
- Cloning: "The process of asexually producing a group of cells (clones), all genetically identical, from a single ancestor" (*BioTech Life Science Dictionary* 1995-97). If an organism is cloned, the clone is genetically identical to the organism it was cloned from.

References

BioTech chronicles. 1997. **www.gene.com/ae**

CD Chronology. 2000. **www.colba.net/~synthifi/cdchrono.htm**

Davidson, J.W., and Batchelor, J.E. 1986. *The American nation.* Englewood Cliffs, NJ: Prentice-Hall.

Gortmaker, S.L. 1990. National health examination survey, 1967-70. Unpublished data.

Gortmaker, S.L. 1990. National longitudinal survey of youth. Unpublished data.

Hagedorn, S.A. *BioTech life science dictionary.* **biotech.icmb.utexas.edu/search/dict-search.html**

The history of computing, Department of Computer Science, Virginia Tech. **ei.cs.vt.edu/~history/index.html**

Hoyle, M. 1994. Computers: From the past to present. Lecture at University at Regina.

Park, R. 1992. Human energy expenditure from *Australopithecus afarensis* to 4-minute mile: Exemplars and case studies. *Exercise Science and Sports Medicine Review* 20: 185-220.

Saltus, R. 1997. The cloning focus is on specialized animals. *Boston Globe,* July 14.

Soundsite, Inc. 1996. A brief history of sound recording and broadcasting technology of film, videos, and television. **www.soundsite.com**

U.S. Department of Health and Human Services. 2000. Healthy People 2010, conference edition, vols. I and II. **www.health.gov/healthypeople**

Van Dam, Laura. 1997. Wild in the streets. *Sanctuary,* May/June.

Zakon, R.H. 1993. *Hobbes' Internet timeline.* **info.isoc.org/guest/zakon/Internet/History/HIT.html**

▶▶ Answer Key

Selected Answers to Activity 1

Table 1

The answers for table 1 will vary, but should be available in most social studies textbooks.

Choose two types of people listed below and explain how one of the inventions or industries listed in table 1 impacted the lives of these individuals.

Answers will vary.

Influence of the cotton gin on Southern planters: They were able to supply more cotton to Northern factories which resulted in great economic success for these individuals. They bought more land and slaves to meet the increasing Northern factory demands. As a result, Southern plantations stretched as far west as Texas, the number of slaves in the United States increased sharply in the 1800s, and the planters depended on Europe and the North for finished goods. Many plantation owners felt they were enslaved to the products of Northern industry.

Influence of the cotton gin on Southern slaves: It reduced the number of slaves that were needed to clean the cotton (one person could do the work of 1,000 people). However, most slaves continued to do back-breaking labor in the fields.

Influence of the steam-powered engine, sewing machine, cotton gin, and new transportation vehicles on mill owners: All of these inventions resulted in an expansion of industry in the North. Mill owners built bigger factories, hired more workers, and grew wealthy.

Influence of advances in textile finishing machinery and transportation on homemakers: Finished textile products became more readily available to the homemaker.

Growth of the mills and factories: Increased the number of jobs available to **young women, children, urban lower class,** and **recent immigrants.** Entire families worked in factories. They needed all their earnings to pay for food and housing. Young women did most of the work in textile mills. Children cleaned debris out of machines and changed spindles. The hours were long, the wages were poor, and the working conditions were unsafe.

Influence of the steel plow on farmers: Made farming the prairie practical. Its sharp blades easily cut through prairie grass roots. Before this technology, farmers depended on huge, unwieldy iron and wooden plows which had to be pulled by six oxen and guided by three men. One man and two horses could operate the steel plow. In 1833, there were no farms in Iowa. By 1860, the steel plow had made it possible for farmers to produce 42,411,000 bushels of corn in Iowa.

Imagine what life was like for one of the two individuals. Describe a typical day's physical activity for the person. What did they do? How many hours a day did they work? Did it change as a result of the invention/industry? How much free time did they have, and what did they do with it?

Factory workers of all ages: Work began at 4 A.M. and ended at 7:30 P.M. Workers took a break for breakfast at 7:30 A.M. and again at noon for lunch. The work was tedious and dangerous (poor ventilation and lighting, unsafe machinery). Any free time they had would have been spent maintaining their homes and resting.

Slaves: Most did hard labor in the fields. "Teenagers worked alongside adults in the field. Children pulled weeds, picked insects from crops and carried water to other workers" (Davidson and Batchelor, 1986). Some worked as many as 16 hours a day.

Older slaves worked in the planter's house cooking, cleaning, and doing other chores. They did not have much free time.

Small Northern and Southern farmers: All members of their families would have spent 10–12-hour days planting and doing household and farm chores. The little free time that they had may have been spent going to church, relaxing, or for children in unstructured play.

Planters: "They entertained lavishly, dressing and behaving like the nobility of Europe . . . They had to make decisions about when to plant and harvest their crops . . . They devoted many hours to local and state politics [and] . . . hired overseers to run the plantation . . . Women were involved in overseeing the house slaves, raising the children, and entertaining" (Davidson and Batchelor, 1986). Children in this group had time for education and much more time for socializing and unstructured play.

Table 2

The answers for table 2 will vary.

Impact of cloning adult sheep: Researchers want to extend the sheep-cloning method to cattle, pigs, and goats. Using these animals they hope to make billions of dollars producing drug proteins, tailor-made tissues, and clones of prize-winning bulls and top milk-producing cows. This technique will impact the economy and medical treatment. It also has stimulated ethical questions about the technique and prompted calls for legislation to regulate its use.

How do the computer, TV, Internet, and VCR affect the daily physical activity of children your age?

See Teacher Resources.

Compare your physical activity (amount and type) to the physical activity of children (11- to 14 years old) living in the early 1800s. How do you account for the difference?

In the 1800s most children were required to spend a large portion of their day doing chores or working in factories. They also had to walk long distances to school or work. Wealthy children had more time for leisure activities, and therefore engaged in less physical activity. Children today are required to do fewer chores and are frequently transported by car or bus. Most of their day is spent doing school work. They also engage in a lot of inactive leisure activities. Advances in technology and the passing of child labor laws, as well as interest in TV, have done much to decrease the physical activity of children.

Compare your free time (amount and uses of it) to the free time of children (11- to 14 years old) living in the early 1800s. How do you account for the difference?

Children have more free time now. (See the answer above for a discussion of why.)

Part I: 1780–1890

The 1800s brought the Industrial Revolution to the United States. Inventions sparked the growth of new industries. Complete the table below by explaining why the new technologies were important, and how they affected two of the following: the economy, geography, politics, travel, environment, or everyday life of people living during that time.

Invention or industry	Inventor	Importance/impact on society
Cotton gin (1793)	Eli Whitney	
Steel plow (1837)	John Deere	
Mechanical reaper (1848)	Cyrus McCormick	
Steam-powered Engine (1782)	James Watt	
Boat (1803)	Robert Fulton	
Train engine (1829)	G. Stephenson	
Telegraph (1840)	Samuel F.B. Morse	
Mills and factories (U.S. 1790)	Moses Brown	
Clipper ships (1845)	John Griffith	

Choose two types of people listed below and explain how one of the inventions or industries listed in table 1 impacted the lives of these individuals (use separate paper).

Southern planter	Southern slave	20-year-old female city dweller
Northern farmer	Northern mill owner	12-year-old northern city dweller
Urban poor	Recent immigrant	Homemaker

Imagine what life was like for one of the two individuals. Describe a typical day's physical activity for the person. What did he or she do? How many hours a day did this person work? Did this person's life change as a result of an invention or advance in the industry? How much free time did he or she have, and what did he or she do with it? Use separate paper if you need more room.

Part II: 1925–1997

Advances in technology, especially in computers, communication, and biotechnology, are currently taking place at a rapid pace. Complete the table below by explaining why the technologies are important and how they are influencing **one** of the following: the economy, politics, medicine, the justice system, the environment, education, communication, or everyday life.

Invention or industry	Inventor	Importance/impact on society
Personal computers available to the general public (1977)	Apple Radio Shack	
Television (1925)	John Logie Baird	
VCR available to the general public (1975)	Sony*	
Internet access available to the general public (1995)	Compuserve* America Online Prodigy	
Compact discs (1983)	Sony* Phillips	
Genetic cloning of an adult sheep (1993)	Dr. Ian Wilmut	
DNA fingerprinting (1978-1980)	David Botstein** Kary Mallis	

*These inventions were the work of groups of scientists who built upon the ideas and inventions of earlier work in the field. They were marketed by the company listed.

**Several different laboratory techniques have been developed.

The rapid advances in technology at the beginning of the 1800s sparked the Industrial Revolution. Do you think that we are in the midst of another revolution? Explain.

What do you think historians will call this revolution?

How do the computer, TV, Internet, and VCR affect the daily physical activity of children your age?

Compare your **physical activity** (amount and type) to the physical activity of children (11- to 14 years old) living in the early 1800s. Give several details to support your answer. How do you account for the difference?

Compare your **free time** (amount and uses of it) to the free time of children (11- to 14 years old) living in the early 1800s. How do you account for the difference?

How is your lifestyle different from that of your grandparents when they were your age?

Directions

Interview a grandparent, great aunt/uncle, neighbor, or friend of the family who was 11-14 years old during the 1920s, 1930s, or 1940s. Ask the questions listed below. Record the answers and your answers to the same questions in the table.

Question When you were 11-14 years old . . .	Adult response	Your response
During what years were you this age?		
Did you walk to school? If yes, how far did you walk		
Did you walk home for lunch?		
What time did school get out?		
How much free time did you have?		
What did you do after school?		
What did you do for fun in the summer?		
What kind of chores did you have to do?		
Did your family own a car? How did you get around?		
Did school offer competitive sports? What kinds? Were their any competitive girls' teams?		
Did you have a job? What was it?		
What kinds of games did you play? Where did you play them?		
How old were you the first time you watched TV? Owned a TV?		
How much TV do you currently watch on a typical day?		

Compare your responses to those of the adult you interviewed. Which of you had (has) a more active lifestyle at 11-14 years old? How do you explain the differences?

Food Rituals and Society

Through class discussion as well as a group activity, students will learn that in addition to its nutritional value, food is often associated with religious and secular (nonreligious) traditions or ethnic celebrations. Special dishes that may include expensive or hard-to-get ingredients, used once a year, are often prepared. This lesson is designed to infuse information about everyday foods and sometimes foods into a classroom unit on food rituals.

▶▶ Behavioral Objective

To understand that "sometimes" foods can be eaten on special occasions.

▶▶ Learning Objectives

Students will be able to:

1. examine the association between food and various religious, secular (nonreligious), and ethnic traditions,

2. give examples of religious and secular food traditions, and

3. state that food rituals often include *sometimes foods* (foods that should be eaten in moderation because they are high in total fat, saturated fat, trans fat, or sugar or low in vitamins and minerals).

▶▶ Materials

- Student resource 1 *Food Rituals and Celebrations*
- Activity 1 *Food Rituals*
- *Optional:* Student resource 1 *What's the Rap on Fat?* (lesson 49, page 335)

▶▶ Procedure

1. (5-8 minutes) Review Teacher Resources. Talk about 5-A-Day and fat guidelines and say explicitly these are not meant to disrupt traditional practices. Some may choose to make lower-fat alternatives, but others may not. Discuss with students some customs and rituals associated with food. In addition, discuss the role of *everyday foods* and *sometimes foods* in the diet. Highlight examples of religious holidays celebrated with special foods. Mention that "sometimes foods" are okay, important, and appropriate for special times.

2. (5-8 minutes) Discuss student resource 1 *Food Rituals and Celebrations*. Ask students where in the Food Guide Pyramid some of the ritual and celebration foods are located. Many foods like pumpkin pie and latkes will belong in the pyramid tip.

Emphasize that there is no minimum recommendation for the foods in the tip of the pyramid, and these foods should be consumed in moderation. For example, eat them during celebrations and traditional meals but on most days, choose foods low in saturated fat and trans fat, and moderate in total fat. Try to make grains, especially whole grains, fruits, and vegetables the main components of your meals.

3. (15 minutes) Distribute activity 1 *Food Rituals*. Allow students to work in small groups of four or five using worksheets to examine their own experience of food rituals.

4. (15 minutes) Group representatives report their findings to the class.

▶▶ Extension Activities

Have a multicultural celebration. Ask students to bring in foods their families typically serve at holiday celebrations. Label each dish with the name of the holiday the food is served at and the category or categories it would fit into on the Food Guide Pyramid. You may wish to ask students to research the historical significance of the food. For example, why is turkey a favorite Thanksgiving food?

▶▶ Teacher Resources

General Background Material

In preparing for this lesson, you may want to refer to the following resources:

- *Time to Take Five*
- *Nutrition and Your Health: Dietary Guidelines for Americans*

See appendix A for information on how to obtain these resources.

- *Fat: Where It's At, page 252*

Specific Background Material

Sometimes Foods

Some of the foods eaten during special celebrations are *sometimes foods*. *Sometimes foods* is a simple way to describe foods that should be eaten in moderation because they are high in total fat, saturated fat, trans fat, or sugar; are low in nutrients; or are not nutrient dense (i.e., the ratio of nutrients to calories is low). Examples of *sometimes foods* are corn chips or potato chips (both high in fat, low in nutrients), sausage (high in fat), and most candy bars and cakes (high in fat and sugar, low in nutrients).

The student resource includes foods associated with some religious and secular celebrations. Sometimes foods are in italics. A list of ingredients and the method of preparation for some of the sometimes foods have been included. Note that in the west, Judaism, Christianity, and Islam are the most prevalent religions, but Hinduism and Buddhism are more prevalent in the east.

Everyday Foods

Everyday foods describes foods like grains, fruits, vegetables, lean cuts of meat, and low-fat dairy products that can be eaten daily because they provide plenty of nutrition and adequate amounts of fat and calories for health.

Healthy Eating (5-A-Day and Fat Guidelines)

To build a healthy eating pattern, make grains (especially whole grains), fruits, and vegetables the foundation of your meals. Encourage students to eat at least two servings of fruit and at least three servings of vegetables (with at least one serving of a dark green or orange vegetable) for a total of five servings a day. Choose a diet low in saturated fat (10% of total calories) and moderate in total fat (30% of total calories).

Not All Fat Is Created Equal

The fat in foods contains a mixture of saturated and unsaturated (monounsaturated and polyunsaturated) fatty acids (commonly called fats). Many animal-based foods, such as fatty meat, whole milk, butter, and lard, are high in saturated fat. This kind of fat typically is solid at room temperature. Eating too much saturated fat increases the risk of developing heart disease. Therefore, the *Dietary Guidelines for Americans* recommends a diet low in saturated fat (less than 10% of calories). Most of the fat you eat should be unsaturated since substituting unsaturated fat for saturated fat in your diet decreases the risk of developing heart disease. Most plant fats or oils are high in unsaturated fat and generally are liquid at room temperature. Vegetable oils (olive, canola, corn, peanut), most nuts, olives, and avocados are good sources of unsaturated fat. However, eating lots of any kind of fat may not be healthy, so try to get no more than 30% of your calories from total fat (unsaturated, saturated fat, and trans fat).

There are exceptions to the rule. Not all plant fats are healthy. Through a commercial process called hydrogenation, plant oils can be converted into solids called trans fat (also called partially hydrogenated vegetable oil). This is how some margarines are made. Not surprisingly, foods high in trans fat have been found to increase the risk of heart disease also. To avoid these fats, check the ingredient lists on packaged foods like cookies and crackers for partially hydrogenated vegetable oil. Also watch out for coconut oil and palm oil since these oils are naturally high in saturated fat.

Also, not all animal foods are high in saturated fat. Some ocean fish, such as salmon, mackerel, and tuna, are high in a polyunsaturated fat—called omega-3 fatty acid—that may protect against heart disease. So choose to eat fish when you get the chance.

Tips for Lowering Saturated Fat Intake

It's okay to eat high-fat foods once in a while. However, if you were to eat meals solely composed of the foods in the tip of the pyramid, you could exceed the recommended total fat intake (30% of total calories) or saturated fat intake (10% of total calories) perhaps in only one meal. The *Dietary Guidelines for Americans* offers these tips on how to lower your intake of saturated fat:

- Cook with vegetable oil instead of butter.
- Read food labels; choose foods lower in saturated fat.
- Trim fat from meat and remove the skin from poultry.
- Choose fat-free or low-fat milk, yogurt, and cheese.
- Choose fruit for dessert.
- Limit intake of processed meats like sausage, salami, and hot dogs.
- Limit intake of candy, cookies, cake, and chips.
- Eat plenty of grains, especially whole grains, fruits, and vegetables.
- Choose two to three servings of fish or other lean meats daily.
- Choose dried beans, peas, or lentils often.

References

Cheung L., Gortmaker, S., and Dart, H. 2001. *Eat well & keep moving.* Champaign, IL: Human Kinetics.

Milford, S. 1992. *Hands around the world: 365 ways to build cultural awareness and global respect.* Charlotte, VT: Williamson.

U.S. Committee on UNICEF. 1985. *Joy through the world.* New York: Dodd, Mead.

U.S. Department of Agriculture and U.S. Department of Health and Human Services. 2000. *Nutrition and your health: Dietary guidelines for Americans* 2000, 5th edition. **www.usda.gov/cnpp**

Willett, W. 2000. Got fat? Exploding nutrition myths. *World Health News.* **www.worldhealthnews. harvard.edu**

Some of the foods eaten during special celebrations are *sometimes foods*. Sometimes foods is a simple way to describe foods that should be eaten in moderation because they are high in total fat, saturated fat, or sugar or low in vitamins and minerals. These foods can be found in the tip of the Food Guide Pyramid. If you were to eat meals solely composed of the foods in the tip of the pyramid, you could exceed the recommended total fat intake (30% of total calories) or saturated fat intake (10% of total calories) perhaps in only one meal. Remember that it's okay to eat high-fat foods once in a while (e.g., fried potato pancakes or chocolate cake), and consider the lower-fat alternatives (e.g., baked potato, fruit, or a low-fat snack) most of the time. Also, be sure to get your daily intake of five or more fruits and vegetables!

The following are examples of secular (nonreligious) and religious celebrations. *Sometimes foods* are listed in italics.

Secular

St. Valentine's Day (February 14) has been dedicated to St. Valentine since he was martyred on that day in AD 269. This special day has ties to the ancient Roman lovers' festival called Lupercalia. Today, lovers and friends exchange affectionate cards as well as *candies*, flowers, and *chocolates*.

Birthdays are celebrated with the Happy Birthday song, which is about 100 years old and is the most popular song in the world. *Birthday cake* originated in Germany a few hundred years ago. Items such as coins and thimbles were baked into the cake. The party guest with the coin in his or her slice would have great wealth, and the person with the thimble would never marry. Many people enjoy *chocolate cakes* on their birthday. *Chocolate cakes* contain flour, baking powder, salt, sugar, spices, unsweetened chocolate, butter, sugar, eggs, milk, and vanilla. Birthday candles, now used in most parts of the world, are another German tradition. The candle's smoke was originally believed to carry prayers and wishes to the heavens.

Around the world, **weddings** frequently include large feasts often with elaborate meals and ornate layered *wedding cakes* and music.

Thanksgiving is a festival held the last Thursday in November celebrating a harvest that kept the Pilgrims alive in their new home. Foods commonly consumed include turkey, squash, *pumpkin pie*, cranberry sauce, and mashed potatoes. *Pumpkin pie* includes pie dough, pumpkin, evaporated milk, sugar, spices, and eggs. It is baked and is often served with *whipped cream*.

Religious

Chanukah (or **Hanukkah**) is the Jewish "feast of the dedication" and falls on the 25th of the Jewish month of Kislev (November/December). Celebrated for eight days, it commemorates the Jewish recapture of Judas Maccabaeus in 165 BC from the Syrian Greeks. The Jews had only a day's supply of sanctified oil to light the temple. Miraculously, the oil lasted for eight days. Frying food in oil is a way of celebrating this miracle. Foods eaten include pea soup, chicken, vegetables, salads, *pound cakes*, *cheese strudels*, *cheesecakes*, and *latkes*. *Latkes*, the most special Chanukah food, are prepared by grating potatoes and mixing them with eggs, flour, salt, and grated onion. They are fried in cooking oil.

Christmas is the Christian commemoration of the birth of Jesus Christ, observed on December 25. Holiday meals vary, but often include roast turkey or ham, vegetables, bread, and hot punch. Two traditional Christmas desserts are the French *buche de Noel*, a rich cake shaped like a Yule log, and British *plum pudding*. In British superstition everyone must take turns stirring the unbaked pudding clockwise (the direction the sun was assumed to rotate around the earth) and make a wish. Stirring counterclockwise was bound to bring trouble! *Eggnog*, also served at Christmas, is a rich beverage prepared with chilled *cream*, eggs, *sugar*, and vanilla.

During **Ramadan**, the ninth month of the Islamic calendar, Muslims customarily invite guests to break the sunrise to sunset fast and dine in the evening. This is traditionally regarded as the month when the first revelation of the Koran was made to Mohammed. Sweets are enjoyed such as *vermicelli pudding* with dried fruits, lamb, special rice with meat and vegetables (biryani), dried fruits, olives, and nanns (bread).

Diwali, the feast of the lights, is a Hindu New Year's celebration held in the fall. Clay lamps are lit to welcome King Rama who returned home after 14 years in the forest. Foods eaten include *halvah* (a candy made from sesame seeds), snacks made from deep-fried legumes, special rice dishes and breads including pooris (puffed breads), and *gulab jaman sweets*. *Gulab jaman* consist of cottage cheese balls fried in ghee (ghee is butter with the milk solids removed, also known as clarified butter) and dipped in sugar.

Name _____

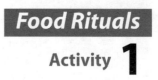

Break into small groups and complete this worksheet as a group. Then select two people from the group to briefly present your findings to the class. (Continue on the other side of this sheet if necessary.)

Student Names _____   _____

_____   _____

1. Discuss rituals and traditions at your homes that involve special foods or meals. Try to list four rituals or traditions from the group.

2. Select one of these rituals and list special foods associated with it.

3. List the sometimes foods associated with the ritual mentioned in question 2.

Appendix **A**

Nutrition Resources

American Heart Association. 1996. *Dietary Guidelines for Healthy American Adults.* Find this resource online at **www.americanheart.org/Heart_and_Stroke_A_Z_Guide/ dietg.html** or write the American Heart Association, National Center, 7272 Greenville Ave., Dallas, TX 75231.

National Dairy Council. 1997. *Daily Food Guide Pyramid.* (See page 485.) This handout features photographs of foods in the five food groups and explains the nutrient composition of combination foods. It will help students determine which food groups they are eating when they eat foods like pizza or chicken stir-fry. **www. nationaldairycouncil.org**

National Dairy Council. 1994. *Guide to Good Eating.* (See page 487.) This handout features photographs of foods in the five food groups and emphasizes the importance of eating a variety of foods from each group every day. **www.nationaldairycouncil.org**

National Dairy Council. 1996. *Seven Ways to Size up Your Servings.* (See page 489.) This handout provides easy ways to measure serving size. **www.nationaldairycouncil.org**

National Institutes of Health and National Cancer Institute. 1995. *Time to Take Five: Eat 5 Fruits and Vegetables a Day.* NIH publication 95-3862. (See page 490.) This pamphlet discusses the health rationale for eating five fruits and vegetables each day. You can order up to 20 copies of this free pamphlet online at publications.nci.nih.gov or contact the National Cancer Institute, Publications Ordering Service, P.O. Box 24128, Baltimore, MD 21227 or call 1-800-4-CANCER (1-800-422-6237), Monday through Friday, 9:00 AM to 4:00 PM EST.

Washington State Dairy Council. No date. *Fat: Where it's at.* From *Fat: A Balancing Act.* These easy-to-read charts show the fat content of many popular foods sorted by food group. The "extras" group contains many typical snack foods. These charts have been adapted into student resource 2 of lesson 42 (pages 252-256).

Dietary Guidelines for Americans

U.S. Department of Agriculture and U.S. Department of Health and Human Services. 2000. *Nutrition and Your Health: Dietary Guidelines for Americans, 2000.* 5th ed.

In 2000, the U.S. Department of Agriculture and the U.S. Department of Health and Human Services released the fifth edition of the *Dietary Guidelines for Americans.* The new dietary guidelines pinpoint three basic messages to improve health and well-being, the ABC's for health:

1. **Aim** for fitness.
   - Aim for a healthy weight.
   - Be physically active each day.
2. **Build** a healthy base.
   - Let the Food Guide Pyramid guide your food choices.
   - Choose a variety of grains daily, especially whole grains.

- Choose a variety of fruits and vegetables daily.
- Keep food safe to eat.

3. **Choose** sensibly.
- Choose a diet low in saturated fat and cholesterol and moderate in total fat.
- Choose beverages and foods to moderate your intake of sugars.
- Choose and prepare foods with less salt.
- If you drink alcoholic beverages, do so in moderation.

This general guide to making healthy choices includes information on interpreting the Food Guide Pyramid, moderating fat intake, establishing healthy eating habits, engaging in physical activity, and avoiding unhealthy behaviors. The *Dietary Guidelines for Americans* can be found online at **www.usda.gov/cnpp/DietGd.pdf** (accessed July 21, 2000; requires Adobe Acrobat to download). You can contact the U.S. Department of Health and Human Services at 200 Independence Avenue SW, Washington, D.C. 20201; 202-619-0257 (toll free 1-877-696-6775). Contact the U.S. Department of Agriculture at 14th & Independence Avenue SW, Washington, D.C. 20250; 202-720-2791.

DAILY FOOD GUIDE PYRAMID

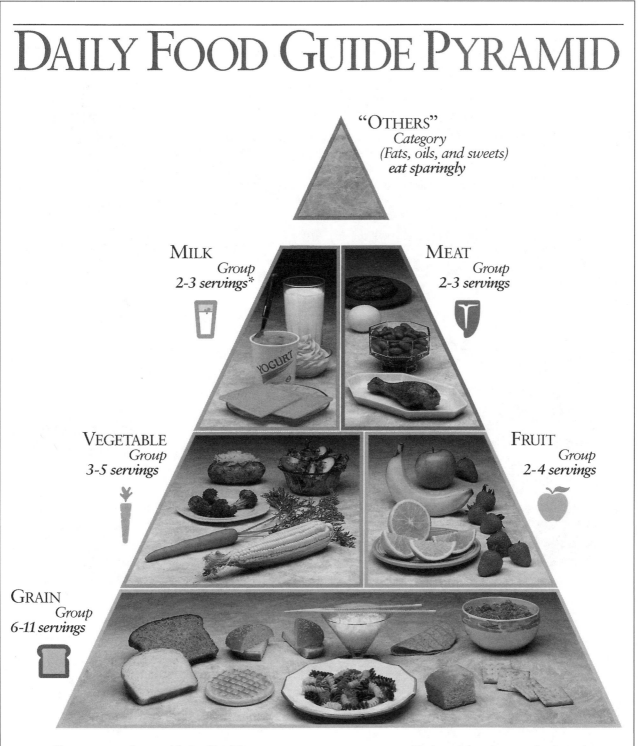

"OTHERS"
Category
(Fats, oils, and sweets)
eat sparingly

MILK
Group
2-3 servings*

MEAT
Group
2-3 servings

VEGETABLE
Group
3-5 servings

FRUIT
Group
2-4 servings

GRAIN
Group
6-11 servings

*Preteens, teens, and young adults (age 11 to 24)
and pregnant and lactating women need 4 servings from
the Milk Group to meet their increased calcium needs.

Need more information on serving sizes or the
variety of foods in each food group? Ask for a copy
of Dairy Council®'s **GUIDE to GOOD EATING.**™

COMBINATION FOODS ARE NUTRITIOUS

Pizza...
   Lasagna...
      Chicken Stir fry!
Where do they fit on the Pyramid?

These mixed dishes—"Combination Foods"—are made by combining foods from the Five Food Groups. So, they fit in several parts of the pyramid.

Combinations count as full or partial servings of two or more food groups. So, they help you meet the recommended number of servings listed on the Daily Food Guide Pyramid.

Key

MILK *Group* — MEAT *Group*
VEGETABLE *Group* — FRUIT *Group*
GRAIN *Group*

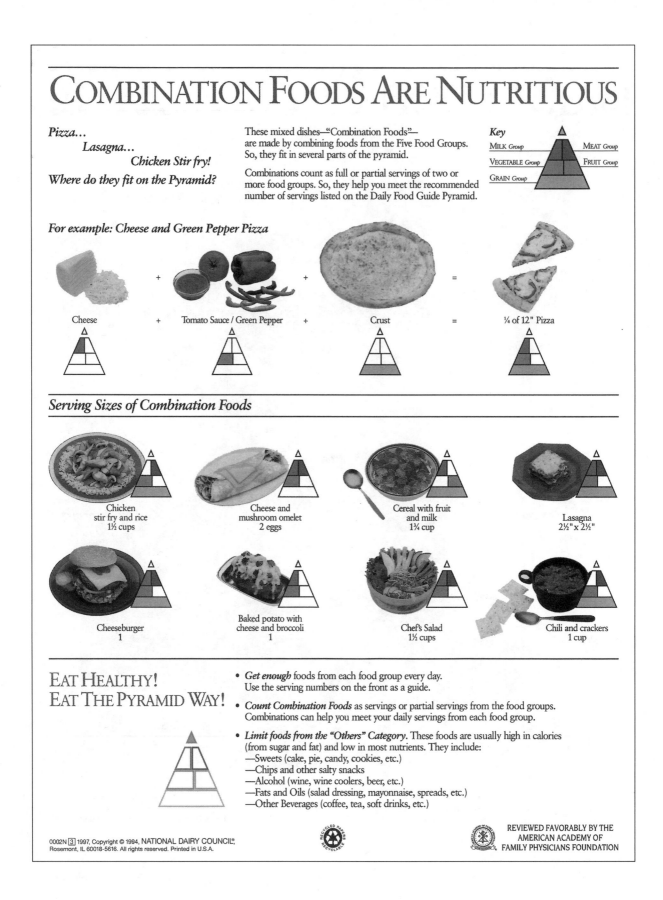

For example: Cheese and Green Pepper Pizza

Cheese + Tomato Sauce / Green Pepper + Crust = ¼ of 12" Pizza

---

Serving Sizes of Combination Foods

Chicken stir fry and rice
1½ cups

Cheese and mushroom omelet
2 eggs

Cereal with fruit and milk
1¾ cup

Lasagna
2½" x 2½"

Cheeseburger
1

Baked potato with cheese and broccoli
1

Chef's Salad
1½ cups

Chili and crackers
1 cup

EAT HEALTHY!
EAT THE PYRAMID WAY!

- **Get enough** foods from each food group every day. Use the serving numbers on the front as a guide.

- **Count Combination Foods** as servings or partial servings from the food groups. Combinations can help you meet your daily servings from each food group.

- **Limit foods from the "Others" Category**. These foods are usually high in calories (from sugar and fat) and low in most nutrients. They include:
  —Sweets (cake, pie, candy, cookies, etc.)
  —Chips and other salty snacks
  —Alcohol (wine, wine coolers, beer, etc.)
  —Fats and Oils (salad dressing, mayonnaise, spreads, etc.)
  —Other Beverages (coffee, tea, soft drinks, etc.)

0002N [3] 1997, Copyright © 1994, NATIONAL DAIRY COUNCIL®, Rosemont, IL 60018-5616. All rights reserved. Printed in U.S.A.

RECYCLED PAPER
RECYCLABLE

REVIEWED FAVORABLY BY THE
AMERICAN ACADEMY OF
FAMILY PHYSICIANS FOUNDATION

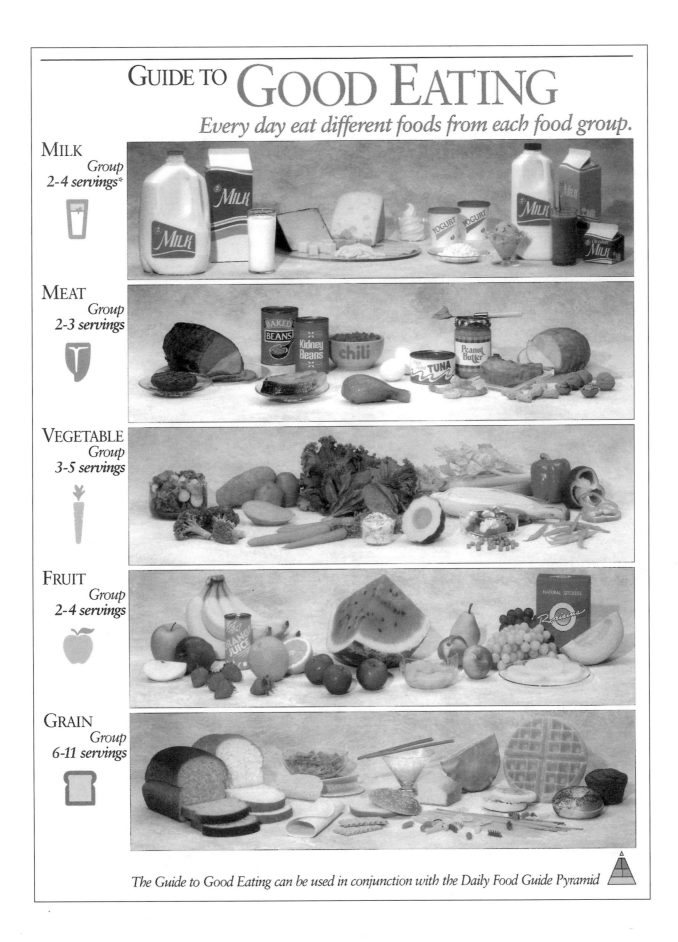

GUIDE TO GOOD EATING

Every day eat different foods from each food group.

MILK
Group
*2-4 servings**

MEAT
Group
2-3 servings

VEGETABLE
Group
3-5 servings

FRUIT
Group
2-4 servings

GRAIN
Group
6-11 servings

The Guide to Good Eating can be used in conjunction with the Daily Food Guide Pyramid

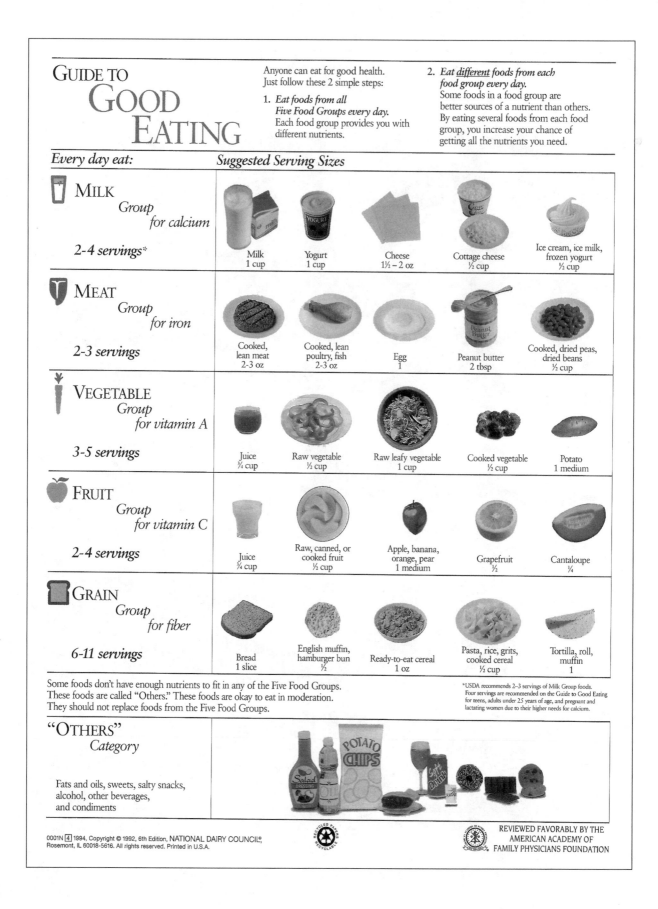

GUIDE TO GOOD EATING

Anyone can eat for good health. Just follow these 2 simple steps:

1. **Eat foods from all Five Food Groups every day.** Each food group provides you with different nutrients.

2. **Eat _different_ foods from each food group every day.** Some foods in a food group are better sources of a nutrient than others. By eating several foods from each food group, you increase your chance of getting all the nutrients you need.

Every day eat: Suggested Serving Sizes

MILK Group for calcium
2-4 servings*

| Milk 1 cup | Yogurt 1 cup | Cheese 1½ – 2 oz | Cottage cheese ½ cup | Ice cream, ice milk, frozen yogurt ½ cup |

MEAT Group for iron
2-3 servings

| Cooked, lean meat 2-3 oz | Cooked, lean poultry, fish 2-3 oz | Egg 1 | Peanut butter 2 tbsp | Cooked, dried peas, dried beans ½ cup |

VEGETABLE Group for vitamin A
3-5 servings

| Juice ¾ cup | Raw vegetable ½ cup | Raw leafy vegetable 1 cup | Cooked vegetable ½ cup | Potato 1 medium |

FRUIT Group for vitamin C
2-4 servings

| Juice ¾ cup | Raw, canned, or cooked fruit ½ cup | Apple, banana, orange, pear 1 medium | Grapefruit ½ | Cantaloupe ¼ |

GRAIN Group for fiber
6-11 servings

| Bread 1 slice | English muffin, hamburger bun ½ | Ready-to-eat cereal 1 oz | Pasta, rice, grits, cooked cereal ½ cup | Tortilla, roll, muffin 1 |

Some foods don't have enough nutrients to fit in any of the Five Food Groups. These foods are called "Others." These foods are okay to eat in moderation. They should not replace foods from the Five Food Groups.

*USDA recommends 2–3 servings of Milk Group foods. Four servings are recommended on the Guide to Good Eating for teens, adults under 25 years of age, and pregnant and lactating women due to their higher needs for calcium.

"OTHERS" Category

Fats and oils, sweets, salty snacks, alcohol, other beverages, and condiments

0001N 4 1994, Copyright © 1992, 6th Edition, NATIONAL DAIRY COUNCIL®, Rosemont, IL 60018-5616. All rights reserved. Printed in U.S.A.

REVIEWED FAVORABLY BY THE AMERICAN ACADEMY OF FAMILY PHYSICIANS FOUNDATION

YS TO SIZE UP YOUR SERVINGS

...ou know exactly how much food you're eating
...uring cups aren't handy, you can still estimate your portion. Remember:

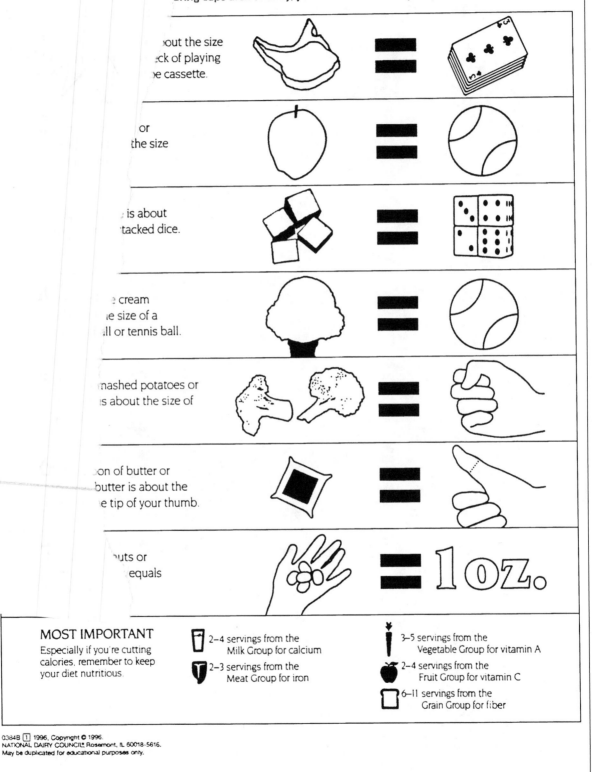

...out the size
...ck of playing
...e cassette.
=

...or
...the size
=

...is about
...tacked dice.
=

...e cream
...e size of a
...ll or tennis ball.
=

...nashed potatoes or
...is about the size of
=

...on of butter or
...butter is about the
...e tip of your thumb.
=

...uts or
...equals
= 1 oz.

MOST IMPORTANT
Especially if you're cutting
calories, remember to keep
your diet nutritious.

2–4 servings from the
Milk Group for calcium

2–3 servings from the
Meat Group for iron

3–5 servings from the
Vegetable Group for vitamin A

2–4 servings from the
Fruit Group for vitamin C

6–11 servings from the
Grain Group for fiber

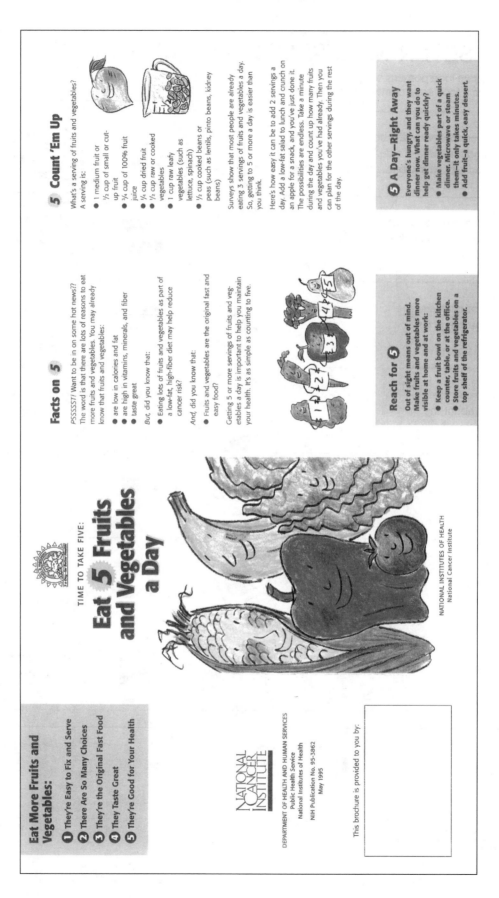

Eat More Fruits and Vegetables:

1. They're Easy to Fix and Serve
2. There Are So Many Choices
3. They're the Original Fast Food
4. They Taste Great
5. They're Good for Your Health

NATIONAL CANCER INSTITUTE

DEPARTMENT OF HEALTH AND HUMAN SERVICES
Public Health Service
National Institutes of Health

NIH Publication No. 95-3862
May 1995

This brochure is provided to you by:

TIME TO TAKE FIVE:

Eat 5 Fruits and Vegetables a Day

Facts on 5

PSSSSST! Want to be in on some hot news?? The word is that there are lots of reasons to eat more fruits and vegetables. You may already know that fruits and vegetables:

- are low in calories and fat
- are high in vitamins, minerals, and fiber
- taste great

But, did you know that:

- Eating lots of fruits and vegetables as part of a low-fat, high-fiber diet may help reduce cancer risk?

And, did you know that:

- Fruits and vegetables are the original fast and easy food?

Getting 5 or more servings of fruits and vegetables a day is important to help you maintain your health. It's as simple as counting to five.

NATIONAL INSTITUTES OF HEALTH
National Cancer Institute

---

5 Count 'Em Up

What's a serving of fruits and vegetables? A serving is:

- 1 medium fruit or ½ cup of small or cut-up fruit
- ¾ cup of 100% fruit juice
- ¼ cup dried fruit
- ½ cup raw or cooked vegetables
- 1 cup raw leafy vegetables (such as lettuce, spinach)
- ½ cup cooked beans or peas (such as lentils, pinto beans, kidney beans)

Surveys show that most people are already eating 3 servings of fruits and vegetables a day. So, getting to 5 or more a day is easier than you think.

Here's how easy it can be to add 2 servings a day. Add a low-fat salad to lunch and crunch on an apple for a snack, and you've just done it. The possibilities are endless. Take a minute during the day and count up how many fruits and vegetables you've had already. Then you can plan for the other servings during the rest of the day.

Reach for 5

Out of sight means out of mind. Make fruits and vegetables more visible at home and at work:

- **Keep a fruit bowl on the kitchen counter, table, or at the office.**
- **Store fruits and vegetables on a top shelf of the refrigerator.**

---

5 A Day–Right Away

Everyone's hungry, and they want dinner now. What can you do to help get dinner ready quickly?

- **Make vegetables part of a quick dinner. Microwave or steam them—it only takes minutes.**
- **Add fruit—a quick, easy dessert.**

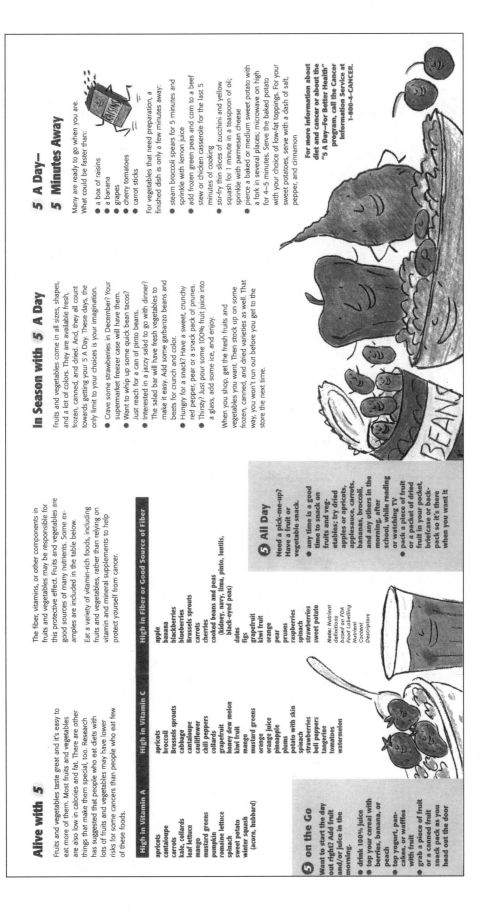

Alive with 5

Fruits and vegetables taste great and it's easy to eat more of them. Most fruits and vegetables are also low in calories and fat. There are other things that make them special, too. Research has suggested that people who eat diets with lots of fruits and vegetables may have lower risks for some cancers than people who eat few of these foods.

The fiber, vitamins, or other components in fruits and vegetables may be responsible for this protective effect. Fruits and vegetables are good sources of many nutrients. Some examples are included in the table below.

Eat a variety of vitamin-rich foods, including fruits and vegetables, rather than relying on vitamin and mineral supplements to help protect yourself from cancer.

High in Vitamin A	High in Vitamin C	High in Fiber or Good Source of Fiber
apricots	apricots	apple
cantaloupe	broccoli	banana
carrots	Brussels sprouts	blackberries
kale, collards	cabbage	blueberries
leaf lettuce	cantaloupe	Brussels sprouts
mango	cauliflower	carrots
mustard greens	chili peppers	cherries
pumpkin	collards	cooked beans and peas
romaine lettuce	grapefruit	(kidney, navy, lima, pinto, lentils,
spinach	honey dew melon	black-eyed peas)
sweet potato	kiwi fruit	dates
winter squash	mango	figs
(acorn, hubbard)	mustard greens	grapefruit
	orange	kiwi fruit
	orange juice	orange
	pineapple	pear
	plums	prunes
	potato with skin	raspberries
	spinach	spinach
	strawberries	strawberries
	bell peppers	sweet potato
	tangerine	
	tomatoes	Note: Nutrient
	watermelon	definitions
		based on FDA
		Food Labelling
		Nutrient
		Content
		Descriptors

5 on the Go

Want to start the day out right? Add fruit and/or juice in the morning.

● drink 100% juice
● top your cereal with berries, banana, or peach
● top yogurt, pancakes, or waffles with fruit
● grab a piece of fruit or a canned fruit snack pack as you head out the door

In Season with 5 A Day

Fruits and vegetables come in all sizes, shapes, and a lot of colors. They are available fresh, frozen, canned, and dried. And, they all count towards getting your 5 A Day. These days, the only limit to your choices is your imagination.

● Crave some strawberries in December? Your supermarket freezer case will have them.
● Want to whip up some quick bean tacos? Just reach for a can of pinto beans.
● Interested in a jazzy salad to go with dinner? The salad bar will have fresh vegetables to make it easy. Add some garbanzo beans and beets for crunch and color.
● Hungry for a snack? Have a sweet, crunchy red pepper, pear or a snack pack of prunes.
● Thirsty? Just pour some 100% fruit juice into a glass, add some ice, and enjoy.

When you shop, get the fresh fruits and vegetables you want. Then stock up on some frozen, canned, and dried varieties as well. That way, you won't run out before you get to the store the next time.

5 All Day

Need a pick-me-up? Have a fruit or vegetable snack.

● any time is a good time to snack on fruits and vegetables; try dried apples or apricots, applesauce, carrots, bananas, broccoli, and any others in the morning, after school, while reading or watching TV
● pack a piece of fruit or a packet of dried fruit in your pocket, briefcase or backpack so it's there when you want it

5 A Day—5 Minutes Away

Many are ready to go when you are. What could be faster than:

● a box of raisins
● a banana
● grapes
● cherry tomatoes
● carrot sticks

For vegetables that need preparation, a finished dish is only a few minutes away:

● steam broccoli spears for 5 minutes and sprinkle with lemon juice
● add frozen green peas and corn to a beef stew or chicken casserole for the last 5 minutes of cooking
● stir-fry thin slices of zucchini and yellow squash for 1 minute in a teaspoon of oil; sprinkle with parmesan cheese
● pierce a baked or medium sweet potato with a fork in several places; microwave on high for 4–5 minutes. Serve the baked potato with your choice of low-fat toppings. For your sweet potatoes, serve with a dash of salt, pepper, and cinnamon

For more information about diet and cancer or about the "5 A Day—For Better Health" program, call the Cancer Information Service at 1-800-4-CANCER.

Appendix 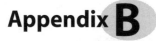 B

Physical Activity Resources

Government Resources

Centers for Disease Control and Prevention Fact Sheets on Physical Activity. **www.cdc.gov/nccdphp/sgr/fact.htm** (accessed May 22, 2000). The fact sheets *Adolescents and Young Adults* and *The Link Between Physical Activity and Morbidity and Mortality* provide information on physical activity levels among youth and list the health benefits of physical activity. For more information, contact the Centers for Disease Control and Prevention, National Center for Chronic Disease Prevention and Health Promotion, Division of Nutrition and Physical Activity, MS K-46, 4770 Buford Highway NE, Atlanta, GA 30341-3724; 1-888-CDC-4NRG or 1-888-232-4674 (toll-free).

Television Resources

Gortmaker, Steven L., Aviva Must, Arthur M. Sobol, Karen Peterson, Graham A. Colditz, and William H. Dietz. 1996. Television viewing as a cause of increasing obesity among children in the United States, 1986–1990. *Archives of Pediatrics & Adolescent Medicine.* 150: 356–362. This article provides evidence that excessive TV viewing contributes to obesity and suggests that decreasing TV time can help prevent this health condition.

Physical Activity Guidelines

Ainsworth, Barbara E., William L. Haskell, Arthur S. Leon, David R. Jacobs, Jr., Henry J. Montoye, James F. Sallis, and Ralph S. Paffenbarger, Jr. 1993. Compendium of physical activities: Classification of energy costs of human physical activities. *Medicine and Science in Sports and Exercise.* 25:71–80. (See the following section.) This journal article contains an appendix that lists MET values (rate of energy expenditure) for many activities.

U.S. Department of Health and Human Services. 2000. *Healthy People 2010.* Conference edition. **www.health.gov/healthypeople.** This report describes national goals for health promotion, protection, prevention, and surveillance.

Compendium of Physical Activities: Classification of Energy Costs of Human Physical Activities

Barbara E. Ainsworth, William L. Haskell, Arthur S. Leon, David R. Jacobs, Jr., Henry J. Montoye, James F. Sallis, and Ralph S. Paffenbarger, Jr. (see reference above)

Abstract

A coding scheme is presented for classifying physical activity by rate of energy expenditure, i.e., by intensity. Energy cost was established by a review of published and unpublished data. This coding scheme employs five digits that classify activity by purpose (i.e., sports, occupation, self-care), the specific type of activity, and its intensity as the ratio of work metabolic rate to resting metabolic rate (METs). Energy expenditure in kilcalories or kilocalories per kilogram body weight can be estimated for all activities, specific activities, or activity types. General use of this coding system would enhance the comparability of results across studies using self reports of physical activity.

METs for Selected Activities

Activity	METs	Activity	METs
Bicycling		**Conditioning**	
< 10 mph	4.0	Calisthenics, moderate effort	4.5
10-11.9 mph, light effort	6.0	Calisthenics, vigorous effort	8.0
12-13.9 mph, moderate effort	8.0	Weightlifting, light effort	3.0
14-15.9 mph, vigorous effort	10.0	Weightlifting, vigorous effort	6.0
Dancing		**Lawn and garden**	
General	4.5	Mowing lawn, general	5.5
Aerobic, general	6.0	Mowing lawn, power mower	4.5
Aerobic, low impact	5.0	Raking leaves	4.0
Aerobic, high impact	7.0	Shoveling snow	6.0
Home activities (chores)		**Running**	
Cleaning house, general	3.5	Jogging, general	7.0
Washing dishes	2.3	Running, cross-country	9.0
Cooking or food preparation	2.5	Running, general	8.0
Child care	3.5	Running up stairs	15.0
Walking		**Sports**	
Hiking, cross-country	6.0	Basketball, game	8.0
Race walking	6.5	Rope jumping, moderate	10.0
Walking, moderate pace	3.5	Skating, roller	7.0
Walking, vigorous pace	4.0	Soccer, general	7.0
Winter activities		**Water activities**	
Skating, ice, general	7.0	Canoeing, rowing, moderate effort	7.0
Skiing, cross-country	7.0	Canoeing, rowing, vigorous effort	12.0
Skiing, downhill, moderate effort	6.0	Swimming laps, moderate effort	8.0
Skiing, downhill, vigorous effort	8.0	Swimming laps, vigorous effort	10.0
Inactivity		**Miscellaneous**	
Watching TV	0.9	Sitting, reading	1.3
Sleeping	0.9	Sitting, writing	1.8
Reading	1.0	Siting, studying	1.8
Talking on phone	1.0	Sitting, in class	1.8

Ainsworth et al., 1993

Appendix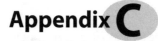

Social Studies Resources

Massachusetts Resources

The following resources are specific to Massachusetts but can be used to provide an example of how a state makes a law. You should be able to find government resources for your own state at your state's web page. To obtain the following resources, contact the Secretary of the Commonwealth, Tours and Government Education Division, State House Room 194, Boston, MA 02133 (phone 617-727-3676), or visit the listed websites.

- *The Ladybug Story: A Story About Lawmaking.* This resource on lawmaking for students tells how a second grade class worked to have the ladybug named the official Massachusetts state bug. **www.magnet.state.ma.us/sec/trs/trslbs/lbsidx.htm**

- *Lawmaking in Massachusetts.* This resource on lawmaking for the teacher provides a more detailed description of the lawmaking process and includes a glossary of important terms. **www.magnet.state.ma.us/sec/trs/trslaw/lawidx.htm**

Appendix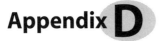

Charting TV Viewing Time

This lesson encourages students to keep TV, video, and computer game time to less than 2 hours per day. Students track and graph their own viewing time and try to decrease it for 1 week. This lesson is designed to infuse information about increasing physical activity and decreasing TV viewing into a math, science, or health class. Optional activities are also included for other subject areas.

▶▶ Behavioral Objective

For students to keep their TV viewing and video-game playing time to less than 2 hours per day.

▶▶ Learning Objectives

Students will be able to

1. chart TV watching and video-game playing for a 2-week period,
2. create bar graphs, line graphs, or pie charts of their TV viewing time and video-game playing time,
3. discuss the advantages and disadvantages of using the different types of graphs to represent data,
4. discuss the importance of accurate gathering and reporting of data,
5. calculate the amount of time they have spent watching TV and playing video games in their lifetime, and
6. discuss the importance of increasing activity and decreasing TV viewing and video-game playing to no more than 2 hours per day.

▶▶ Materials

- Graph paper, rulers, magic markers, poster paper, tape, protractor, and a compass
- Activity 1 *TV Viewing* charts (weeks 1 and 2)
- Activity 2 *Interpreting Week 1 Data*
- Activity 3 *Interpreting Week 2 Data*
- Overhead transparency 1
- Student resource 1 *Graphing Data*
- Optional: *Class Data* charts (weeks 1 and 2)

The unit can also be implemented using a computer. Enter data into spreadsheets, then create charts and graphs.

▶▶ Procedure

Week 1 (Day 1)

1. (3 minutes) Ask students to estimate how many hours per day they spend watching TV and videos and playing video games. What is their hypothesis; how much TV do they think they watch?

Throughout this activity when we refer to TV viewing, we mean watching TV or videos or playing computer and TV video games.

2. (5 minutes) Show overhead transparency 1. Point out the variables plotted on the *x*- and *y*-axis. Ask students the following:

- In 1967-70, how much TV was the largest group of children watching?
- What about in 1990?
- Where do you think you fall on this graph compared with children in 1990?

3. (2 minutes) Explain the following:

- During the next 2 weeks you will record the actual time you spend on screen time: watching TV, movies, and videos, and playing computer games and TV video games.
- During the first week you should track your regular viewing pattern.
- During the second week you will try to decrease your viewing time.
- The purpose of this activity is for you to become aware of the time you spend in these sedentary activities and then to decrease that time.
- You will have an exciting opportunity to participate in a scientific study, and accurate, honest reporting is as important as decreasing screen time. Statistics involves collecting, analyzing, and presenting data in an accurate manner. If you do not give honest information, the results won't be accurate.

4. (5 minutes) Hand out the TV viewing charts. Have students record their estimated viewing hours at the top of the chart for week 1. Explain that they should record their viewing daily for the next 7 days on the top half of the chart. Remind them to round to the nearest half hour and to express numbers as fractions: 2-1/2 hours, for example. We highly recommend that the extension activity 1 be included during this week. Mention the first of the ten Power Down Tips. You may choose to write a different one on the chalkboard every day or show them on an overhead. (See Teacher Resources.)

End of Week 1

1. (5 minutes) At the end of the first week, ask students to calculate their total number of viewing hours for the week as well as their daily average.

2. (20 minutes) Have students graph their data. Student resource 1 *Graphing Data* gives examples of types of graphs they might choose to construct. However, you may wish to (1) ask students to brainstorm what types of graphs they think would best represent their data, or (2) assign students different types of graphs so that they can compare the advantages and disadvantages of representing data using bar graphs, pie charts, and line graphs.

3. (10 minutes) Have students complete activity 2 *Interpreting Week 1 Data*. This activity asks them to estimate the amount of time they have spent watching TV in their lifetime. It also asks them to interpret their graphs and brainstorm some alternative activities they might do in week 2 to replace some of their screen time. You could assign this for homework.

4. (5 minutes) Explain that during the second Power Down week, students should try to limit their viewing time to a maximum of 2 hours per day, as recommended by the American Academy of Pediatrics. Ask students why they think reducing viewing time is important. Refer them to their responses on activity 1.

5. After eliciting student ideas, emphasize the following:

- Students should be active every day. Decreasing viewing time may encourage an increase in more active forms of entertainment.
- Activity is required for health. Children need activity to develop cardiovascular fitness, muscular strength, flexibility, and confidence in their physical ability.
- Just a small increase in physical activity can generate genuine health benefits. Refer to Teacher Resources for further discussion of this topic.

Week 2

1. During week 2, have students record their viewing time on the bottom half of the TV viewing charts.

2. (5 minutes) Have the class brainstorm some alternative activities to replace watching TV (they should refer to the ideas they generated in activity 2). Record their suggestions on a large piece of paper that can be displayed in the classroom. We strongly recommend that extension activity 1 be included during week 2.

End of Week 2

1. (15 minutes) At the end of the second week, have students calculate the number of hours watched per day and per week and graph their data.

2. (10 minutes) Students should compare their week 1 and week 2 graphs and use activity 3 *Interpreting Week 2 Data* to help them analyze their results.

3. (5 minutes) Put students into groups of four. Have students share their graphs and results. Students should calculate the average change in TV viewing time for their group and report their findings to the class. If students used different types of graphs to display their data, they should discuss and record the advantages and disadvantages of each type of graphic representation.

4. (10 minutes) Have the groups report their findings to the class.

5. Ask students the following:

- What conclusions can you draw from the class findings?
- Did the class as a whole meet the goal of watching TV and playing computer games for 2 hours or less per day?
- What recommendations about TV viewing patterns can you make?

▶▶ Extension Activities

Activity 1

1. During week 1 and week 2, students should record their daily total viewing time on the *Class Data* charts. Having students record their data as they enter the classroom each day will help remind them of their assignment. (Consider making this an anonymous activity by assigning each student a number, so that children don't feel inclined to fabricate their data.)

2. At the end of week 1, ask several volunteers to calculate the class daily average for week 1 and to construct a bar graph of the results.

3. At the end of week 2, ask several volunteers to calculate the class daily average for week 2 and to add this information to last week's bar graph.

4. Collaborate with other classes to construct a display of the class graphs from all the classrooms participating in Power Down. Calculate the school-wide average for weeks 1 and 2.

Activity 2

As a class, create a histogram that shows the frequency of total hours of screen time, comparing week 1 to week 2 of Power Down. Collect weekly totals for week 1 and week 2. Put the number of students on the vertical axis and the total range of hours on the horizontal axis. Separate the total number of viewing hours into 5-hour ranges, beginning with 0-5 hours and ending with 20 hours or more. Shade your bars for week 1 to contrast them with week 2.

Activity 3

Ask older relatives or friends what they did as children to entertain themselves. They are likely to suggest good non-TV activities.

Activity 4

Make a poster or collage of activities you could do instead of watching TV.

Activity 5

Create a symbol, poster, or logo for the campaign.

Activity 6

Give parents copies of the TV viewing charts and have them keep track of their viewing time.

▶▶ Writing Activities

Activity 1

Ask students to write a report summarizing the purpose of the study, their hypothesis, graphs, calculations, and analysis questions on activities 1 and 2.

Activity 2

Write an essay about what life would be like without TV.

▶▶ Teacher Resources

General Background Material

In preparing for this lesson, you may want to refer to the following resources:

- *Television Viewing as a Cause of Increasing Obesity Among Children in the United States, 1986–1990*
- *Physical Activity Guidelines for Adolescents: Consensus Statement*

See appendix B for information on how to obtain these resources.

Specific Background Material

Planet Health endorses the American Academy of Pediatrics recommendation to limit TV viewing to no more than 2 hours per day.

Planet Health's Activity Message: Physical activity promotes health and well-being, and offers opportunities to socialize and have fun. Adolescents should be moderately active for at least 30 minutes every day or nearly every day as part of play, games, sports, chores, transportation, or planned exercise, AND they should aim for at least three sessions per week of vigorous physical activity lasting 20 minutes or more.

Included in the concept of TV time are the following: TV shows, videos, movies at theaters, and computer and video games. Students should aim for a daily average of 2 hours or less for all of these sources of "screen time" combined. Computer time spent doing homework is not targeted for reduction by Power Down.

Power Down Tips

These are simple messages focused on decreasing TV viewing. You can write a different one on the chalkboard every day or use an overhead transparency.

Did You Know?

1. The average child spends more time watching TV than any other activity except sleeping.
2. Kicking the TV habit gets easier as time passes.
3. You don't have to sit still while watching TV—you can be dancing, cleaning, cooking, or doing something else.

Strive to Decrease TV Time.

1. The percentage of 12-17 year olds watching TV for 5 or more hours per day has increased greatly, from 13% in 1967-70 to 43% in 1990.
2. One easy way to cut down on TV time is to take the TV out of the room where you sleep (if applicable). If you don't want to physically take it out of the room, you can just unplug it.
3. During Power Down week, post TV tracking reminders on refrigerators, bulletin boards, and near TV sets.
4. Watch TV only if your favorite show is on.

Trade TV Time for Active Time

1. Watching less than 2 hours of TV each day can help you get fit!
2. Take note of the times when you watch TV but you aren't really interested—when you channel surf or watch reruns. Take this as an opportunity to be physically active instead.
3. Physical activity builds fitness, is fun, and helps release energy! Just a small increase in physical activity can generate genuine benefits.

Hours of TV viewed per day in US youth aged 12-17 in 1967-70 vs. youths in 1990

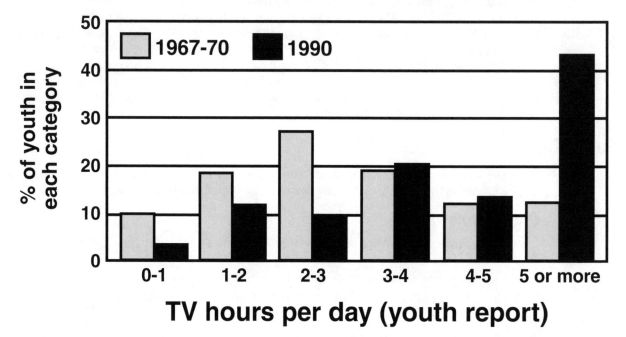

Source: Gortmaker, S.L. Unpublished data. National Health Examination Survey, 1967-70, and National Longitudinal Survey of Youth, 1990.

Name _____

Choose one of the following types of graphs (pie chart, line graph, or histogram) to represent your TV viewing hours.

Pie Chart

How much of time do you spend watching TV and videos and playing computer games?

- Take a *typical* day from week 1 and a *typical* day from week 2 (Power Down week).
- Create a pie chart for each week with the following categories: school, TV/computer games/video games, sleeping, eating, homework, physical activity, going to/from school, and other. Round to the nearest half hour.
- Use a different color for each sector.

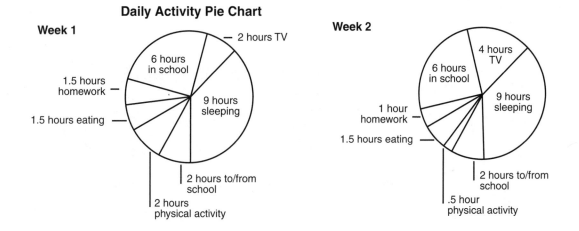

Daily Activity Pie Chart

Optional: Calculate the central angle of the sector for each activity. (Remember that the whole pie has 360 degrees.) Calculate the circumference and the area of your circle. Record your findings next to the pie charts.

Line Graph

Create a line graph (or coordinate graph) comparing TV viewing time in week 1 and week 2 (Power Down week).

- Put the number of hours of TV watched on the vertical axis and the days of the week on the horizontal axis.
- Plot the hours per day you spent watching TV and videos and playing computer games.
- Use a solid line to connect week 1 data points and a dashed line to connect week 2 data points.

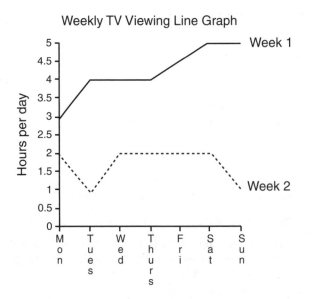

Weekly TV Viewing Line Graph

Histogram

Create a histogram that compares the number of hours you spent watching TV during week 1 to week 2.

- Put the number of hours of TV watched per day on the vertical axis and the days of the week on the horizontal axis.

- Create one bar for each day you spent watching TV and videos and playing computer games. Do **not** shade week 1 bars.

- Add a shaded or colored bar next to each of your week 1 bars to represent your TV viewing for week 2. (See example.)

- At the far right of the horizontal axis graph your week 1 and week 2 averages

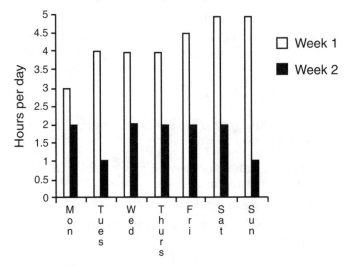

Weekly TV Viewing Histogram

Optional: Chart the week 2 weekly averages as individuals and as a class.

Name _____

Start date _____

Television Viewing Chart
Week 1

Estimated daily average prior to doing this activity:				
Day of week	**TV and videos on TV**	**Movies at the cinema**	**Computer/video games**	**Total time**
	(list time spent in each activity, rounded to the nearest half hour)			(add times across)
Saturday				
Sunday				
Monday				
Tuesday				
Wednesday				
Thursday				
Friday				
Weekly average:			**Weekly total:**	

Television Viewing Chart
Week 2

Day of week	**TV and videos on TV**	**Movies at the cinema**	**Computer/video games**	**Total time**
	(list time spent in each activity, rounded to the nearest half hour)			(add times across)
Saturday				
Sunday				
Monday				
Tuesday				
Wednesday				
Thursday				
Friday				
Weekly average:			**Weekly total:**	

Answer the following questions based on the results of your week 1 TV viewing charts and graphs.

Graph Interpretation

1. On which days did you spend the most time in front of a TV, movie screen, or computer? Why did you watch more on those days?

2. On which days did you spend the least time on these activities? Why did you watch less on those days?

3. How did your daily *estimate* compare to your *actual* daily average?

4. How much higher or lower was your average daily viewing compared to the national recommendations?

5. Using your week 1 total viewing time as a weekly average, how much time have you spent on these activities in your lifetime? Explain how you came up with the answer.

Questions for Reflection

1. What is the role of TV and computers in your life?

2. Why is it important to limit your TV viewing and other screen time?

3. Compared to last year at this time, are you more or less active? Why do you think that your activity level went up or down?

4. Brainstorm five activities you enjoy doing that could replace screen time.

Answer the following questions based on the results of your week 1 and week 2 TV viewing charts and graphs.

Graph Interpretations

1. Describe how your viewing pattern changed during week 2.

2. How much higher or lower was your average daily viewing in week 2 compared to the national recommendations?

3. Using your week 2 total viewing time as a weekly average, how much time have you spent on these activities in your lifetime? Explain how you came up with the answer. (Complete this on the reverse side.)

4. What is the difference between the total lifetime viewing calculated above and the total you calculated using week 1 data?

Student name	Sunday	Monday	Tuesday	Wednesday	Thursday	Friday	Saturday	Weekly total
1.								
2.								
3.								
4.								
5.								
6.								
7.								
8.								
9.								
10.								
11.								
12.								
13.								
14.								
15.								
16.								
17.								
18.								
19.								
20.								
21.								
22.								
23.								
24.								
25.								
26.								

Student name	Sunday	Monday	Tuesday	Wednesday	Thursday	Friday	Saturday	Weekly total
1.								
2.								
3.								
4.								
5.								
6.								
7.								
8.								
9.								
10.								
11.								
12.								
13.								
14.								
15.								
16.								
17.								
18.								
19.								
20.								
21.								
22.								
23.								
24.								
25.								
26.								

Appendix 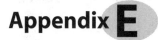 E

Massachusetts Curriculum Frameworks

The following curriculum frameworks will help you select lessons that best suit your curriculum objectives. *Planet Health* lessons meet Massachusetts Department of Education learning standards in health, English language arts, math, science and technology, and history and social science.

Language Arts

Lesson	Theme	Area	Learning standard/strand
32 Pyramid Power	Balanced diet	Health	Personal and physical health strand/content area nutrition
		Language arts	Learning standard 1 (language strand)
		Language arts	Learning standard 2 (language strand)
		Language arts	Learning standard 3 (language strand)
		Language arts	Learning standard 9 (literature strand)
		Language arts	Learning standard 19 (composition strand)
		Language arts	Learning standard 23 (composition strand)
33 Carbohydrates: Energy Food	Balanced diet	Health	Personal and physical health strand/content area nutrition
		Language arts	Learning standard 1 (language strand)
		Language arts	Learning standard 2 (language strand)
		Language arts	Learning standard 4 (language strand)
		Language arts	Learning standard 9 (literature strand)
		Language arts	Learning standard 13 (literature strand)
		Language arts	Learning standard 19 (composition strand)
		Language arts	Learning standard 23 (composition strand)

Lesson	Theme	Area	Learning standard/strand
34 The Language of Food	Fruits and vegetables	Health	Personal and physical health strand/content area nutrition
		Language arts	Learning standard 1 (language strand)
		Language arts	Learning standard 2 (language strand)
		Language arts	Learning standard 4 (language strand)
		Language arts	Learning standard 9 (literature strand)
		Language arts	Learning standard 10 (literature strand)
		Language arts	Learning standard 11 (literature strand)
		Language arts	Learning standard 15 (literature strand)
		Language arts	Learning standard 20 (composition strand)
35 Keep it Local	Fruits and vegetables	Health	Personal and physical health strand/content area nutrition
		Health	Community and environmental health strand/content area group and community health
		Language arts	Learning standard 1 (language strand)
		Language arts	Learning standard 2 (language strand)
		Language arts	Learning standard 3 (language strand)
		Language arts	Learning standard 4 (language strand)
		Language arts	Learning standard 9 (literature strand)
		Language arts	Learning standard 10 (literature strand)
		Language arts	Learning standard 13 (literature strand)
		Language arts	Learning standard 15 (literature strand)
		Language arts	Learning standard 20 (composition strand)
36 Write a Fable: Important Messages About Activity	Activity	Health	Personal and physical health strand/content area physical activity and fitness
		Language arts	Learning standard 1 (language strand)
		Language arts	Learning standard 2 (language strand)
		Language arts	Learning standard 4 (language strand)
		Language arts	Learning standard 9 (literature strand)
		Language arts	Learning standard 10 (literature strand)
		Language arts	Learning standard 20 (composition strand)
		Language arts	Learning standard 22 (composition strand)

(continued)

(continued)

Lesson	Theme	Area	Learning standard/strand
37 Go for the Goal	Activity	Health	Personal and physical health strand/content area physical activity and fitness
		Language arts	Learning standard 1 (language strand)
		Language arts	Learning standard 2 (language strand)
		Language arts	Learning standard 4 (language strand)
		Language arts	Learning standard 9 (literature strand)
		Language arts	Learning standard 11 (literature strand)
38 Lifetime Physical Activities: Research One, Describe One, Try One!	Lifestyle	Health	Personal and physical health strand/content area physical activity and fitness
		Language arts	Learning standard 1 (language strand)
		Language arts	Learning standard 2 (language strand)
		Language arts	Learning standard 3 (language strand)
		Language arts	Learning standard 4 (language strand)
		Language arts	Learning standard 9 (literature strand)
		Language arts	Learning standard 19 (composition strand)
		Language arts	Learning standard 22 (composition strand)
39 Choosing Healthy Foods	Lifestyle	Health	Personal and physical health strand/content area nutrition
		Language arts	Learning standard 1 (language strand)
		Language arts	Learning standard 2 (language strand)
			Learning standard 2 (language strand)
		Language arts	Learning standard 3 (language strand)
		Language arts	Learning standard 4 (language strand)
		Language arts	Learning standard 9 (literature strand)
		Language arts	Learning standard 28 (media strand)

Math

Lesson	Theme	Area	Learning standard/strand
40 Problem Solving: Making Healthy Choices	Balanced diet	Health	Personal and physical health strand/content area nutrition
		Language arts	Learning standard 1 (language strand)
		Language arts	Learning standard 2 (language strand)
		Language arts	Learning standard 3 (language strand)
		Language arts	Learning standard 4 (language strand)
		Language arts	Learning standard 9 (literature strand)
		Mathematics	Learning standard 1.6 (number sense strand: number and number relationships)
		Mathematics	Learning standard 1.8 (number sense strand: computation and estimation)
		Mathematics	Learning standard 2.4 (patterns, relations, and functions strand: patterns and functions)
41 Figuring Out Fat	Balanced diet	Health	Personal and physical health strand/content area nutrition
		Language arts	Learning standard 1 (language strand)
		Language arts	Learning standard 2 (language strand)
		Language arts	Learning standard 4 (language strand)
		Language arts	Learning standard 9 (literature strand)
		Mathematics	Learning standard 1.6 (number sense strand: number and number relationships)
		Mathematics	Learning standard 1.8 (number sense strand: computation and estimation)
		Mathematics	Learning standard 2.4 (patterns, relations, and functions strand: patterns and functions)
42 Looking for Patterns: What's for Lunch?	Balanced diet	Health	Personal and physical health strand/content area nutrition
		Language arts	Learning standard 1 (language strand)
		Language arts	Learning standard 2 (language strand)
		Language arts	Learning standard 3 (language strand)
		Language arts	Learning standard 4 (language strand)
		Language arts	Learning standard 9 (literature strand)

(continued)

511

(continued)

Lesson	Theme	Area	Learning standard/strand
		Mathematics	Learning standard 2.5 (patterns, relations, and functions strand: algebra)
		Mathematics	Learning standard 4.2 (statistics and probability strand: statistics
43 Apples, Oranges, and Zucchini: An Algebra Party	Fruits and vegetables	Health	Personal and physical health strand/content area nutrition
		Language arts	Learning standard 1 (language strand)
		Language arts	Learning standard 2 (language strand)
		Language arts	Learning standard 4 (language strand)
		Language arts	Learning standard 9 (literature strand)
		Mathematics	Learning standard 2.5 (patterns, relations, and functions strand: algebra)
44 Plotting Coordinate Graphs: What Does Your Day Look Like?	Activity	Health	Personal and physical health strand/content area physical activity and fitness
		Language arts	Learning standard 1 (language strand)
		Language arts	Learning standard 2 (language strand)
		Language arts	Learning standard 4 (language strand)
		Language arts	Learning standard 9 (literature strand)
		Mathematics	Learning standard 2.4 (patterns, relations, and functions strand: algebra)
		Mathematics	Learning standard 2.5 (patterns, relations, and functions strand: algebra)
45 Survey the Class	Activity	Health	Personal and physical health strand/content area physical activity and fitness
		Language arts	Learning standard 1 (language strand)
		Language arts	Learning standard 2 (language strand)
		Language arts	Learning standard 4 (language strand)
		Language arts	Learning standard 9 (literature strand)
		Mathematics	Learning standard 4.2 (statistics and probability strand: statistics)

Lesson	Theme	Area	Learning standard/strand
46 Circle Graphs: Where Did the Day Go?	Lifestyle	Health	Personal and physical health strand/content area physical activity and fitness
		Language arts	Learning standard 1 (language strand)
		Language arts	Learning standard 2 (language strand)
		Language arts	Learning standard 4 (language strand)
		Language arts	Learning standard 9 (literature strand)
		Language arts	Learning standard 19 (composition strand)
		Mathematics	Learning standard 1.6 (number sense strand: number and number relationships)
		Mathematics	Learning standard 2.4 (patterns, relations, and functions strand: patterns and functions)
		Mathematics	Learning standard 3.4 (geometry and measurement strand: measurement)
47 Energy Equations	Lifestyle	Health	Personal and physical health strand/content area nutrition
		Language arts	Learning standard 1 (language strand)
		Language arts	Learning standard 2 (language strand)
		Language arts	Learning standard 4 (language strand)
		Language arts	Learning standard 9 (literature strand)
		Language arts	Learning standard 19 (composition strand)
		Mathematics	Learning standard 1.6 (number sense strand: number and number relationships)
		Mathematics	Learning standard 2.4 (patterns, relations, and functions strand: patterns and functions)
		Mathematics	Learning standard 4.2 (statistics and probability strand: statistics)

Science

Lesson	Theme	Area	Learning standard/strand
48 Mighty Minerals: Calcium and Iron	Balanced diet	Health	Personal and physical health strand/content area nutrition
		Health	Community and environmental health strand/content area disease prevention and control
		Language arts	Learning standard 1 (language strand)
		Language arts	Learning standard 2 (language strand)
		Language arts	Learning standard 4 (language strand)
		Language arts	Learning standard 9 (literature strand)
		Language arts	Learning standard 19 (composition strand)
		Science and technology	Strand 1: Inquiry
		Science and technology	Strand 2: Domains of science–Life sciences
49 Fat Functions	Balanced diet	Health	Personal and physical health strand/content area nutrition
		Language arts	Learning standard 1 (language strand)
		Language arts	Learning standard 2 (language strand)
		Language arts	Learning standard 4 (language strand)
		Language arts	Learning standard 9 (literature strand)
		Science and technology	Strand 1: Inquiry
		Science and technology	Strand 2: Domains of science–Life sciences
50 Smart Snacks	Balanced diet	Health	Personal and physical health strand/content area nutrition
		Language arts	Learning standard 1 (language strand)
		Language arts	Learning standard 2 (language strand)
		Language arts	Learning standard 4 (language strand)
		Language arts	Learning standard 9 (literature strand)
		Science and technology	Strand 1: Inquiry
		Science and technology	Strand 2: Domains of science–Life sciences

Lesson	Theme	Area	Learning standard/strand
51 The Plants We Eat	Fruits and vegetables	Health	Personal and physical health strand/content area nutrition
		Language arts	Learning standard 1 (language strand)
		Language arts	Learning standard 2 (language strand)
		Language arts	Learning standard 4 (language strand)
		Language arts	Learning standard 9 (literature strand)
		Science and technology	Strand 1: Inquiry
		Science and technology	Strand 2: Domains of science–Life sciences
52 Foods for Energy	Activity	Health	Personal and physical health strand/content area nutrition
		Language arts	Learning standard 1 (language strand)
		Language arts	Learning standard 2 (language strand)
		Language arts	Learning standard 4 (language strand)
		Language arts	Learning standard 9 (literature strand)
		Science and technology	Strand 1: Inquiry
		Science and technology	Strand 2: Domains of science–Life sciences
53 Muscle Mysteries	Activity	Health	Personal and physical health strand/content area physical activity and fitness
		Language arts	Learning standard 1 (language strand)
		Language arts	Learning standard 2 (language strand)
		Language arts	Learning standard 4 (language strand)
		Language arts	Learning standard 9 (literature strand)
		Science and technology	Strand 1: Inquiry
		Science and technology	Strand 2: Domains of science–Life sciences
54 The Human Heart	Lifestyle	Health	Personal and physical health strand/content area physical activity and fitness
		Language arts	Learning standard 1 (language strand)
		Language arts	Learning standard 2 (language strand)
		Language arts	Learning standard 4 (language strand)
		Language arts	Learning standard 9 (literature strand)

(continued)

(continued)

Lesson	Theme	Area	Learning standard/strand
		Science and technology	Strand 1: Inquiry
		Science and technology	Strand 2: Domains of science–Life sciences
55 How Far Can You Jump?	Lifestyle	Health	Personal and physical health strand/content area physical activity and fitness
		Language arts	Learning standard 1 (language strand)
		Language arts	Learning standard 2 (language strand)
		Language arts	Learning standard 4 (language strand)
		Language arts	Learning standard 9 (literature strand)
		Science and technology	Strand 1: Inquiry
		Science and technology	Strand 2: Domains of science–Life sciences

Social Studies

Lesson	Theme	Area	Learning standard/strand
56 Food Through the Ages	Balanced diet	Health	Personal and physical health strand/content area nutrition
		Language arts	Learning standard 1 (language strand)
		Language arts	Learning standard 2 (language strand)
		Language arts	Learning standard 4 (language strand)
		Language arts	Learning standard 9 (literature strand)
		Language arts	Learning standard 19 (composition strand)
		History and social science	Learning standard 1 chronology and cause (history strand)
		History and social science	Learning standard 3 research evidence and point of view (history strand)
57 Democracy and Diet	Balanced diet	Health	Personal and physical health strand/content area nutrition
		Language arts	Learning standard 1 (language strand)
		Language arts	Learning standard 2 (language strand)
		Language arts	Learning standard 4 (language strand)
		Language arts	Learning standard 9 (literature strand)
		Language arts	Learning standard 19 (composition strand)
		History and social science	Learning standard 18 principles and practices of American government (civics and government strand)
		History and social science	Learning standard 19 citizenship (civics and government strand)
58 Global Foods	Fruits and vegetables	Health	Personal and physical health strand/content area nutrition
		Language arts	Learning standard 1 (language strand)
		Language arts	Learning standard 2 (language strand)
		Language arts	Learning standard 4 (language strand)
		Language arts	Learning standard 9 (literature strand)
		Language arts	Learning standard 19 (composition strand)
		History and social science	Learning standard 9 the effects of geography (geography strand)

(continued)

(continued)

Lesson	Theme	Area	Learning standard/strand
59 Around the World With Five a Day	Fruits and vegetables	Health	Personal and physical health strand/content area nutrition
		Language arts	Learning standard 1 (language strand)
		Language arts	Learning standard 2 (language strand)
		Language arts	Learning standard 3 (language strand)
		Language arts	Learning standard 4 (language strand)
		Language arts	Learning standard 9 (literature strand)
		Language arts	Learning standard 19 (composition strand)
		History and social science	Learning standard 1 chronology and cause (history strand)
		History and social science	Learning standard 3 research evidence and point of view (history strand)
		History and social science	Learning standard 8 places and regions of the world (geography strand)
60 Map Maker	Activity	Health	Personal and physical health strand/content area physical activity and fitness
		Language arts	Learning standard 1 (language strand)
		Language arts	Learning standard 2 (language strand)
		Language arts	Learning standard 4 (language strand)
		Language arts	Learning standard 9 (literature strand)
		Language arts	Learning standard 19 (composition strand)
		History and social science	Learning standard 7 physical spaces of the earth (geography strand)
61 Free to be Fit	Activity	Health	Personal and physical health strand/content area physical activity and fitness
		Language arts	Learning standard 1 (language strand)
		Language arts	Learning standard 2 (language strand)
		Language arts	Learning standard 4 (language strand)
		Language arts	Learning standard 9 (literature strand)
		Language arts	Learning standard 19 (composition strand)
		History and social science	Learning standard 17 the founding documents (civics and government strand)
		History and social science	Learning standard 19 citizenship (civics and government strand)

Lesson	Theme	Area	Learning standard/strand
62 Impact of Technology	Lifestyle	Health	Personal and physical health strand/content area physical activity and fitness
		Language arts	Learning standard 1 (language strand)
		Language arts	Learning standard 2 (language strand)
		Language arts	Learning standard 4 (language strand)
		Language arts	Learning standard 9 (literature strand)
		Language arts	Learning standard 19 (composition strand)
		History and social science	Learning standard 1 chronology and cause (history strand)
		History and social science	Learning standard 6 interdisciplinary learning: natural science, mathematics, and technology in history (history strand)
		History and social science	Learning standard 9 the effects of geography (geography strand)
		History and social science	Learning standard 10 human alteration of environments (geography strand)
		History and social science	Learning standard 13 the economy of the United States (economic strand)
63 Food Rituals and Society	Lifestyle	Health	Personal and physical health strand/content area nutrition
		Language arts	Learning standard 1 (language strand)
		Language arts	Learning standard 2 (language strand)
		Language arts	Learning standard 3 (language strand)
		Language arts	Learning standard 4 (language strand)
		Language arts	Learning standard 9 (literature strand)
		Language arts	Learning standard 19 (composition strand)
		History and social science	Learning standard 5 interdisciplinary learning: religion, ethics, philosophy, and literature in history (history strand)
		History and social science	Learning standard 8 places and regions of the world (geography strand)

Health

Personal and Physical Health Strand/Content Area Nutrition: Students will gain the knowledge and skills to select a diet that supports health and reduces the risk of illness and future chronic diseases.

Personal and Physical Health Strand/Content Area Physical Activity and Fitness: Students will acquire the principles of training and conditioning and will apply the concept of wellness to their lives.

Community and Environmental Health Strand/Content Area Disease Prevention and Control: Students will learn signs, symptoms, and treatment of chronic diseases, and gain skills related to health promotion, disease prevention and health maintenance.

Community and Environmental Health Strand/Content Area Group and Community Health: Students will learn the influence of social, cultural, and economic factors on health and will gain skills to promote health and collaborate with others to facilitate healthy, safe, and supportive communities.

Language Arts

Learning Standard 1 (Language Strand): Students will use agreed-upon rules for informal and formal discussion in small and large groups.

Learning Standard 2 (Language Strand): Students will pose questions, listen to the ideas of others, and contribute their own information or ideas in group discussions and interviews in order to acquire new knowledge.

Learning Standard 3 (Language Strand): Students will make oral presentations that demonstrate appropriate consideration of audience, purpose, and information to be conveyed.

Learning Standard 4 (Language Strand): Students will acquire and use correctly an advanced reading vocabulary of English words.

Learning Standard 9 (Literature Strand): Students will identify the basic facts and essential ideas in what they have read and heard.

Learning Standard 10 (Literature Strand): Students will identify, analyze, and apply knowledge of the characteristics of different genres.

Learning Standard 11 (Literature Strand): Students will identify, analyze, and apply knowledge of theme in literature and poetry and provide evidence from the text to support their understanding.

Learning Standard 13 (Literature Strand): Students will apply knowledge of the structure, elements and meaning of informational material and provide evidence from the text to support their understanding.

Learning Standard 15 (Literature Strand): Students will identify and analyze how an author's choice of words sets tone and appeals to the senses.

Learning Standard 19 (Composition Strand): Students will write with a clear focus, logically developed ideas and adequate detail.

Learning Standard 20 (Composition Strand): Students will select and use appropriate genres when writing for different audiences and rhetorical purposes.

Learning Standard 22 (Composition Strand): Students will use knowledge of standard English conventions to edit their writing.

Learning Standard 23 (Composition Strand): Students will use self-generated questions, note-taking, summarizing, precis writing, and outlining (concept mapping) to enhance learning when reading and writing.

Learning Standard 28 (Media Strand): Students will design and create coherent media productions with a clear controlling idea, adequate detail, and appropriate consideration of audience, purpose, and medium.

Mathematics

Learning Standard 1.6 (Number Sense Strand: Number and Number Relationships): Students engage in problem solving, communicating, reasoning and connecting to apply proportions and percents; to investigate and describe the relationships among fractions, decimals and percents; to represent numerical relationships in one- and two-dimensional graphs; and to apply ratios, proportions and percents.

Learning Standard 1.8 (Number Sense Strand: Computation and Estimation): Students engage in problem solving, communicating, reasoning and connecting to compute with whole numbers and fractions, use computation, estimation, and proportions to solve problems, and develop and explain procedures for computing, estimating and solving problems.

Learning Standard 2.4 (Patterns, Relations, and Functions Strand: Patterns and Functions): Students engage in problem solving, communicating, reasoning and connecting to describe and represent relationships with models, tables, graphs, and sentences.

Learning Standard 2.5 (Patterns, Relations, and Functions Strand: Algebra): Students engage in problem solving, communicating, reasoning and connecting to know and apply algebraic procedures for solving equations and inequalities; to understand and apply the concepts of variable, expression, and equation; to apply algebraic methods to solve a variety of real-world and theoretical problems; to construct expressions or equations that model problems; to represent situations and number patterns with graphs; to analyze tables and graphs to identify properties and relationships.

Learning Standard 3.4 (Geometry and Measurement Strand: Measurement): Students engage in problem solving, communicating, reasoning and connecting to select appropriate units and tools to measure the degree of accuracy required in a particular situation; to describe the meaning of angle measure; and to develop and apply formulas and procedures for determining measures to solve problems.

Learning Standard 4.2 (Statistics and Probability Strand: Statistics): Students engage in problem solving, communicating, reasoning and connecting to collect, organize and describe data systematically; to construct, read, and interpret tables, charts and graphs; to make inferences and convincing arguments that are based on data analysis; and to develop and explain why statistical methods are powerful aids to decision making.

Science and Technology

Strand 1 Inquiry: Note and describe relevant details and patterns. Apply personal knowledge and knowledge to make predictions. Describe trends in data even when patterns in the data are not exact. Note and describe relevant details. Represent data and findings using tables and pictorial demonstrations. Use more complex tools to make observations and gather and represent quantitative data. Communicate the idea that there is usually more than one solution to a problem. Design an investigation specifying problem specifying variables to be changed, controlled, and measured. Reformulate ideas based on evidence.

Strand 2 Domains of Science Life Sciences: Investigate and explain that complex multi-cellular organisms are interacting systems of cells, tissues and organs that fulfill life processes through mechanical, electrical, and chemical means, including procuring and manufacturing food. Explore and describe plants as a major category of living organisms.

History and Social Science

Learning Standard 1 Chronology and Cause (History Strand): Students will understand the chronological order of historical events and recognize the complexity of historical cause and effect, including the interaction of forces from different spheres of human activity.

Learning Standard 3 Research Evidence and Point of View (History Strand): Students will acquire the ability to frame questions that can be answered by historical study and research; to collect, evaluate, and employ information from primary and secondary sources, and to apply it in oral and written presentations.

Learning Standard 5 Interdisciplinary Learning: Religion, Ethics, Philosophy, and Literature in History (History Strand): Students will learn and compare basic tenets of world religions and their influence on individual and public life as well as the course of history.

Learning Standard 6 Interdisciplinary Learning Natural Science, Mathematics, and Technology in History (History Strand): Students will describe and explain major advances, discoveries, and inventions over time and will explain some of their effects and influences in the past and present on human life.

Learning Standard 7 Physical Spaces of the Earth (Geography Strand): Students will describe, visualize and map the earth's physical characteristics.

Learning Standard 8 Places and Regions of the World (Geography Strand): Students will identify and explain the location and features of geographical places.

Learning Standard 9 The Effects of Geography (Geography Strand): Students will learn how physical environments have influenced particular cultures and how geographic factors have affected such things as agriculture. Students understand how technology has increased human capacity for modifying the environment and acquiring resources, and analyze the impact of increased technology on the environment.

Learning Standard 10 Human Alteration of Environments (Geography Strand): Students recognize the intended and unintended consequences of technological advances on the environment.

Learning Standard 13 The Economy of the United States (Economic Strand): Students comprehend the major stages of economic change in the United States from 1600s to 1877.

Learning Standard 17 The Founding Documents (Civics and Government Strand): Students will learn in progressively greater detail the content and the history of the Founding Documents of the United States – *The Declaration of Independence* and *The Constitution of the United States*.

Learning Standard 18 Principles and Practices of American Government (Civics and Government Strand): The students will describe and compare the basic legislative process at all levels; how lobbyists, individuals, and other interest groups can influence policy makers and legislative agenda.

Learning Standard 19 Citizenship (Civics and Government Strand): Students learn the ways in which individuals participate in the political process and in civic life.

About the Authors

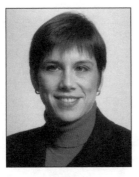

Jill Carter, MA, EdM, is a project coordinator for the Harvard Prevention Research Center on Nutrition and Physical Activity. From 1996 to 1997 she was the curriculum development coordinator for the School-Based Wellness Initiative in the department of health and social behavior at the Harvard School of Public Health. Carter's years of experience as a high school and middle school science teacher provided her with the experience to design a curriculum that encourages active, inquiry-based learning across multiple disciplines. She earned her master of education degree in teaching and curriculum from Harvard University and her master of arts degree in exercise physiology from the University of Iowa.

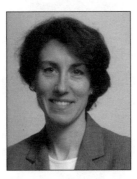

Jean Wiecha, PhD, serves as deputy director at the Harvard Prevention Research Center on Nutrition and Physical Activity. From 1994 to 1997, as a project director for the School-Based Wellness Initiative in the department of health and social behavior at the Harvard School of Public Health, she managed the federal research grant to develop, implement, and evaluate *Planet Health*. Dr. Wiecha earned her doctoral and master of science degrees in human nutrition from Tufts University.

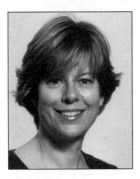

Karen E. Peterson, RD, ScD, is an associate professor of nutrition in the departments of maternal and child health and nutrition at the Harvard School of Public Health as well as co-investigator at the Harvard Prevention Research Center. She draws from 15 years of experience counseling and administering nutrition services for children in clinical, community, and state health care settings. Dr. Peterson was co-principal investigator of the *Planet Health* intervention trial. She earned her doctorate in nutrition from the Harvard School of Public Health.

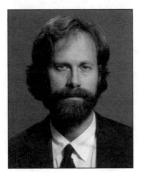

Steven L. Gortmaker, PhD, is a senior lecturer in the department of health and social behavior at the Harvard School of Public Health and principal investigator and director of the Harvard Research Prevention Center. He was also principal investigator of the *Planet Health* intervention trial. For the past 20 years, he has researched and practiced in the areas of children's nutrition and physical activity and has published more than 80 research articles. He was involved in early studies to document the increase of obesity in young people and television viewing as a cause of obesity. He earned his doctorate in sociology from the University of Wisconsin at Madison.